Immunosuppressant Analogs
in Neuroprotection

Immunosuppressant Analogs in Neuroprotection

Edited by

Cesario V. Borlongan, PhD
National Institute on Drug Abuse, Baltimore, MD

Ole Isacson, Dr Med Sci
Neuroregeneration Laboratories,
McLean Hospital/Harvard Medical School
Belmont, MA

Paul R. Sanberg, PhD, DSc
University of South Florida College of Medicine, Tampa, FL

Foreword by
Solomon H. Snyder, MD *and Bahman Aghdasi*, PhD
Johns Hopkins University School of Medicine, Baltimore, MD

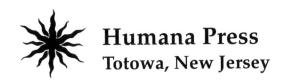

Humana Press
Totowa, New Jersey

Due diligence has been taken by the publishers, editors, and authors of this book to assure the accuracy of the information published and to describe generally accepted practices. The contributors herein have carefully checked to ensure that the drug selections and dosages set forth in this text are accurate and in accord with the standards accepted at the time of publication. Notwithstanding, as new research, changes in government regulations, and knowledge from clinical experience relating to drug therapy and drug reactions constantly occurs, the reader is advised to check the product information provided by the manufacturer of each drug for any change in dosages or for additional warnings and contraindications. This is of utmost importance when the recommended drug herein is a new or infrequently used drug. It is the responsibility of the treating physician to determine dosages and treatment strategies for individual patients. Further it is the responsibility of the health care provider to ascertain the Food and Drug Administration status of each drug or device used in their clinical practice. The publisher, editors, and authors are not responsible for errors or omissions or for any consequences from the application of the information presented in this book and make no warranty, express or implied, with respect to the contents in this publication.

This publication is printed on acid-free paper. ∞
ANSI Z39.48-1984 (American Standards Institute) Permanence of Paper for Printed Library Materials.

Cover illustration: (A) (Background on cover) From Fig. 3 D in Chapter 4 "Effects of Neuroimmunophilin Ligands on Parkinson's Disease and Cognition," by Joseph P. Steiner et al. (B) (Foreground on cover) From Fig 2 A, B in Chapter 13 "Immunosuppressants in Traumatic Brain Injury," by David O. Okonkwo and John T. Povlishock.
Cover design by Patricia F. Cleary

For additional copies, pricing for bulk purchases, and/or information about other Humana titles, contact Humana at the above address or at any of the following numbers: Tel.: 973-256-1699; Fax: 973-256-8341; E-mail: humana@humanapr.com or visit our website at http://www.humanapress.com

Photocopy Authorization Policy:
Authorization to photocopy items for internal or personal use, or the internal or personal use of specific clients, is granted by Humana Press Inc., provided that the base fee of US $20.00 per copy, is paid directly to the Copyright Clearance Center at 222 Rosewood Drive, Danvers, MA 01923. For those organizations that have been granted a photocopy license from the CCC, a separate system of payment has been arranged and is acceptable to Humana Press Inc. The fee code for users of the Transactional Reporting Service is: [0-89603-944-7/03 $20.00].

Printed in the United States of America. 10 9 8 7 6 5 4 3 2 1

Library of Congress Cataloging in Publication Data

Immunosuppressant analogs in neuroprotection / edited by Cesario V. Borlongan, Ole
Isacson, Paul R. Sanberg ; foreword by Solomon H. Snyder and Bahman Aghdasi.
   p. ; cm.
  Includes bibliographical references and index.
  ISBN 0-89603-944-7 (alk. paper); e-ISBN 1-59259-315-1
   1. Nervous system—Degeneration—Chemoprevention. 2. Immunosuppressant agents. 3.
Nervous system—Regeneration. I. Borlongan, Cesario V. II. Isacson, Ole. III. Sanberg,
Paul R.
   [DNLM: 1. Immunosuppressive Agents—therapeutic use. 2. Immunophilins. 3.
Neuroprotective Agents—pharmacology. QW 920 I326 2002]
  RC365.I46 2002
  616.8′0611—dc21   2002190244

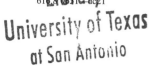

To Christine and Mia
(Cesar)

To patients with neurological diseases and their families
(Ole)

To my brothers and sisters: Steven, Susan, Donald, and Jennifer
(Paul)

Foreword
Why are Immunophilin Ligands Neurotrophic?

Solomon H. Snyder and Bahman Aghdasi

Scientists are too compartmentalized. Each of us is an expert in our own microdomain yet ignorant of advances in nearby fields. The immunophilin story elegantly exemplifies this situation. Cyclosporin A was introduced into clinical use in the 1970s, revolutionizing organ transplantation, while FK506 appeared in the 1980s. By 1990 cyclophilins and the FKBPs were identified as receptors respectively for cyclosporin A and FK506. In the vast majority of studies the only tissues examined were lymphocytes or comparable cells of the immune system *(1)*. Though immunophilins were one among the hottest areas of research in immunology, most neuroscientists had never heard of their existence. Such was the status of the field when one of us (SHS) read the elegant paper by Siekierka et al. *(2)* identifying FKBP12 as the receptor for the actions of FK506 based on its binding [^{3}H] FK506 with high affinity and selectivity. Using an experimental sample of [^{3}H] FK506 from NEN-DuPont, Joseph Steiner in our lab examined its binding to a wide range of rat tissues and discovered marked regional variations within the brain with some areas displaying FKBP12 densities up to 50 times more than those of immune tissues *(3)*. We noted dramatic augmentation of FKBP12 expression in the facial nucleus of the brain stem in rats subjected to facial nerve crush *(4)*. The time course of these changes closely mimicked similar alterations in GAP-43, a protein known to be involved in neural regrowth. This led to our demonstration that FK506, rapamycin, and cyclosporin A all stimulate neurite outgrowth in cultures of PC12 cells as well as in sensory ganglia *(5)*. Subsequently, we and others observed neurotrophic effects of immunosuppressant drugs in multiple systems in intact animals *(6–9)*. The observation that nonimmunosuppressant ligands of the immunophilins were just as neurotrophic as the immunosuppressant drugs *(10)* led to the development of nonimmunosuppressant molecules substantially smaller than classic immunosuppressant drugs that augment the regrowth of damaged peripheral and central neurons in intact animals. These drugs are also neuroprotective in conditions such as stroke *(11)*.

The beneficial effects of immunophilin ligands in most models of neuronal damage may lead to utility in neurodegenerative diseases. Previous efforts to stimulate neuronal regrowth clinically have employed neurotrophic proteins such as nerve growth factor. Delivery of such proteins into the central nervous system presents major hurdles. By contrast, immunophilin ligands in current clinical trial are water-soluble small molecules that readily penetrate the blood–brain barrier. Moreover, whereas neurotrophic proteins stimulate normal as well as damaged neurons, which can lead to adverse effects [such as hyperalgesia elicited by nerve growth factor *(12)*], the immunophilin ligands appear to act only on damaged neurons.

Influences of immunophilin ligands in multiple models of neurologic disease are the focus of the various chapters in *Immunosuppressant Analogs in Neuroprotection*. This essay will attempt to explicate challenges in trying to understand the molecular mechanisms whereby neurotrophic effects are achieved. Whether neuroprotective actions in cerebral ischemia and traumatic brain injury involve the same or similar mechanisms is unclear. Interestingly, neurotrophic proteins can also be neuroprotective. Since cerebral ischemia can be elicited via an extraordinary array of biochemical alterations, potential mechanisms for neuroprotection are comparably diverse. By contrast, there are only a limited number of known mechanisms for stimulating nerve growth, and so we will focus on the neurotrophic side of the story.

A unitary hypothesis for neurotrophic actions of immunophilin ligands must explain several phenomena. For instance, all three classes of immunosuppressants have been shown to be neurotrophic, including cyclosporin A, FK506, and rapamycin. Accordingly, both cyclophilins and FKBPs must presumably play a role in neurotrophic effects. Immunosuppressive effects of these drugs stem from the drug–immunophilin complex binding to and inhibiting calcineurin. FK506 and cyclosporin derivatives that bind to the immunophilins but fail to inhibit calcineurin are neurotrophic, which rules out calcineurin as a mediator. One of the reasons for positing an immunosuppressant target downstream of the immunophilins was the need to invoke a gain-of-function to account for the great potency of immunosuppressants. Thus, FKBP12 and cyclophilin concentrations in most tissues are extremely high, up to 1% of soluble protein, so that low nanomolar concentrations of drugs could only occupy a small percentage of tissue immunophilin *(1)*. Though cyclophilin and FKB12 show no similarity in amino acid sequence, they both share peptide prolylisomerase activity, which is inhibited by immunosuppressant drugs providing an initial hypothesis for immunosuppressant effects. However, at therapeutic concentrations of the drug, one would inhibit only a small fraction of the total tissue content of immunophilin-mediated isomerase activity. By contrast, a drug could bind to a minor percentage of total tissue immunophilin, but the drug–immunophilin complex could still exert a crucial influence on calcineurin activity. Utilizing the analogy with calcineurin inhibition, one might expect neurotrophic actions to employ a molecular target providing a similar gain of function, especially as low nanomolar concentrations of drugs stimulate neurite outgrowth. Such a target would presumably respond to the rapamycin–FKBP12 complex as well as to immunophilin complexes with cyclosporin A and FK506. Rapamycin binds with high affinity to FKBP12, but the drug–immunophilin complex does not interact with calcineurin. Instead, the complex binds to a unique target protein designated FRAP (FK506 and rapamycin activated protein), RAFT (rapamycin and FK506 target), or mammalian TOR (target of rapamycin)*(1,6)*. Crystallographic studies show how FK506 interacting with FKBP12 facilitates secondary interactions with calcineurin, interactions not feasible in the presence of rapamycin. One would have to propose a different sort of binding mechanism for a neurotrophic target that could accommodate rapamycin in the same way as FK506. Alternatively, one could argue that rapamycin might act differently than FK506. There are two components to neurotrophic effects. One involves inhibition of cell division and the second involves neurite extension. Rapamycin was first developed as a cancer chemotherapeutic agent, as it potently inhibits cell division through RAFT and protein translational targets of RAFT such as p70S6 kinase. Such actions could account for neurotrophic actions of rapamycin, at least in culture models *(13)*.

In searching for potential neurotrophic targets, one should bear in mind proteins that are already known to bind to immunophilins. These include the inositol 1,4,5-trisphosphate (IP$_3$) receptor (II) as well as the ryanodine receptor *(14,15)*, both of which are major intracellular calcium channels. FKBP12 appears to be a physiologic subunit of the channels stabilizing their conductance state. Stripping FKBP12 off the channels makes them more "leaky" to calcium. Such leakiness would presumably adversely affect cellular function. Accordingly, FK506, which causes FKBP12 to dissociate from the channels, would be expected to worsen neurotoxicity. On the other hand, once the channel is open, the ability of FKBP12 to increase its inertia would make it more difficult to close so that FK506 might decrease calcium release from the damaged cell. However, micromolar concentrations of FK506 are required to dissociate FKBP12 *(14)*. Moreover, cyclophilins have not yet been demonstrated to be associated with any calcium channels so that one would not be able to explain neurotrophic effects of cyclosporin A. Members of the TGFβ receptor are also "targets" of FKBP12. Other members of the family include receptors for bone morphogenetic protein (BMP), activin, and inhibin as well as proteins such as ALK-7 for which there is not yet a known physiologic ligand *(16–19)*. FKBP12 appears to be a physiologic subunit of these receptors that normally inhibits signaling *(17,20)*. Members of the TGFβ family can be neurotrophic as well as neuroprotective *(21)*. FK506 causes the dissociation of FKBP12 from members of the TGFβ receptor family leading to augmented signaling. Some members of the FK506 family elicit this dissociation at concentrations as low as 10 nM, consistent with potencies relevant to neurotrophic effects *(20,22)*.

One component of neurotrophic actions is turning off the cell cycle. Interestingly, we recently demonstrated that targeted deletion of FKBP12 leads to cell cycle arrest in the G1 phase *(23)*. This is a direct consequence of loss of FKBP12 as the effect is rescued by transfection with FKBP12. The arrest arises from up-regulation of p21 whose activity is well known to cause growth arrest. The p21 stimulation derives from overactivity of TGFβ receptor signaling secondary to loss of the inhibitory actions of FKBP12. TGFβ signals primarily through three pathways: SMAD, p38 kinase, and MAP kinase. Cell cycle arrest is attributed to overactivation of p38 kinase in the FKBP12 deficient cells, because it is selectively prevented by an inhibitor of p38 kinase, whereas inhibitors of other pathways have no effect.

Since several members of the TGFβ receptor family have been associated with neurotrophic actions, any given one of them might be a target for actions of FKBP12 ligands. However, none are known to be associated with cyclophilin, so this particular model cannot explain the neurotrophic effects of such drugs.

One complication in any model attempting to explain neurotrophic actions of immunophilin ligands is the sheer multiplicity of the immunophilins. There exist at least 15 discrete members of the FKBP12 family and a comparable number of cyclophilins *(2,24–32)*. These vary markedly in their intracellular localization, molecular weight, and association with other proteins. Though we know a great deal about FKBP12 and cyclophilin A, few functions have been clarified for the other immunophilins.

Elucidating the molecular mechanisms for the neurotrophic actions of drugs will certainly enhance greatly our understanding of what causes neurons to grow normally and to regrow following damage. Such insights will likely lead to new generations of therapeutic agents. Unfortunately, at the present time no single theory can adequately explain the neurotrophic effects of these agents.

ACKNOWLEDGMENTS

Supported by USPHS grant DA00266 and Research Scientist Award DA-00074 to SHS.

REFERENCES

1. Schreiber, S. L., and Crabtree, G. R. (1995) Immunophilins, ligands, and the control of signal transduction. Harvey Lect **91**, 99–114.
2. Siekierka, J. J., Hung, S. H., Poe, M., Lin, C. S., and Sigal, N. H. (1989) A cytosolic binding protein for the immunosuppressant FK506 has peptidyl-prolyl isomerase activity but is distinct from cyclophilin. Nature **341**, 755–757.
3. Steiner, J. P., Dawson, T. M., Fotuhi, M., Glatt, C. E., Snowman, A. M., Cohen, N., and Snyder, S. H. (1992) High brain densities of the immunophilin FKBP colocalized with calcineurin. Nature **358**, 584–587.
4. Lyons, W. E., Steiner, J. P., Snyder, S. H., and Dawson, T.M. (1995) Neuronal regeneration enhances the expression of the immunophilin FKBP-12. J Neurosci **15**, 2985–2994.
5. Lyons, W. E., Steiner, J. P., Snyder, S. H., and Snyder, S. H. (1994) Immunosuppressant FK506 promotes neurite outgrowth in cultures of PC12 cells and sensory ganglia. Proc Natl Acad Sci USA **91**, 3191–3195.
6. Snyder, S. H., Lai, M. M., and Burnett, P. E. (1998) Immunophilins in the nervous system. Neuron **21**, 283–294.
7. Steiner, J. P., and Hamilton, G. S., Ross, D. T., Valentine, H. L., Guo, H., Connolly, M. A., Liang, S., Ramsey, C., Li, J. H., Huang, W., Howorth, P., Soni, R., Fuller, M., Sauer, H., Nowotnik, A. C., and Suzdak, P. D. (1997) Neurotrophic immunophilin ligands stimulate structural and functional recovery in neurodegenerative animal models. Proc Natl Acad Sci USA **94**, 2019–2024.
8. Gold, B. G., Katoh, K. & Storm-Dickerson, T. (1995) The immunosuppressant FK506 increases the rate of axonal regeneration in rat sciatic nerve. J Neurosci **15**, 7509–7516.
9. Gold, B. G., Zeleny-Pooley, M., Wang, M. S., Chaturvedi, P., and Armistead, D. M. (1997) A nonimmunosuppressant FKBP-12 ligand increases nerve regeneration. Exp Neurol **147**, 269–278.
10. Steiner, J. P., Connolly, M. A., Valentine, H. L., Hamilton, G. S., Dawson, T. M., Hester, L., and Snyder, S. H. (1997) Neurotrophic actions of nonimmunosuppressive drugs FK 506, rapamycin and cyclosporin A. Nat Med **3**, 421–428.
11. Sharkey, J. and Butcher, S. P. (1994) Immunophilins mediate the neuroprotective effects of FK506 in focal cerebral ischaemia. Nature **371**, 336.
12. Shu, X. Q. and Mendell, L. M. (1999) Neurotrophins and hyperalgesia. Proc Natl Acad Sci USA **96**, 7693–7696.
13. Mark, M. D. and Storm, D. R. (1997) Coupling of epidermal growth factor (EGF) with the antiproliferative activity of cAMP induces neuronal differentiation. J Biol Chem **272**, 17238–17244.
14. Cameron, A. M., Steiner, J. P., Roskams, A. J., Ali, S. M., Ronnett, G. V., and Snyder, S. H. (1995) Calcineurin associated with the inositol 1, 4, 5-triphosphate receptor-FKBP12 complex modulates Ca2+ flux. Cell **83**, 463–472.
15. Brillantes, A. B., Ondrias, K., Scott, A., Kobrinsky, E., Ondriasova, E., Moschella, M. C., Jayaraman, T., Landers, M., Ehrlich, B. E., and Marks, A. R. (1994)

Stabilization of calcium release channel (ryanodine receptor) function by FK506-binding protein. Cell **77**, 513–523.

16. Piek, E., Heldin, C. H., and Ten Dijke, P. (1999) Specificity, diversity, and regulation in TGF-beta superfamily signaling. Faseb J **13**, 2105–2124.

17. Massague, J. (1998) TGF-beta signal transduction. Annu Rev Biochem **67**, 753–791.

18. Watanabe, R., Yamada, Y., Ihara, Y., Someya, Y., Kubota, A., Kagimoto, S., Kuroe, A., Iwakura, T., Shen, Z. P., Inada, A., Adachi, T., Ban, N., Miyawaki, K., Sunaga, Y., Tsuda, K., and Seino, Y. (1999) The MH1 domains of smad2 and smad3 are involved in the regulation of the ALK signals. Biochem Biophys Res Commun **254**, 707–712.

19. Jornvall, H., Blokzijl, A., ten Dijke, P., and Ibanez, C. (2001) The orphan receptor serine/threonine kinase ALK7 signals arrest of proliferation and morphological differentiation in a neuronal cell line. J. Biol. Chem **276**, 5140–5146.

20. Wang, T., Li, B. Y., Danielson, P. D., Shah, P. C., Rockwell, S., Lechleider, R. J., Martin, J., Manganaro, T., and Donahoe, P. K. (1996) The immunophilin FKBP12 functions as a common inhibitor of the TGF beta family type I receptors. Cell **86**, 435–444.

21. Ho, T. W., Bristol, L. A., Coccia, C., Li, Y., Milbrandt, J., Johnson, E., Jin, L., Bar-Peled, O., Griffin, J. W., and Rothstein, J. D. (2000) TGFbeta trophic factors differentially modulate motor axon outgrowth and protection from excitotoxicity. Exp. Neurol **161**, 664–675.

22. Okadome, T., Oeda, E., Saitoh, M., Ichijo, H., Moses, H. L., Miyazono, K., and Kawabata, M. (1996) Characterization of the interaction of FKBP12 with the transforming growth factor-beta type I receptor in vivo. J Biol Chem **271**, 21687–21690.

23. Aghdasi, B., Ye, K., Resnick, A., Ha, H. C., Gou, X., Dawson, T. M., Dawson, V. L. & Snyder, S. H. (2001) FKBP12, 12-kDa FK506-binding Protein, is a Physiologic Regulator of the Cell Cycle. Proc Natl Acad Sci USA **98**, 2425–2430.

24. Harding, M. W., Galat, A., Uehling, D. E., and Schreiber, S. L. (1989) A receptor for the immunosuppressant FK506 is a cis-trans peptidyl-prolyl isomerase. Nature **341**, 758–760.

25. Lam, E., Martin, M. M., Timerman, A. P., Sabers, C., Fleischer, S., Lukas, T., Abraham, R. T., O'Keefe, S. J., O'Neill, E. A., and Wiederrecht, G. J. (1995) A novel FK506 binding protein can mediate the immunosuppressive effects of FK506 and is associated with the cardiac ryanodine receptor. J Biol Chem 270, 26,511–26,522.

26. Jin, Y. J., Albers, M. W., Lane, W. S., Bierer, B. E., Schreiber, S. L. & Burakoff, S. J. (1991) Molecular cloning of a membrane-associated human FK506- and rapamycin-binding protein, FKBP-13. Proc Natl Acad Sci USA **88**, 6677–6681.

27. Jin, Y. J. and Burakoff, S. J. (1993) The 25-kDa FK 506-binding protein is localized in the nucleus and associates with casein kinase II and nucleolin. Proc Natl Acad Sci USA **90**, 7769–7773.

28. Pedersen, K. M., Finsen, B., Celis, J. E., and Jensen, N. A. (1999) mu FKBP38: a novel murine immunophilin homolog differentially expressed in Schwannoma cells and central nervous system neurons in vivo. Electrophoresis **20,** 249–255.
29. Baughman, G., Wiederrecht, G. J., Campbell, N. F., Martin, M. M., and Bourgeois, S. (1995) FKBP51, a novel T-cell-specific immunophilin capable of calcineurin inhibition. Mol Cell Biol. **15,** 4395–4402.
30. Smith, D. F., Albers, M. W., Schreiber, S. L., Leach, K. L., and Deibel, M. R. (1993) FKBP54, a novel FK506-binding protein in avian progesterone receptor complexes and HeLa extracts. J Biol Chem **268,** 24,270–24,273.
31. Tai, P. K., Albers, M. W., Chang, H., Faber, L. E., and Schreiber, S. L. (1992) Association of a 59-kilodalton immunophilin with the glucocorticoid receptor complex. Science **256,**1315–1318.
32. Davis, E. C., Broekelmann, T. J., Ozawa, Y., and Mecham, R. P. (1998) Identification of tropoelastin as a ligand for the 65-Kd FK506-binding protein, FKBP65, in the secretory pathway. J Cell Biol **140,** 295–303.

Preface

The most widely used immunosuppressant drug therapy in organ and neural transplantation is cyclosporin-A(CsA). CsA was isolated from soil fungus in 1976, and was shown to block T-cell proliferation by inhibiting cytokine transcription via binding to calcium-calmodium-dependent phosphatase, calcineurin (Figs. 1 and 2). CsA was subsequently marketed by Sandoz Pharmaceuticals Inc. in 1979. To date, there are 250,000 organ and 300 neural transplant recipients who have benefited form CsA adjunctive treatment. Though structurally different, another calcineurin inhibitor FK-506 (also known as tacrolimus) has been shown to produce similar immunosuppressive effects. Over the last five years, accumulating evidence suggests that both CsA and FK-506 can be neuroprotective, in addition to their primary immunosuppressive effects (Table 1 and Fig. 3). Although mainly used as immunosuppressants, newly identified nonimmunosuppressive properties of CsA and KF-506 suggest their potential as therapeutic agents for neurological disorders. Four major CNS actions of CsA and FK-506 could promote neuropro-tection. First, inhibition of calcium-phosphatase calcineurin by these immunosuppressants can prevent calcium-dependent enzyme disturbances and can reduce nitric oxide production. Because calcium channel blockers and nitric oxide synthase inhibitors have been shown to alleviate neurobehavioral deficits in models of neurological disorders, similar beneficial effects may be rendered by these calcineurin inhibitors. Second, blockade of the mitochondrial permeability transition pore (which is an inducer of cell death) by these immunosuppressants has been shown to retard neurodegeneration. Opening of the mitochondrial permeability transition pore triggers release of apoptotic factors that can initiate cascades leading to cell death. Such upregulation of apoptotic markers has been noted in many neurological disorders. Accordingly, this inhibition of the opening of the mitochondrial permeability transition pore can block apoptotic cell death. Third, CsA and FK-506 can promote neurotrophic factor support. In primary cultures of dopaminergic cells, enhanced elongation of neurites was observed after treatment with immunosuppressants or their analogs. Similar neurite outgrowth or regrowth following exposure to immunosuppressants has been noted in normal or damaged sciatic, cortical cholinergic, and serotonergic neurons. Immunosuppressant treatment thus offers neurotrophic factor support to many neurotransmitter

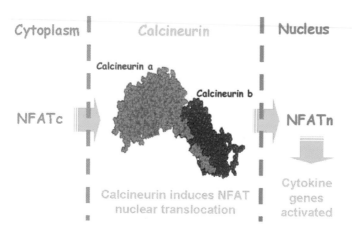

Fig. 1. T-cell activation. Nuclear factor of activated T-cells (NFGAT) predominantly resides in the cytoplasm (NFATc), and is translocated into the nucleus via calcium/calmodulin-dependent serine/threonine phosphatase, calcineurin (composed of a catalytic subunit called calcineurin A, and a regulatory subunit calcineurin B). Once NFAT reaches the nucleus (NFATn), cytokine genes are activated, resulting in IL-2 production during T-cell activation.

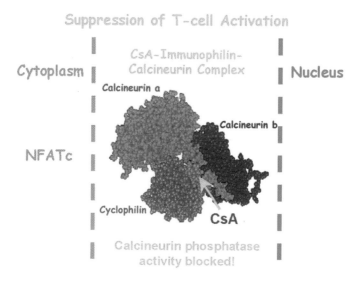

Fig. 2. Suppression of T-cell activation. Calcineurin is the target of immunosuppresive drugs CsA and FK-506. When an immunosuppressive drug binds with its specific immunophilin and the calcineurin complex, NFAT cannot translocate from the cytoplasm into the nucleus. Accordingly, the blockade of the calcineurin phosphatase activity leads to suppression of T-cell activation.

Table 1
Neural Actions of Immunosuppressants and Their Analogs

Inhibition of calcineurin
Blockade of mitochondrial permeability transition pore opening
Promotion of neurotrophic factor effects
Scavenging of free radicals

Note. Accumulating evidence in recent years suggests that immunosuppressants and structurally similar drugs can modulate CNS functions,
which may promote neuroprotection, in addition to their primary immunosuppressive functions.

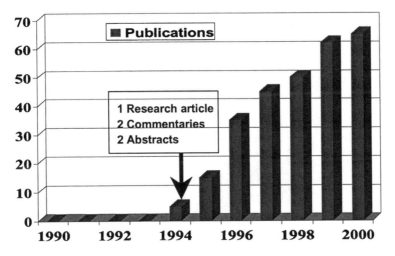

Fig. 3. Scientific literature, 1990–2000. Neuroprotective effects of immunosuppressants
and their analogs have recently been demonstrated, with a surge in peer-reviewed publications
over the last five years.

systems. Fourth, immunosuppressants or structurally similar drugs can block
formation of free radicals, thereby inhibiting lipid peroxidation. Because free
radical scavengers have been shown to protect against models of neuronal
death, the potential of these drugs to prevent increased production of free
radicals may lead to similar protective effects. Though it is not clear whether
these factors initiate events causing cell death or consequences of the disease
process, experimental therapeutic efforts aimed at preventing or at least delay-
ing disease progression by blocking calcium channels, restoring mitochondrial energy metabolism, providing neurotrophic factors, and scavenging
excess free radicals have shown beneficial effects. In this regard, CsA and FK-

506, by targeting calcium channels and the mitochondria permeability transition pore, promoting neurotrophic factor support, and inhibiting free radicals may be considered multiple site-of-action therapeutic drugs.

The observations that immunophilins and structurally similar ligands possess neurotrophic and neuroprotective properties in addition to their immunosuppressive effects suggest that immunosuppressant therapy may have dual beneficial effects for transplant recipients by promoting graft survival and function, as well as inhibiting graft rejection. *Immunosuppressant Analogs in Neuroprotection* focuses on recent preclinical evidence that demonstrates neurotrophic/neuroprotective effects of immunosuppressants when administered alone or when combined with neural transplantation therapy in animal models of neurological disorders. The Foreword by Drs. Snyder and Aghdasi introduces the reader to the evolution of immunosuppressants as neuroprotective agents, and discusses the impetus for developing immunosuppressant analogs, called neuroimmunophilins, as neuroprotective agents for neurological disorders. Part I (Chapter 1: Introduction, Keep et al.) provides the scientific rationale for initiating investigations into the neurotrophic/ neuroprotective effects of immunosuppressants. The succeeding chapters are then divided into six sections that correspond to specific animal models of neurological disorders.

Part II deals with the use of immunosuppressants and similar drugs without immunosuppressive primary action in Parkinson's disease animal models, including MPTP and 6-OHDA (Chapter 2, Ogawa and Tanaka). Because differential positive effects of immunosuppressants have been attributed to minimal access of these compounds to cross the blood–brain barrier, a chronic and a high dosage (>10 mg/kg) drug treatment coupled with a compromised blood–brain barrier may be needed to promote the neuroprotective effects of immunosuppressants. However, high dosage and chronic immunosuppressant regimens produce such negative side effects as nephrotoxicity and hallucination among others. Analogs of immunosuppressants have been developed to avoid these risk factors including elimination of the immunosuppressive property of the drug, but retaining its neurotrophic feature. These non-immunosuppressant analogs, neuroimmunophilins are discussed in detail in Chapters 3 (Costantini and Isacson) and 4 (Steiner et al.). The effects of immunosuppressants in parkinsonian animals that have received dopaminergic transplant are discussed in detail in Chapter 5 (Castilho et al.). The blockade of the mitochondrial permeability transition pore and how it relates to the protective effects of immunosuppressants in Parkinson's disease are presented in Chapter 6 (Korlipara and Schapira).

Most neurological disorders are characterized by cognitive dysfunctions, in addition to motor abnormalities. Part III presents laboratory findings showing the therapeutic efficacy of drugs resembling immunosuppressants or even immunosuppressants themselves in two major neurological disorders, namely Alzheimer's disease (Chapter 7, Mattson) and Huntington's disease (Chapter 8, Leventhal and Kordower).

Neurological disorders may be characterized by progressive neurodegeneration, as tackled in Parts II and III. Other neurological disorders are characterized by severe brain insults, such as stroke and traumatic brain injury, and are accompanied by more debilitating effects. Part IV provides evidence of similar beneficial effects of immunosuppressants in animal models of stroke (Chapter 9, Gogvadze and Richter; Chapter 10, Wakita and colleagues; Chapter 11, Ogawa and colleagues; Chapter 12, Sharkey and colleagues), and traumatic brain injury (Chapter 13, Okonkwo and Povlishock).

Part V provides positive effects of immunosuppressants in spinal cord injury (Chapter 14, Ibarra and Diaz-Ruiz; Chapter 15, Palladini and Caronti); Part VI presents their utility in sciatic nerve injury (Chapter 16, Gold; Chapter 17, Steiner et al.); Part VII discusses potential use of immunosuppressants in other disorders of the central nervous system (ALS: Chapter 18, Keep et al.; Drug addiction: Chapter 19, Watanabe).

Although we have categorized the chapters according to the type of neurological disorders that the authors have used to demonstrate beneficial effects of immunosuppressants and/or their analogs, most of the chapters offer novel hypotheses on the mechanisms of neuroprotection. For example, Chapters 6, 9, 13, and 18 support the blockade of mitochondrial permeability transition pore hypothesis, Chapters 2–5, 12, and 15–17 provide proof of neurotrophic effects, and Chapter 13 proposes the free radical scavenging effects of immunosuppressants. In addition, one may note that chapters dealing with CsA or FK-506 (2, 5, 6, 8, 10, 11, 13–16, and 19) demonstrate the therapeutic efficacy of these immunosuppressants based on their unique property of inhibiting calcineurin, whereas chapters on neuroimmunophilin (3, 4, 12, 17, and 18) argue that calcineurin inhibition (i.e., immunosuppressive property) is not necessary for neuroprotection.

These preclinical observations indicate that CsA and FK-506, and their analogs, exert neuroprotective effects on their own. In addition to providing immunosuppression to the transplanted tissues, immunosuppressants may also enhance the survival of the grafts and the damaged host tissue via their trophic factor effect and other survival-promoting features. We have pointed out above that neuroprotection with immunosuppressant treatment may only be consistently achieved with chronic and high doses and a compromised blood–brain barrier. The advent of immunosuppressant analogs, such as the neuroimmuno-philins, may be an equally potent alternative to deliver these agents into the central nervous system and one that can promote neuroprotection.

The goal of *Immunosuppressant Analogs in Neuroprotection* is to advance the use of immunosuppressants and their analogs as a new breed of neuroprotective agents. Because the majority of these agents have been used in the clinic as immunosuppressants for many years now, we believe that their new clinical application as neuroprotective agents will be expedited, such as other experimental drugs (e.g., antioxidants, anti-apoptotic agents, bioenergetic supplements, etc.) used for the treatment of neurological disorders.

Cesario V. Borlongan, PhD
Ole Isacson, Dr Med Sci
Paul R. Sanberg, PhD, DSc

Contents

Contributors

BAHMAN AGHDASI • Department of Neuroscience, Johns Hopkins University School of Medicine, Baltimore, MD

ICHIRO AKIGUCHI • Department of Neurology, Faculty of Medicine, Kyoto University, Sakyo-ku, Kyoto, Japan

T. E. ALLSOPP • Fujisawa Institute of Neuroscience in Edinburgh, University of Edinburgh, Edinburgh, UK

M. ASANUMA • Department of Neuroscience, Institute of Molecular and Cellular Medicine, Okayama University Medical School, Okayama, Japan

CESARIO V. BORLONGAN • National Institute on Drug Abuse, National Institute of Health, Baltimore, MD and Department of Neurology and Institute of Molecular Medicine and Genetics, Medical College of Georgia and Research and Affiliations Service Line, Augusta Veterans Medical Center, Augusta, GA

PATRIK BRUNDIN • Section for Neuronal Survival, Wallenberg Neuroscience Center, Lund, Sweden

BRUNELLA CARONTI • Department of Neurological Sciences, University La Sapienza, Rome, Italy

ROGER F. CASTILHO • Departamento de Patologia Clínica, Faculdade de Cíencias Médicas, Universidade Estadual De Campinas, Campinas, Brazil

LAUREN C. COSTANTINI • Neuroregeneration Laboratories, McLean Hospital, Harvard Medical School, Belmont, MA; currently at Titan Pharmaceuticals Inc., South San Francisco, CA

KATALIN CSISZAR • Laboratory of Matrix Pathobiology, Pacific Biomedical Research Center, University of Hawaii, Honolulu, HI

ARACELI DIAZ-RUIZ • Neuroimmunology Department, Proyecto Camina, A.C., Mexico City, Mexico

ESKIL ELMÉR • Experimental Brain Research, Wallenberg Neuroscience Center, Lund University, Sweden and Maas Biolab, LLC, Albuquerque, NM

KEITH S. K. FONG • Laboratory of Matrix Pathobiology, Pacific Biomedical Research Center, University of Hawaii, Honolulu, HI

VLADIMIR GOGVADZE • Institute of Theoretical and Experimental Biophysics, Pushchino, Russia

BRUCE G. GOLD • Center for Research on Occupational and Environmental Toxicology (CROET), and the Department of Cell and Developmental Biology, Oregon Health and Science University, Portland, OR

GREGORY HAMILTON • Department of Research, Guilford Pharmaceuticals Inc., Baltimore, MD

OSKAR HANSSON • Section for Neuronal Survival, Wallenberg Neuroscience Center, Lund, Sweden

ANTONIO IBARRA • Neuroimmunology Department, Proyecto Camina, A.C., Mexico City, Mexico

OLE ISACSON • Neuroregeneration Laboratories, McLean Hospital, Harvard Medical School, Belmont, MA

P. A. JONES • Fujisawa Institute of Neuroscience in Edinburgh, University of Edinburgh, Edinburgh, UK

MARCUS F. KEEP • Division of Neurosurgery, University of New Mexico, Albuquerque, New Mexico and Maas Biolab, LLC, Albuquerque, NM

JEFFREY H. KORDOWER • Department of Neurological Sciences, Rush Presbyterian Medical Center, Chicago, IL

L. V. P. KORLIPARA • University Department of Clinical Neurosciences, Royal Free and University College, London, UK

LIZA LEVENTHAL • Department of Neurological Sciences, Rush Presbyterian–St. Luke's Medical Center, Chicago, IL

MARK P. MATTSON • Laboratory of Neurosciences, National Institute on Aging, Bethesda, MD

J.F. MCCARTER • Fujisawa Institute of Neuroscience in Edinburgh, University of Edinburgh, Edinburgh, UK

A.L. MCGREGOR • Fujisawa Institute of Neuroscience in Edinburgh, UK

THERESA MORROW • Department of Research, Guilford Pharmaceuticals Inc., Baltimore, MD

DAVID O. OKONKWO • Departments of Neuroscience and Neurosurgery, University of Virginia, Charlottesville, VA

NORIO OGAWA • Department of Neuroscience, Institute of Molecular & Cellular Medicine, Okayama, Japan

GUIDO PALLADINI • Department of Neurological Sciences, University "La Sapienza," Rome, Italy

JOHN T. POVLISHOCK • Department of Anatomy, Medical College of Virginia, Virginia Commonwealth University, Richmond, VA

CHRISTOPH RICHTER • Institute of Biochemistry, Swiss Federal Institute of Technology (ETH), Zurich, Switzerland

DOUGLAS T. ROSS • Department of Research, Guilford Pharmaceuticals Inc., Baltimore, MD

PAUL R. SANBERG • Division of Neurological Surgery, University of South Florida College of Medicine, Tampa, FL

HANSJORG SAUER • Department of Research, Guilford Pharmaceuticals Inc., Baltimore, MD

A. H. V. SCHAPIRA • University Department of Clinical Neurosciences, Royal Free and University College Medical School, London, UK

JOHN SHARKEY • Fujisawa Institute of Neuroscience in Edinburgh, University of Edinburgh, Edinburgh, UK

SOLOMON H. SNYDER • Department of Neuroscience, Johns Hopkins University School of Medicine, Baltimore, MD

JOSEPH P. STEINER • Department of Neurobiology, Guilford Pharmaceuticals, Baltimore, MD

KEN-ICHI TANAKA • Department of Neuroscience, Institute of Molecular and Cellular Medicine, Okayama University Medical School, Okayama, Japan

HIDEKAZU TOMIMOTO • Department of Neurology, Faculty of Medicine, Kyoto University, Sakyo-Ko, Tokyo, Japan and Maas Biolab, LLC, Honolulu, HI

HIROYUKI UCHINO • Department of Anesthesiology, Tokyo Medical College, Shinjuki-ku, Tokyo, Japan; and Maas BiolAB, LLC, Albuquerque, NM

HEATHER VALENTINE • Department of Research, Guilford Pharmaceuticals Inc., Baltimore, MD

HIDEAKI WAKITA • Department of Neurology, Faculty of Medicine, Kyoto University, Kyoto, Japan

SHIGERU WATANABE • Department of Psychology, Keio University, Tokyo, Japan

I

IMMUNOSUPPRESSANTS, NEUROLOGIC DISORDERS, AND NEUROPROTECTION

Introduction: Immunosuppressants as Neuroprotective Agents

Marcus F. Keep, Hiroyuki Uchino, and Eskil Elmér

INTRODUCTION

The discovery that the two most powerful immunosuppressants, cyclosporin A and FK506, are also the most effective neuroprotectants known is profoundly important to neurology. Two drugs that revolutionized the field of organ transplantation as immunosuppressants are beginning to have an even greater impact on medicine in their new role as neuroprotectants. The elucidation of the mechanisms of action of these drugs in ischemia, trauma, and neurodegeneration has enhanced our understanding of some of the complexities of neuronal death and survival.

EARLY IMMUNOSUPPRESSANTS: RADIATION, AZATHIOPRINE, AND CORTICOSTEROIDS

The earliest immunosuppressants, ionizing radiation and especially corticosteroids, also have neuroprotective properties. Radiation was the first immunosuppressive used in the 1950s (1–3). Total-body ionizing radiation is immunosuppressive by inducing death of rapidly dividing immune cells via production of free radicals and direct DNA damage and works well for recipients of closely matched sibling donors (2), but was abandoned because of lethal infections and bone marrow toxicity. Radiation was found to be neuroprotective at low doses in the early 1990s. Irradiation eliminated reactive astrocytes at the site of brain trauma, reduced tissue degeneration, increased structural healing, and rescued some axonotomized neurons (4). Recent studies show reduced tissue damage and improved behavioral outcomes with radiation of traumatized rat spinal cords (5). An effect beyond local immunosuppression may be involved and warrants further exploration.

While azathioprine immunosuppression is useful in true autoimmune neurological diseases such as myasthenia gravis (6), it does not have its own

From: *Immunosuppressant Analogs in Neuroprotection*
Edited by: C. V. Borlongan, O. Isacson, and P. R. Sanberg © Humana Press Inc., Totowa, NJ

direct neuroprotective effect. Azathioprine is a less toxic mustard gas variant *(7,8)*, first used for transplant immunosuppression in the early 1960s, and is still used today *(9)*. Azathioprine induces immunosuppression by inhibiting DNA and RNA synthesis in rapidly proliferating immune cells.

Corticosteroids were first used to treat rejection in 1960 *(10)* in a radiated patient and remain a pillar of modern immunosuppression. Corticosteroids impair especially the cellular or T-cell immune system, prevent antigen–T-cell receptor-induced lymphocyte proliferation by blocking cytokine gene activation of interleukin 2 (IL-2) in particular *(11)*. Other effects of steroids include increased susceptibility to infections, cushingoid appearance, avascular bone necrosis, heart disease, diabetes, and neoplasia through lost immunosurveillance.

Immunosuppression with both azathioprine and corticosteroids *(12,13)* was the standard for 20 yr *(14)*, allowing transplantation to include other organs, such as liver *(15)*, lung *(16)*, pancreas *(17)*, and heart *(18)*. Modest, but definite, improved recovery from spinal cord injury was found in 1990 with high-dose corticosteroid treatment [methylprednisolone (Solu-Medrol, Pharmacia & Upjohn)]—30 mg/kg the first hour, 5.4 mg/kg/h for 23 h, started within 8 h of injury. Then this treatment became the clinical standard of care for spinal cord injury neuroprotection *(19,20)*. Corticosteroids have a neuroprotective membrane-stabilizing and free-radical-inhibiting effect separate from their immunosuppressive and catabolic activity. While high-dose corticosteroids are not currently consistently used in traumatic brain injury or stroke, there remains interest in examining the high doses used successfully in spinal cord injury *(21–23)*.

Catabolism and immunosuppression have prompted a search for side effect-free neuroprotectant steroid analogs. These analogs are called lazaroids, in reference to the described resuscitation of the apparently dead Lazarus by the healer Jesus in the early first century (John 11:38–44, *New Testament, The Bible*; 5.110. *The Koran*). Lazaroids have been studied especially for neural transplantation to increase survival of fetal dopamine neurons *(24)*. The first lazaroid used in therapy for human use is a nonimmunosuppressive 21-aminosteroid conjugated with vitamin E, tirilazad mesylate, or Freedox (Pharmacia & Upjohn). Lazaroids, like corticosteroids, inhibit lipid peroxidation, scavenge free radicals, and stabilize membranes, but without the same side effects. Lazaroids are used clinically in Europe for neuroprotection against vasospasm-induced ischemia *(25)* and human neural transplantation to enhance grafted fetal dopaminergic cell survival in patients with Parkinson's disease *(26,27)*, but these analogs have not been consistently effective in a variety of stroke and traumatic brain

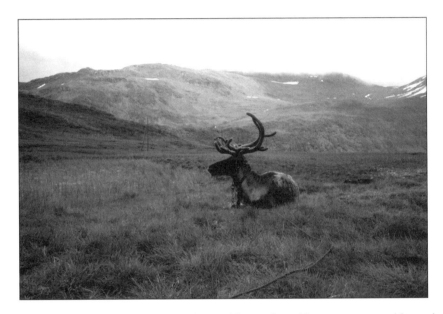

Fig. 1. The Hardanger Vidda is located in southern Norway, traversed by train between Oslo and Bergen, with its waterfalls plunging down to the Hardanger Fjord along the western flank. Its dramatic primal Scandinavian terrain is one of treeless, windswept survival at over 1000 m. The Vidda is inhabited by reindeer, grasses, lichens, mosses, and the cyclosporin-producing soil fungus *Tolypocladium inflatum Gams*. Photograph by Anette Elmér.

injury protocols *(28,29)*. Corticosteroid neuroprotection led not only to the development of the first clinical neuroprotection protocol for spine injury and the development of nonimmunosuppressive lazaroid analogs, but also helped inspire researchers to look at other immunosuppressants as possible neuroprotectants.

The Modern Era of Immunosuppression and Neuroprotection: Neuroimmunophilin Ligands Cyclosporin A, FK506, and Rapamycin

Immunosuppressive Effects of Cyclosporin A

Cyclosporin A (CsA) is a cyclic undecapeptide isolated from the fungus species *Tolypocladium inflatum Gams*, grown from a soil specimen from Hardanger Vidda, Norway *(30)* (Fig. 1). CsA was isolated by Sandoz (now Novartis) in 1969. J. F. Borel and coworkers *(31)* found it to have remarkable immunosuppressive properties in 1972. For an exciting historical coverage *see* refs. *32* and *33*. CsA was used for the first time clinically by R. Y.

Calne and coworkers *(34)* in the late 1970s, and since that time it has been the workhorse of transplantation immunosuppression, giving better graft and patient survival than was previously possible. CsA binds a number of proteins in various subcellular compartments, including its endogenous intracytoplasmic high-affinity receptor cyclophilin A, with which it creates a structural binary relationship *(35–37)*. Cyclophilin A is plentiful in many tissues, especially immune cells and neurons which explains its focused effect in these two systems.

The CsA–cyclophilin complex initiates immunosuppression by binding to and inhibiting the protein phosphatase calcineurin *(38–40)*. Inhibition of phosphatase activity keeps the "cytoplasmic nuclear factor of activated T cells" (NF-AT) phosphorylated, so that the NF-AT cannot enter the nucleus where it would induce the genes for IL-2 and the IL-2 receptor *(41,42)*. Decreased expression of IL-2 prevents T-cell activation *(41,43)*. CsA also inhibits cyclophilin's other function as a rotamase, which is a peptidylprolyl-*cis-trans*-isomerase-facilitating tertiary protein folding and unfolding *(44,45)*. Rotamase inhibition is not related to immunosuppression, but may be responsible for immunophilin neurotrophism *(46,47)*.

Several cyclophilin isoforms are located in specific organelles, with cyclophilins B and C found within the endoplasmic reticulum *(48)*. Cyclophilin D is mainly located within the mitochondria, which plays an important role, not in immunosuppression, but in neuroprotection. Another cyclophilin is cyclophilin-40 with binding sites for three classes of immunosuppressants: steroids, CsA, and macrolides, and NK-TR, the tumor recognition complex *(49)*. CsA is, in addition, a substrate for and noncompetitive inhibitor of the *p*-glycoprotein transporter in the brain capillary endothelium. This transport mechanism keeps bilirubin and certain drugs, including CsA itself, from crossing the blood–brain barrier, which explains in part why its neuroprotective effect was not discovered during decades of clinical use for transplantation.

CsA effects include immunosuppression, nephrotoxicity, hypertension, hepatoxicity, neurotoxicity, and increased incidence of B-cell lymphomas *(50–52)*. Around 40% of patients may have some type of central nervous system effect, with minor tremor being the most common. A few patients who receive transplants experience severe neurotoxicity manifested as confusion, hallucinations, weakness, ataxia, dysphasia, cortical blindness, posterior leukoencephalopathy, and seizures *(53)*. The neurotoxicity may not be completely caused by CsA, because associated risk factors in these patients include hyponatremia, hypomagnesemia, hypocalcemia, hypoglycemia, infections, hypertension, polypharmacy, hepatic encephalopathy

(51,54,55), graft malfunction, and aluminum overload *(56)*. Symptoms resolve in most cases spontaneously or with dose reduction. CsA, when it crosses the blood–brain barrier, has remarkable neuroprotectant qualities.

Immunosuppressive Effects of FK506

FK506 (tacrolimus; Prograf, Fujisawa) is a macrolide lactone with a hemiketal-masked α,β-diketoamide in a 23-member ring isolated from *Streptomyces tsukubaensis*, a soil fungus found in Tsukuba, Japan. Its immunosuppressive properties were identified in 1984 *(57–59)*. FK506 is 50 to 100 times a more potent immunosuppressant than CsA, and was championed by Starzl who sought a drug more effective and less toxic than CsA (T. E. Starzl, personal communication to M. Keep, 1986). FK506 began clinical use in 1989 for liver transplantation for which it now is the immunosuppressant of choice, although it shares many of the major side effects of CsA. It is also used in renal, heart, small bowel *(60)*, and multiorgan transplantation. Recent hand transplantation using FK506 immunosuppression *(61)* returns us to the surgeons Cosmas and Damian *(62)* who were reported in the third century to have grafted, without rejection, an unrelated cadaveric donor leg onto a recipient.

FK506 binds to abundant FK-binding proteins (e.g., FKBP-12) in the cytoplasm of T cells. The FK506–FKBP-12 complex (like the CsA–cyclophilin complex) inhibits the phosphatase activity of calcineurin, blocks the transfer of NF-AT to the nucleus and thus prevents the formation of IL-2 and related factors *(42,43)*. The result is inhibition of T-cell clonal proliferation and immunosuppression *(63)*. Like cyclophilins, FKBPs are rotamases, and FK506 inhibition of FKBP rotamase activity is not related to immunosuppression, but may be responsible for immunophilin neurotrophism *(64,65)*. FK506 has no difficulty crossing the blood–brain barrier, and has remarkable neuroprotectant properties.

Immunosuppressive Effects of Rapamycin

Rapamycin (sirolimus; Rapamune, Wyeth-Ayerst) is a macrocyclic triene antibiotic produced by *S. hygroscopicu*, isolated from soil samples from Easter Island (*Rapa Nui* in Polynesian, hence rapamycin) *(66,67)*. It is a 31-member macrocyclic lactone whose similar structure to FK506 led to its discovery as an immunosuppressant. It binds to a different FK binding protein, FKBP-25, which complex does not inhibit calcineurin and so has no effect on IL-2 production. Sirolimus induces immunosuppression, however, by blocking downstream-activation cascades of IL-2 and IL-6 pathways, *(68,69)*, which then inhibits T-cell clonal proliferation *(63,70)*. Toxicities of rapamycin include immunosuppression, and a dose-limiting thrombocytopenia *(71)*. Because of its this latter effect, sirolimus is used primarily as an adjuvant to CsA or FK506 immunosuppression. Rapamycin is not neuroprotective, and even competitively inhibits FK506 (but not CsA) neuroprotection. However, it does have neurotrophic properties that may be useful in neuroregeneration. (*See* Chapter 16)

The Future of Immunosuppression

CsA, FK506, corticosteroids, and azathioprinelike drugs will remain at the helm of transplant immunosuppression for the extended present. Rapamycin is in trials as an add-on drug. Future predictable developments in transplantation and immunosuppression include tolerance-induction, engineered xenografts, cloned and stem-cell autografts, and semisynthetic organs.

NEUROIMMUNOPHILINS AS NEUROPROTECTANTS

Events Leading to the Discovery of FK506 Neuroprotection

While CsA was the earlier immunosuppressant, FK506 became the lead neuroprotectant and neurotrophin in the early 1990s. It was discovered that FKBPs were concentrated 50 times more in brain than T cells, and in neurons at higher concentrations than glia, giving the first indications that the immunophilins might be involved in neural function. Cyclophilins and FKBPs, first categorized as immunophilins, now became known as neuroimmunophilins *(72)*. FKBP was found in highest concentrations in the hippocampus, striatonigral, and cerebellar granule cells, colocalizing with calcineurin *(72,73)*. Concurrently, researchers from Dawson's group in 1994 *(74)* showed glutamate neurotoxicity to be blunted by nitric oxide synthase (NOS) inhibitors. Neural cultures with FK506 showed protection from glutamate toxicity, surmised to be through inhibition of calcineurin and inhibition of NOS *(75,76)*. NOS is in its active form only when dephosphorylated by calcineurin, so when calcineurin is inhibited by FK506-FKBP, nitric oxide levels remain low, and neuroprotection from glutamate toxicity is possible *(77)*. Rapamycin in turn blocked FK506 from inhibiting calcineurin, thereby blocking the neuroprotective effect of FK506. Thus calcineurin inhibition, and the resultant NOS inhibition, was thought to induce neuroprotection.

Adding to FK506's appeal as a neuroprotection candidate was that it blocks the release of presynaptic glutamate induced by a NMDA-challenge *(78)*, while CsA seemed less promising since treated synaptosomes had enhanced potentially toxic glutamate release when challenged by K^+ channel blockers *(79)*. It was shown, however, 4 yr later, that FK506 did not protect in vivo neurons against NMDA neurotoxicity *(76)*. More recent studies, while confirming FK506 neuroprotection in ischemia, have brought the NOS inhibition mechanism of neuroprotection partially into question *(80)*.

Neuroimmunophilins as Neurotrophins

The neurotrophic effects of immunophilin ligands are a related, but distinct, effect from neuroprotection. The neurotrophism is discussed briefly in this chapter, and fully for FK506 and FKBPs in Chapter 16 and for CsA in Chapter 15.

In 1993 Teichner and associates *(81)* demonstrated that CsA exerts neurotrophic effects on transected rat spinal cords, with a robust sprouting of descending axons across the glial scar, which was confirmed in their 1996 follow-up study *(82)*. The authors, however, felt that CsAs inhibition of NOS should block regeneration, and not have its own neurotrophic effect and attributed the sprouting to immunosuppression blocking autoimmunity. Cell culture work from the same group in 1995 failed to show CsA neurotrophism, perhaps due to the cell line chosen, continuing their impression of the importance of autoimmunity blocking regeneration *(83)*. In light of predating work showing CsA neurotrophism and neurite outgrowth in PC12 cells and sensory ganglia, it is not clear why there was no effect. Palladini does not mention the blood–brain barrier, and does not refer to the reported neurotrophic effects by Lyons and coworkers in 1994 *(84)*. In hindsight, a likely explanation for the observed axon sprouting is less the effect of blocked autoimmunity, and more that the spinal transection opened the blood–brain barrier, allowing for CsA neurotrophism.

In 1994 Lyons and coworkers *(84)* showed that all the neuroimmunophilins FK506, rapamycin, and less so CsA promoted neurite outgrowth in PC12 cells and sensory neuron cultures. Furthermore, in 1995 Gold *(85,86)* showed that FK506 promotes neuronal remyelination after sciatic nerve crush injury. FK506 and rapamycin neurotrophism is described in use patents, for example, Lyons and associates at the Johns Hopkins University School of Medicine *(87)*.

It was realized that potentially treating neurodegenerative disease would require chronic administration with the risks of immunosuppression and nephrotoxicity. This led to the development of immunophilin ligands, small, orally active, blood–brain barrier-crossing molecules that retain neurotrophism by docking to FKBP-12 and inhibiting rotamase, but which are nonimmunosuppressive because they lack the calcineurin docking domain *(49,88,89)*. These ligands promote neurite outgrowth in culture and, in vivo, the regeneration of damaged peripheral nerves and central neurons

(90). This led to numerous patents for neurotrophic small-molecule FKBP ligands, [for example, G. S. Hamilton and J. P. Steiner at Guilford Pharmaceuticals Inc. *(91)*; small molecule inhibitors of rotamase enzyme, 1997, US Patent: 5,614,547; D. M. Armistead (Vertex Pharmaceuticals Inc.) *(92)*; methods and compositions for stimulating neurite growth, 2000, US Patent: 6,037,370; Lyons et al. (Johns Hopkins University School of Medicine) *(87)*; stimulating nerve growth with immunophilins, 2000, US Patent: 6,080,753], which are being developed in collaboration with larger pharmaceutical companies. A Guilford small molecule is currently in Phase 2 European Parkinson's trials.

FK506 as a Neuroprotective Agent

FK506 inhibition of NOS, and demonstration of neurotrophic effects, led to the first neuroprotection in vivo ischemia experiments at the Fujisawa Institute of Neuroscience in 1994 (for full details *see* Chapter 12). Sharkey and Butcher demonstrated protection in a middle cerebral artery (MCA) occlusion–reperfusion model of focal ischemia with 46% reduction in cortical infarct volume when FK506 was administered 60 min postocclusion. Rapamycin itself was not neuroprotectant, and even blocked FK506 actions, confirming calcineurin to be a critical step for FK506 neuroprotection. In hindsight, CsA was found ineffective because of a subtherapeutic dose *(93)*. This led to a use patent for FK506 to treat ischemia, J. S. Kelly, S. P. Butcher, and J. Sharkey, Fujisawa Pharmaceutical Co., Ltd. *(94)*: Use of macrolides for the treatment of cerebral ischemia, 1997, US Patent 5,648,351. Researchers in Japan demonstrated that FK506 gave moderate protection to the gerbil CA1 hippocampal region in 5-min forebrain transient global ischemia model with simultaneous *(95)* or 2-h posttreatment *(96)*. This was confirmed by T. Wieloch's group *(97)* the same year in the rat model of 10-min forebrain ischemia, although not as dramatically as CsA *(2)*.

Sharkey and Butcher *(98)* confirmed their focal ischemia finding in 1996 1 min posttreatment, and revealed not only a 60% infarct reduction, but also a quantified improvement in poststroke motor skills. The results were also confirmed in 1996 by Kuroda and Siesjö *(99)* with delayed FK506 administration. Sharkey and Butcher *(76)* made further evaluation in 1997 showing that a higher dose of FK506 (10 mg/kg) reduced cortical damage by 50% up to 2 h posttreatment, although not at 3 h.

Yoshimoto and Siesjö *(100)* confirmed, in a model of focal (MCA occlusion) reperfusion injury, that immediate postinsult intraarterial FK506 reduces infarct volume by 50%, while CsA in the same model reduced infarct volume by 90%. However, Kuroda and coworkers *(101)* looked at the more severe hyperglycemic focal ischemia (30-min MCA occlusion model) and showed FK506 to be equally or trending to slightly more effective than CsA in reducing infarct volume to less than 1/3 of control. In 1998 Friberg and coworkers *(102)* showed no protective effect of FK506 on hypoglycemic coma-induced brain damage, implicating mitochondrial function as a central component of cell death in this insult model.

Continued evaluation by other groups confirms that FK506 has a robust neuroprotective effect against focal ischemia with reperfusion in rat with recent suggestions of FK506's mechanism of neuroprotection being inhibition of release of apoptotic ceramide *(80,103)*. Researchers in arenas beyond ischemia are starting to look at FK506 as a neuroprotectant. Recent work found a moderate neuroprotectant effect on retinal ganglion cells following optic nerve crush injury *(104)*. However, no neuroprotective effect of FK506 was found in a model of traumatic brain injury *(105)* further implicating the role of mitochondrial function in certain types of neuronal cell death.

The ease of FK506 administration, safety, and strength of effect in animal stroke models make human clinical trials desirable. The Fujisawa Institute team in Edinburgh hopes to bring their FK506 ischemia discovery to the aid of patients (J. Kelly, personal communications to M. Keep 1997 and 1998). Fujisawa may soon begin human FK506 stroke trials. While there are some differences in efficacy between FK506 and CsA in different models of stroke and neural insult, just as in transplantation, there will likely be a useful and welcome role for both in clinical neuroprotection.

Cyclosporin A as a Neuroprotective Agent

CsA, Mechanism of Action

The CsA-binding cyclophilins are 20 times more enriched in neurons than T cells, especially in the hippocampus, cortex, substantia nigra, locus ceruleus, caudate-putamen, cerebellum, brainstem motor nuclei, and spinal cord ventral horn *(106,107)*. CsA, in addition to inhibiting calcineurin and rotamase activity, is unique in that it is the only neuroimmunophilin demonstrated to directly block the mitochondrial permeability transition (mPT), and the formation of the mitochondrial "megapore." This profoundly important effect is discussed briefly below, and also in other chapters in this book.

The megapore is a still incompletely defined, large unselective pore between the mitochondrial inner and outer membranes, formed in the combined presence of elevated mitochondrial Ca^{2+} and free radicals *(108–111)*. Inhibitors of mPT include CsA, magnesium ions, protons, ATP, and ADP *(112,113)*. Cyclophilin D's position within the mitochondrial matrix *(114)* permits CsA interaction to inhibit the mPT, thereby both preserving the proton gradient, important for oxidative phosphorylation *(115)*, and blocking release of proapoptotic caspase activators cytochrome *c*, procaspase 9, and apoptosis-inducing factor (AIF). The formation of the mPT has been implicated as the defining penultimate event prior to necrosis and apoptosis.

CsA Immunosuppression for Neurological Autoimmune Diseases

True autoimmune neurological diseases such as myasthenia gravis respond to corticosteroid, azathioprine, plasmapheresis, and also CsA immunosuppression *(6,116)*. While myasthenia gravis showed benefit, multiple sclerosis showed no or modest effect from CsA immunosuppression, overshadowed by side effects *(117–119)*. At the immunosuppressive dose given in those studies, CsA could not cross the blood–brain barrier to contact the central nervous system. It remains to be seen if CsA, when it crosses the blood–brain barrier, will be directly neuroprotective in multiple sclerosis, and is worthy of study.

The role of autoimmunity in amyotrophic lateral sclerosis (ALS) was always controversial, but plasma exchange, intrathecal and systemic steroids, azathioprine, and cyclophosphamide treatments were tried and found ineffective *(117)*. CsA immunosuppression was also attempted, with no difference in outcome was found between CsA and untreated human ALS groups *(120)*. In hindsight, CsA, while suitable for systemic immunosuppression, unfortunately did not cross the blood–brain barrier where it might have had a neuroprotective effect on the motor neurons of the patients. (For a discussion of the transgenic ALS mouse model and intrathecal CsA *see* Chapter 18.

Persistence of the Immunosuppression Paradigm,
and the Importance of Brain Penetration of CsA

Ryba and associates *(121)* in 1991 sought to examine if CsA might blunt the suspected autoimmunologic role in postsubarachnoid hemorrhage (SAH) vasospasm from cerebral aneurysm rupture. They theorized that if an immune-mediated angiopathy and vasospasm of the cerebral arteries could be blocked by CsA, this would prevent the brain from becoming ischemic. They concluded that they had found a better outcome with CsA in their SAH patients. However, the average age of those receiving CsA immunosuppression was 38 yr compared to control patients who were 48 yr *(121)*. The 8-yr age advantage is likely the reason for their apparent better outcome, and not CsA immunosuppression. While Ryba's group did not publish another study on this topic, Manno and coworkers *(122)* in 1997 confirmed that SAH patients had no benefit from simple CsA treatment. SAH is a transient opening of a cerebral aneurysm, letting blood under pressure into the subarachnoid space and directly into contact with brain tissue. As long as there is no rebleeding, the aneurysm is resealed, and any CsA systemically administered post-SAH could not reach the brain to exert neuroprotection. It is not yet known if CsA, when it crosses the blood–brain barrier, will be directly neuroprotective to vasospasm-induced brain ischemia and is worthy of study. On the other hand, if CsA were in the blood prior to the aneurysm rupture, then the blood laden with CsA in the subarachnoid space in contact with the brain could have a neuroprotective effect. This is indicated in the study by Shiga and colleagues where CsA-loaded blood likely inadvertently entered the subarachnoid space at the time of ischemia *(124)*.

In their study, rats were preloaded with CsA. Focal reperfusion ischemia was then induced using a nylon filament passed through the carotid artery, which was left in the MCA for 1 h and then removed to allow for reperfusion. While this method usually causes only rare (2–3%) intracranial hemorrhages *(123)*, the Shiga group excluded 40% of their animals because of intracranial hemorrhage. Among the surviving rats there was a significant reduction in infarct size which they attributed to CsA's immunosuppressive effect *(124)*. It is now known that systemic administration of an immunosuppressive dose of CsA does not give neuroprotection, even with long-term pretreatment, because it is actively excluded from the brain by the intact blood–brain barrier *(3,100–102)*. Shiga's group likely inadvertently disrupted the MCA with the filament technique, as evidenced by the high hemorrhage rate, which allowed the pretreatment CsA that was already in the blood to enter the subarachnoid space to contact the brain and exert a neuroprotective effect. They did not follow up this initial study. Subsequent experiments using similar models, with CsA treatment and no opening of the blood–brain barrier showed no neuroprotective effect *(2,3,100,101)*.

CsA immunosuppression likely has an effect on immune responses to ischemia. However, these immune responses are not responsible for neuronal death or survival. This can be seen in studies of CsA immunosuppression without neuroprotection when the blood–brain barrier is intact. In 1993 and 1995 Ogawa and coworkers *(125,126)* examined CsA immunosuppression on reduction of muscarinic acetylcholine receptors in the hippocampus after 5 min of transient forebrain ischemia, without opening the blood–brain barrier. While they noted that CsA reduced the number of reactive glial cells and acetylcholine receptor binding, they found it had no protective effect on CA1 hippocampal cell survival *(125,126)*. This research was revisited by the Ogawa group in 1999 *(127)*, giving again CsA treatment without opening the blood–brain barrier. While restored receptor binding was detected, they confirmed the negative effect on survival of

CA1 neurons (*see* Chapter 11). In 1995 Wakita and collaborators *(128)* examined the role of T cells and activated microglia in white matter changes of chronic cerebral hypoperfusion and found that CsA immunosuppression reduced activated microglia and macrophages, and white matter rarefaction. There was no loss of neurons in either CsA or control groups so there was no opportunity to observe for neuroprotection or lack of it because of the intact blood–brain barrier *(128)* (*see* Chapter 10).

It is necessary to get CsA to contact the brain to have a neuroprotective effect, but there is a threshold dose. When Sharkey and Butcher *(93)* demonstrated FK506 protection from focal stroke in a MCA endothelin cortical injection occlusion model in 1994, they found CsA ineffective. Even though they physically opened the blood–brain barrier with the endothelin injection into the cortex, they used a subtherapeutic CsA dose (1mg/kg iv), which was insufficient for neuroprotection *(93)*. In 1997, using a higher dose of CsA (20 mg/kg iv), and opening the blood–brain barrier, they demonstrated powerful neuroprotectant effect of CsA and demonstrated it to be at least equal to that of FK506 *(76)*.

Acute and chronic systemic CsA administration at immunosuppressive doses is not neuroprotective with an intact blood–brain barrier, because it does not come into contact with neurons. CsA's potential neuroprotection was missed because of the lack of awareness by neuroscientists that the extremely lipophilic CsA does not cross the blood–brain barrier because of the active extrusion mechanism by the *p*-glycoprotein transporter in the brain capillary endothelium. This led to major confusion and several failures before the realization that CsA is profoundly neuroprotectant when it crosses the blood–brain barrier and comes into contact with neurons.

*Opening the Blood–Brain Barrier, and the Discovery
that CsA is Neuroprotective In Vivo*

It was the progression of organ grafting to include neural transplantation in the 1980s that led to the discovery that the quintessential immunosuppressant CsA is also a very powerful neuroprotective agent. The Departments of Anatomy and Neurology in Lund, Sweden, building on early Swedish advances in imaging the catecholamine system, pursued animal and human work pioneering the grafting of fetal mesencephalic dopamine neurons into rodents and finally humans. The primary immunosuppressive agent used in Lund was CsA *(129)*. This led to a Swedish tradition for CsA immunosuppression in numerous projects involving stereotactic implantation of cells into the rodent central nervous system.

Work involving neurotrophins indicated they might be useful neuroprotectants *(130)* and so were tried in a model of global ischemia by

E. Elmér in 1993 (then at the department of Neurology, Lund University Hospital, Sweden) in a collaboration with H. Uchino. The model was grafting nerve growth factor (NGF)-secreting genetically engineered cells (immortalized HiB5 cells, kindly supplied by Professor A. Björklund, Lund) into the unilateral hippocampus, and then (after 1 wk) animals were subjected to 7 min of global ischemia via carotid clamping and temporary exsanguination. This model consistently produces 70–80% cell loss of hippocampal CA1 neurons. The animal group with neurotrophin-secreting cells deposited near the vulnerable CA1 region was "anticipated" to display reduced cell death, while the control group with nonsecreting HiB5 cells was not expected to display any reduction. To protect the implanted engineered cells from rejection, both experimental and control groups were given daily CsA injections (10 mg/kg ip) from d 1 (implantation) to d 14 (evaluation). When the NGF cells were injected stereotactically into the hippocampal formation, a physical disruption of the blood–brain barrier was made in all rats. The surprise finding was that after the ischemic insult, neither group had any overt hippocampal cell loss!

The operative technique and other general parameters were questioned. Some considerations were unsuccessfully performed ischemia, or a change of supplier of the experimental animals. It was recommended by senior researchers that this particular experiment should be dropped to devote resources to more promising work. However, E. Elmér was certain of the ischemic technique performed by H. Uchino and found normal 70–80% cell death in an added control experiment without HiB5 cells or CsA. The needle insertion itself was removed as the explanation in further central experiments. During late-night discussions it was realized by E. Elmér and H. Uchino that the needle insertion had opened the blood–brain barrier, and in combination with administering CsA, was the critical measure that allowed CsA to actually enter the brain parenchyma, come into contact with neurons, and give neuroprotection. The discovery was confirmed in a further experiment: One group of animals was treated daily with CsA without a needle lesion, ischemia at d 7 and evaluation at d 14. The other group received daily CsA treatment, stereotactic saline injection into the hippocampus at d 1, ischemia at d 7, and evaluation at d 14. The group that both received CsA treatment and saline injection into the hippocampus (opening the blood–brain barrier) displayed neuroprotection, with 90% reduction in neuronal cell death (Fig. 2) *(2,3)*. Rats receiving CsA without a needle lesion (with intact blood–brain barrier) had no benefit from the CsA treatment and displayed the usual 70–80% cell death in the hippocampal CA1 region (Fig. 2) *(2,3)*. This was the first confirmation of the

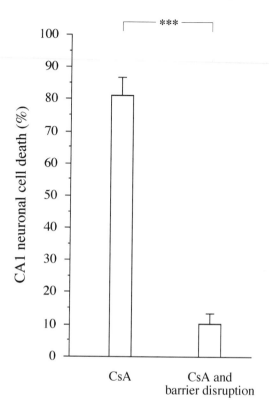

Fig. 2. Histopathological outcome in the CA1 sector of hippocampus at 7 d of recovery following 7 min of ischemia in animals treated with CsA (10 mg/kg). Systemic administration of CsA exerted significant neuroprotection only in combination with disruption of the blood–brain barrier (see text). Damage is given as percent of the total neuronal population in CA1 (at bregma –3.8). ***$p < .001$. For further details *see* refs. *2* and *3*.

discovery that CsA is a powerful neuroprotective agent when it crosses the blood–brain barrier and comes into contact with the brain. In addition, it was also the first in vivo demonstration of a connection between mitochondrial permeability transition and neuronal ischemic cell death. In discussions with M. Keep it was realized that this ischemic neuroprotective effect also extended to a broad spectrum of neural insults, including traumatic brain injury and neurodegeneration. This understanding led to a use patent for CsA as a neuroprotectant *(131)*. Since then, CsA has been confirmed to be a potent neuroprotective agent in animal models of global ischemia *(1,3,132)* with ischemia for as long as 30 min *(133)*, and focal ischemia *(100,101)* when it can cross the blood–brain barrier. One useful finding is that high-dose intracarotid CsA itself autosaturates the *p*-glycoprotein transporter, allowing CsA to cross the blood–brain barrier and protect against embolic stroke with a therapeutic window of up to 6 h *(100)*. In addition, a sufficiently high systemic dose of CsA can autosaturate the *p*-glycoprotein transporter *(134)*. Short-term intravenous CsA doses of 30 mg/kg or more will autosaturate the *p*-glycoprotein transporter and allow CsA to cross the blood–brain barrier for neuroprotection, but it remains to be seen if the side effect profile is acceptable.

FK506 shares the effect of rotamase and calcineurin inhibition with CsA, but not the mitochondrial protection. FK506 is equally or less effective in some stroke models, and is not neuroprotectant in hypoglycemic coma and cortical impact models *(102,135)*, while CsA is. Likely the additional effect of directly protecting the mitochondria, accounts for CsA's added neuroprotection. Despite the mitochondrial protection, just like FK506 and nonimmunosuppressive CsA analogs *(136)*, there is no evidence that CsA is useful in permanent focal ischemia (E. Elmér, M. Keep, and B. Johansson, unpublished observations). There is a theoretical limit to neuroprotection, and permanent complete cessation of blood flow seems to be that limit. Furthermore, the therapeutic time window for any known drug intervention so far has not been extended beyond 6 h.

Extensive and compelling CsA neuroprotection is documented in several rat models of stroke, particularly global and focal embolic ischemia. Based on this, and the favorable safety profile of CsA, human trials are now being planned in Lund, Sweden.

Traumatic Brain Injury

With stroke, the challenge of CsA administration is its delivery across the blood–brain barrier. This is not the case with traumatic brain injury (TBI), which itself opens the blood–brain barrier. Traumatic disruption of cerebral capillaries and vessels making up the blood–brain barrier allows simple intravenous CsA administration. Some TBI patients have intraventricular catheters for intracranial pressure monitoring passed through the brain. This further opens the blood–brain barrier and gives direct access to the cerebrospinal fluid for intraventricular injections of CsA, which would eliminate systemic effects of immunosuppression or nephrotoxicity. There is not a significant cerebrospinal fluid–brain barrier to prevent entry of CsA into neurons. However, any neurotoxicity from intrathecal CsA will need to be defined for short-term administration for TBI.

CsA has been studied in animal models of TBI with numerous recent publications, second only to ischemia (*see* Chapter 13). Using a rat cortical impact model, Okonkwo and colleagues *(137,138)* were the first to administer intrathecal CsA by injection into the cisterna magna, with pre- and 30-min posttreatment showing significant protection from secondary axotomy, and preserved mitochondrial integrity. This confirms that the cerebrospinal fluid–brain barrier does not block CsA entry and that there is a therapeutic window for clinical use *(139)*.

Scheff and Sullivan *(135)* demonstrated in 1999 that systemic administration of CsA protected against cortical damage in a similar open-blood–brain barrier model with administration 15 min after the insult, preserving mitochondrial membrane potential, blocking the mPT *(140)*, and preserving hippocampal synaptic plasticity *(141)*. Continuous posttreatment lasting for 7 d, showed an unprecedented 74% decrease in lesion size *(105)*. This indicates that TBI secondary damage occurs over several days giving an extended window of opportunity for neuronal salvage. FK506 failed to show an effect, suggesting the importance of mitochondrial protection in TBI *(135)*. The first indication that the remarkable CsA neuroprotection found in animals may have human applicability is a German case report describing a 14-yr-old transplant recipient on CsA who suffered severe TBI and made a surprisingly good recovery *(142)*. Based on this compelling animal data, human trials with CsA for TBI are planned at the Medical College of Virginia. (R. M. Bullock, personal communication to M. Keep and E. Elmér).

Neurodegeneration

Evidence is building that FK506, CsA, and the FKBP small molecules are neuroprotective and neurotrophic in the neurodegenerative disease models of Alzheimer's (Chapter 7), Parkinson's (Chapters 2–6), Huntington's (Chapter 8), and amyotrophic lateral sclerosis (Chapter 18). It has been proposed that one of the final common pathways of neuronal cell death in neurodegeneration is the result of mitochondrial dysfunction *(143)*. Various susceptibilities include accumulation of toxic amyloid and senilin proteins and decreased cytochrome oxidase activity in Alzheimer's, disease, decreased electron transport functions in Parkinson's disease *(144)*, CAG repeat huntingtin protein in Huntington's disease *(145,146)* aberrant SOD function in ALS *(147)*, accumulation of intramitochondrial iron in Frederick's ataxia *(148)*, and intramitochondrial copper in Wilson's disease *(149)*.

The additional stress on the mitochondria by increased free radical formation shifts the mitochondria toward formation of the mPT. This increased susceptibility to mPT formation results in specific cell population depletion over time, such as cholinergic septal, dopaminergic substantia nigral, GABAergic striatal, motor, or Purkinje neurons. Both CsA and FK506, as inhibitors of calcineurin and NOS, could indirectly shift the curve back away from mPT formation by reducing free radical formation. However, CsA itself is able to also directly inhibit the mPT, which may confer additional neuroprotection *(150)*.

In Alzheimer's disease there is evidence that abnormal amyloid and senilin proteins make the neurons more susceptible to stress, with mitochondria as targets *(151)*. Important work by Cassarino and colleagues *(152)* demonstrates that CsA helps maintain mitochondrial membrane potential in Alzheimer's cybrids. Borlongan and colleagues *(153)* has led the effort in Alzheimer's, showing a beneficial CsA effect on septal cholinergic neurons in vivo, neurons whose loss is most associated with early memory decline. Down syndrome, a related juvenile neurodegenerative disease, may also respond to the mitochondrial neuroprotective effects of CsA *(154)*.

Parkinson's and Huntington's Diseases

MPTP is a mitochondrial neurotoxin which caused parkinsonism in some humans consuming illicit synthetic narcotics, and joins 6-hydroxydopamine (6-OHDA) in creating animal models of parkinsonism. Despite an early report in 1989 that CsA enhanced MPTP neurotoxicity *(155)* considerable recent evidence shows CsA to strongly protect dopamine neurons in vitro and in vivo from MPTP *(156–160)*. Borlongan and colleagues *(161–163)* has shown that CsA, when it crosses the blood–brain barrier, upregulates dopamine neurons and increases animal motor activity. Huntington's CAG triplet protein appears to be neurotoxic via increased mitochondrial susceptibility *(164,165)*. CsA protects against mitochondrial calcium overload and the mitochondrial toxin 3-nitropropionic acid in vitro and in vivo models of Huntington's disease, implicating the mPT *(166,167)*. It has been suggested that CsA might be useful for treating Huntington's disease and Parkinson's disease *(168)*. Like steroid-derived lazaroids, CsA (and FK506) have been found to be neuroprotective in fetal cell culture of dopamine neurons *(169)* *(see* Chapter 5) and may be added to clinical use in preparing neural tissue for transplantation. This raises the interesting speculation whether human improvement from neural transplants for Parkinson's disease, Huntington's disease, and stroke *(170–182)* is not due only to cell survival from immunosuppression, but also to the extended CsA administration with blood–brain barrier opened by stereotactic needle passes through the brain to deliver grafted cells, similar to the first experiment that lead to the discovery of CsA neuroprotection. This could be easily tested by administering CsA with implanted deep-brain stimulators (Aptiva, Medtronic) used for treating Parkinson's disease, which would open the blood–brain barrier to CsA, without cellular grafts.

Chronic neuroprotection for neurodegeneration requires further study with CsA and FK506. The primary concern with systemic administration for both drugs is immunosuppression and nephrotoxicity, while CsA does not easily cross the blood–brain barrier. These concerns are addressed by developing an intrathecal cerebrospinal fluid delivery of CsA or FK506 through permanent implanted intraventricular access port (Model 8506, Medtronic) with periodic percutaneous injections that would bathe periventricular structures like hippocampus, fornix, septum, caudate–basal ganglia, and mesencephalon to medulla brainstem nuclei, and the spinal central canal down to the conus. Once the CsA or FK506 empties out from the ventricular system into the subarachnoid space, it would further bathe external structures including the cerebral cortex, cerebellar folia, external brainstem, spinal cord, and nerve roots. The vanishingly small doses of CsA or FK506 entering the systemic circulation with cerebrospinal fluid through arachnoid granulations would not cause systemic complications of immunosuppression nor nephrotoxicity. Issues of intraventricular dosing are being defined, and the question of potential neurotoxicity needs to be answered in animal studies.

CONCLUDING REMARKS

Several classic immunosuppressants and their analogs have shown the new and separate effect of neuroprotection, most notably corticosteroids, FK506 and CsA. This is a profound paradigm shift, especially for FK506 and CsA, that are being understood for their immense potential to effectively treat many neurological diseases, which, until now, have been without hope or help. This new understanding of neuroimmunophilin ligand neuroprotection arises from the cross-pollination from visceral graft immunosuppression, neural transplantation, and the calling to save humans from the shipwrecks of neurological disease.

ACKNOWLEDGMENTS

This work was supported by the Victoria S. and Bradley L. Geist Foundation, the Restorative Neurosurgery Foundation, John and Anna-Stina Mattson's fund (E.E.), NHR (E.E.), and Maas BiolAB, LLC. Maas BiolAB, LLC intellectual property includes the use of cyclosporin for neurological indications.

REFERENCES

1. Li P A, Uchino H, Elmér E, Siesjö B K. Amelioration by cyclosporin A of brain damage following 5 or 10 min of ischemia in rats subjected to preischemic hyperglycemia. Brain Res 1997;753:133–140.
2. Uchino H, Elmér E, Uchino K, et al. Cyclosporin A dramatically ameliorates CA1 hippocampal damage following transient forebrain ischaemia in the rat. Acta Physiol Scand 1995;155:469–471.
3. Uchino H, Elmér E, Uchino K, et al. Amelioration by cyclosporin A of brain damage in transient forebrain ischemia in the rat. Brain Res 1998;812: 216–226.
4. Kalderon N, Alfieri AA, Fuks Z. Beneficial effects of x-irradiation on recovery of lesioned mammalian central nervous tissue. Proc Natl Acad Sci USA 1990;87:10,058–10,062.
5. Ridet JL, Pencalet P, Belcram M, et al. Effects of spinal cord x-irradiation on the recovery of paraplegic rats. Exp Neurol 2000;161:1–14.
6. Schalke BCG. Kappos L, Rohrbach E, et al. Cyclosporin a vs azathioprine in the treatment of myesthenia gravis: final results of a randomized, controlled double-blind clinical trial. Neurology 1988;38:135.
7. Hektoen L, Corper HJ. The effects of mustard gas (dichloroethylsulphide) on antibody formation. J Infect Dis 1921;28:279–293.
8. Schwartz R, Dameshek W. Drug-induced immunological tolerance. Nature 1959;183:1682–1683.
9. Calne RY. The development of immunosuppressive therapy. Transplant Proc 1981;13:44–49.
10. Polley HF, Slocumb CH. Behind the scenes with cortisone and ACTH. Mayo Clin Proc 1976;51:471–477.
11. Crabtree GR. Contingent genetic regulatory events in T lymphocyte activation. Science 1989;243:355–361.
12. Goodwin WE, Kaufman JJ, Mims MM., et al. Human renal transplantation. I. Clinical experiences with six cases of renal homotransplantation. J Urol 1963;89:13–24.
13. Starzl TE. Personal reflections in transplantation. Surg Clin North Am 1978;58:879–893.
14. Calne RY. Azathioprine, In: Ginns LCC, Benedict Cosimi A, Morris PJ, eds. Transplantation. Blackwell Science, Malden, MA, 1999, pp. 113–114.
15. Starzl TE, Marchioro TL, Von Kaulla KN, et al. Homotransplantation of the liver in humans. Surg Gynecol Obstet 1963;117:659–676.
16. Hardy JD, Webb WR, Dalton MLJ, Walker GRJ. Lung homotransplantation in man. JAMA 1963;186:1065–1074.
17. Kelly WD, Lillehei RC, Merkel FK, et al. Allotransplantation of the pancreas and duodenum along with the kidney in diabetic nephropathy. Surgery 1967;61:827–837.
18. Barnard CN. The operation. A human cardiac transplant: an interim report of a successful operation performed at Groote Schuur Hospital, Cape Town. S Afr Med J 1967;41:1271–1274.

19. Bracken MB, Shepard MJ, Collins WF, et al. (1990) A randomized, controlled trial of methylprednisolone or naloxone in the treatment of acute spinal-cord injury. Results of the Second National Acute Spinal Cord Injury Study. N Engl J Med 1990;322:1405–1411.
20. Bracken MB, Shepard MJ, Collins WF Jr, et al. Methylprednisolone or naloxone treatment after acute spinal cord injury: 1-year follow-up data. Results of the second National Acute Spinal Cord Injury Study. J Neurosurg 1992;76: 23–31.
21. Segatore M. Corticosteroids and traumatic brain injury: status at the end of the decade of the brain. J Neurosci Nurs 1999;31:239–250.
22. Newell DW, Temkin NR, Bullock R, Choi, S. Corticosteroids in acute traumatic brain injury. BMJ 1998;316:396.
23. Alderson P, Roberts I. Corticosteroids for acute traumatic brain injury. Cochrane Database Syst Rev 2000;CD000196.
24. Frodl EM, Nakao N, Brundin P. Lazaroids improve the survival of cultured rat embryonic mesencephalic neurones. Neuroreport 1994;5:2393–2396.
25. Kassell NF, Haley EC Jr, Apperson-Hansen C, Alves WM. Randomized, double-blind, vehicle-controlled trial of tirilazad mesylate in patients with aneurysmal subarachnoid hemorrhage: a cooperative study in Europe, Australia, and New Zealand. J Neurosurg 1996;84:221–228.
26. Othberg A, Keep M, Brundin P, Lindvall O. Tirilazad mesylate improves survival of rat and human embryonic mesencephalic neurons in vitro. Exp Neurol 1997;147:498–502.
27. Brundin P, Pogarell O, Hagell P, et al. Bilateral caudate and putamen grafts of embryonic mesencephalic tissue treated with lazaroids in Parkinson's disease. Brain 2000;123:1380–1390.
28. The RANTTAS Investigators. A randomized trial of tirilazad mesylate in patients with acute stroke (RANTTAS). Stroke 1996;27:1453–1458.
29. Marshall LF, Maas AI, Marshall SB, et al. A multicenter trial on the efficacy of using tirilazad mesylate in cases of head injury. J Neurosurg 1998;89:519–525.
30. Borel JF. Ciclosporin and its future. Prog Allergy 1986;38:9–18.
31. Borel JF, Feurer C, Gubler HU, Stahelin H. Biological effects of cyclosporin A: a new antilymphocytic agent. Agents Actions 1976;6:468–475.
32. Borel JF Cyclosporine: historical perspectives. Transplant Proc 1983;15: 2219–2229.
33. Borel JF. History of cyclosporin A and its significance in immunology. In: DJG White ed, Cyclosporin A. Elsevier Biomedical Press, Amsterdam, 1982, pp. 5–17.
34. Calne RY, White DJ, Thiru S, et al. Cyclosporin A in patients receiving renal allografts from cadaver donors. Lancet 1978;2:1323–1327.
35. Fruman DA, Burakoff SJ, Bierer BE. Immunophilins in protein folding and immunosuppression. FASEB J 1994;8:391–400.
36. Handschumacher RE, Harding MW, Rice J, et al. Cyclophilin: a specific cytosolic binding protein for cyclosporin A. Science 1984;226:544–547.

37. Schreiber SL, Crabtree GR. The mechanism of action of cyclosporin A and FK506. Immunol. Today 1992;13:136–142.
38. Liu J, Farmer JD Jr, Lane WS, et al. Calcineurin is a common target of cyclophilin-cyclosporin A and FKBP-FK506 complexes. Cell 1991;66: 807–815.
39. Cardenas ME, Muir RS, Breuder T, Heitman J. Targets of immunophilin-immunosuppressant complexes are distinct highly conserved regions of calcineurin A. EMBO J 1995;14:2772–2783.
40. Batiuk TD, Kung L, Halloran PF. Evidence that calcineurin is rate-limiting for primary human lymphocyte activation. J Clin Invest 1997;100:1894–1901.
41. Bram RJ, Hung DT, Martin PK, et al. Identification of the immunophilins capable of mediating inhibition of signal transduction by cyclosporin A and FK506: roles of calcineurin binding and cellular location. Mol Cell Biol 1993;13:4760–4769.
42. Fruman DA, Klee CB, Bierer BE, Burakoff SJ. Calcineurin phosphatase activity in T lymphocytes is inhibited by FK 506 and cyclosporin A. Proc Natl Acad Sci USA 1992;89:3686–3690.
43. Jiang, H., Suguo, H., Takahara, S., et al. Combined immunosuppressive effect of FK 506 and other immunosuppressive agents on PHA- and CD3-stimulated human lymphocyte proliferation in vitro. Transplant Proc 1991;23: 2933–2936.
44. Takahashi N, Hayano T, Suzuki M. Peptidyl-prolyl cis-trans isomerase is the cyclosporin A-binding protein cyclophilin. Nature 1989;337:473–475.
45. Fischer G, Wittmann-Liebold B, Lang K, et al. Cyclophilin and peptidyl-prolyl cis-trans isomerase are probably identical proteins. Nature 1989;337:476–478.
46. Schreiber SL. Chemistry and biology of the immunophilins and their immunosuppressive ligands. Science 1991;251:283–287.
47. Bierer BE, Somers PK, Wandless TJ, et al. Probing immunosuppressant action with a nonnatural immunophilin ligand. Science 1990;250:556–559.
48. Friedman J, Weissman I. Two cytoplasmic candidates for immunophilin action are revealed by affinity for a new cyclophilin: one in the presence and one in the absence of CsA. Cell 1991;66:799–806.
49. Snyder SH, Sabatini DM, Lai MM., et al. Neural actions of immunophilin ligands. Trends Pharmacol Sci 1998;19:21–26.
50. Myers BD. Cyclosporine nephrotoxicity. Kidney Int 1986;30:964–974.
51. Thompson CB, June CH, Sullivan KM, Thomas ED. Association between cyclosporin neurotoxicity and hypomagnesaemia. Lancet 1984;2:1116–1120.
52. Lorber MI, Van Buren CT, Flechner SM, et al. Hepatobiliary and pancreatic complications of cyclosporine therapy in 466 renal transplant recipients. Transplantation 1987;43:35–40.
53. Gijtenbeek JM, van den Bent MJ and Vecht CJ. Cyclosporine neurotoxicity: a review. J Neurol 1999;246:339–346.
54. Appleton RE, Farrell K, Teal P, et al. Complex partial status epilepticus associated with cyclosporin A therapy. J Neurol Neurosurg Psychiatry 1989;52:1068–1071.

55. de Groen PC, Aksamit AJ, Rakela J, et al. Central nervous system toxicity after liver transplantation. The role of cyclosporine and cholesterol. N Engl J Med 1987;317:861–866.
56. Stein DP, Lederman RJ, Vogt DP, et al. Neurological complications following liver transplantation. Ann Neurol 1992;31:644–649.
57. Kino T, Hatanaka H, Miyata S, et al. FK-506, a novel immunosuppressant isolated from a Streptomyces. II. Immunosuppressive effect of FK-506 in vitro. J Antibiot (Tokyo) 1987;40:1256–1265.
58. Kino T, Hatanaka H, Hashimoto M, et al. FK-506, a novel immunosuppressant isolated from a Streptomyces. I. Fermentation, isolation, and physicochemical and biological characteristics. J Antibiot (Tokyo) 1987;40: 1249–1255.
59. Tanaka H, Kuroda A, Marusawa H, et al. Physicochemical properties of FK-506, a novel immunosuppressant isolated from Streptomyces tsukubaensis. Transplant Proc 1987;19:11–16.
60. Todo S, Fung JJ, Starzl TE, et al. Liver, kidney, and thoracic organ transplantation under FK 506. Ann Surg 1990;212:295–305; discussion 306–297.
61. Kanitakis J Jullien D, Nicolas JF, et al. Sequential histological and immunohistochemical study of the skin of the first human hand allograft. Transplantation 2000;69:1380–1385.
62. Cosmas S, Damian S, The Catholic Encyclopedia, Robert Appleton Company, 1908.
63. Bierer BE, Mattila PS, Standaert RF, et al. Two distinct signal transmission pathways in T lymphocytes are inhibited by complexes formed between an immunophilin and either FK506 or rapamycin. Proc Natl Acad Sci USA 1990;87:9231–9235.
64. Siekierka JJ, Hung SH, Poe M, et al. A cytosolic binding protein for the immunosuppressant FK506 has peptidyl-prolyl isomerase activity but is distinct from cyclophilin. Nature 1989;341:755–757.
65. Kay JE. Structure-function relationships in the FK506-binding protein (FKBP) family of peptidylprolyl cis-trans isomerases. Biochem J 1996;314:361–385.
66. Vezina C, Kudelski A, Sehgal SN. Rapamycin (AY-22,989), a new antifungal antibiotic. I. Taxonomy of the producing streptomycete and isolation of the active principle. J Antibiot (Tokyo) 1975;28:721–726.
67. Sehgal SN, Baker H, Vezina C. Rapamycin (AY-22,989), a new antifungal antibiotic. II. Fermentation, isolation and characterization. J Antibiot (Tokyo) 1975;28:727–732.
68. Kahan BD. Immunosuppressive agents acting upon lymphokine synthesis and signal transduction. Clin Transplantation 1993;7:113–125.
69. Kelly PA, Gruber SA, Behbod F, Kahan BD. Sirolimus, a new, potent immunosuppressive agent. Pharmacotherapy 1997;17:1148–1156.
70. Morris RE. Rapamycin: antifungal, antitumor, antiproliferative, and immunosuppressive macrolides. Transplantation Rev 1992;6:39–87.
71. Murgia MG, Jordan S, Kahan BD. The side effect profile of sirolimus: a phase I study in quiescent cyclosporine-prednisone-treated renal transplant patients. Kidney Int 1996;49:209–216.

72. Steiner JP, Dawson TM, Fotuhi M et al. High brain densities of the immunophilin FKBP colocalized with calcineurin. Nature 1992;358:584–587.
73. Dawson TM, Steiner JP, Lyons WE, et al. The immunophilins, FK506 binding protein and cyclophilin, are discretely localized in the brain: relationship to calcineurin. Neuroscience 1994;62:569–580.
74. Dawson VL, Brahmbhatt HP, Mong JA, Dawson TM. Expression of inducible nitric oxide synthase causes delayed neurotoxicity in primary mixed neuronal-glial cortical cultures. Neuropharmacology 1994;33:1425–1430.
75. Dawson TM, Steiner JP, Dawson VL, et al. Immunosuppressant FK506 enhances phosphorylation of nitric oxide synthase and protects against glutamate neurotoxicity. Proc Natl Acad Sci USA 1993;90:9808–9812.
76. Butcher SP, Henshall DC, Teramura Y, et al. Neuroprotective actions of FK506 in experimental stroke: in vivo evidence against an antiexcitotoxic mechanism. J Neurosci 1997;17:6939–6946.
77. Bredt DS, Ferris CD, Snyder SH. Nitric oxide synthase regulatory sites. Phosphorylation by cyclic AMP-dependent protein kinase, protein kinase C, and calcium/calmodulin protein kinase; identification of flavin and calmodulin binding sites. J Biol Chem 1992;267:10,976–10,981.
78. Steiner JP, Dawson TM, Fotuhi M, Snyder SH. Immunophilin regulation of neurotransmitter release. Mol Med 1996;2:325–333.
79. Nichols RA, Suplick GR, Brown JM. Calcineurin-mediated protein dephosphorylation in brain nerve terminals regulates the release of glutamate. J Biol Chem 1994;269:23,817–23,823.
80. Toung TJ, Bhardwaj A, Dawson V L, et al. Neuroprotective FK506 does not alter in vivo nitric oxide production during ischemia and early reperfusion in rats. Stroke 1999;30:1279–1285.
81. Teichner A, Morselli E, Buttarelli FR, et al. Treatment with cyclosporine A promotes axonal regeneration in rats submitted to transverse section of the spinal cord. J Hirnforsch 1993;34:343–349.
82. Palladini G, Caronti B, Pozzessere G, et al. Treatment with cyclosporine A promotes axonal regeneration in rats submitted to transverse section of the spinal cord—II—Recovery of function. J Hirnforsch 1996;37:145–153.
83. Fabrizi NDC, Caronti B, Palladini G. Autoimmunity, central axonal regeneration and CsA A. In vitro observations on the action mechanisms. Rend Fis Acc Lincei 1995;9:87–93.
84. Lyons WE, George EB, Dawson TM, et al. Immunosuppressant FK506 promotes neurite outgrowth in cultures of PC12 cells and sensory ganglia. Proc Natl Acad Sci USA 1994;91:3191–3195.
85. Gold BG, Katoh K, Storm-Dickerson T. The immunosuppressant FK506 increases the rate of axonal regeneration in rat sciatic nerve. J Neurosci 1995;15:7509–7516.
86. Gold BG. FK506 and the role of immunophilins in nerve regeneration. Mol Neurobiol 1997;15:285–306.
87. Lyons WE, George EB, Dawson TM, et al. Stimulating nerve growth with immunophilins, US Patent and Trademark Office, (2000), Patent: 6,080,753, Johns Hopkins University School of Medicine, Baltimore, MD.

88. Steiner JP, Connolly MA, Valentine HL., et al. Neurotrophic actions of nonimmunosuppressive analogues of immunosuppressive drugs FK506, rapamycin and cyclosporin A. Nat Med 1997;3:421–428.
89. Gold BG, Zeleny-Pooley M, Wang MS, et al. A nonimmunosuppressant FKBP-12 ligand increases nerve regeneration. Exp Neurol 1997;147:269–278.
90. Steiner JP, Hamilton GS, Ross DT, et al. Neurotrophic immunophilin ligands stimulate structural and functional recovery in neurodegenerative animal models. Proc Natl Acad Sci USA 1997;94:2019–2024.
91. Hamilton GS, Steiner JP. Small molecule inhibitors of rotamase enzyme, US Patent and Trademark Office, (1997), Patent: 5,614,547, Guilford Pharmaceuticals Inc., Baltimore, MD.
92. Armistead DM. Methods and compositions for stimulating neurite growth, US Patent and Trademark Office, (2000), Patent: 6,037,370, Vertex Pharmaceuticals Incorporated, Cambridge, MA.
93. Sharkey J, Butcher SP. Immunophilins mediate the neuroprotective effects of FK506 in focal cerebral ischemia. Nature 1994;371:336–339.
94. Kelly JS, Butcher SP, Sharkey J. Use of macrolides for the treatment of cerebral ischemia, US Patent and Trademark Office, (1997), Patent: 5,648,351, Fujisawa Pharmaceutical Co., Ltd., Osaka, JP.
95. Tokime T, Nozaki K, Kikuchi H. Neuroprotective effect of FK506, an immunosuppressant, on transient global ischemia in gerbil. Neurosci Lett 1996;206:81–84.
96. Ide T, Morikawa E, Kirino T. An immunosuppressant, FK506, protects hippocampal neurons from forebrain ischemia in the mongolian gerbil. Neurosci Lett 1996;204:157–160.
97. Drake M, Friberg H, Boris-Möller F, et al. The immunosuppressant FK506 ameliorates ischaemic damage in the rat brain. Acta Physiol Scand 1996;158:155–159.
98. Sharkey J, Crawford JH, Butcher SP, Marston HM. Tacrolimus (FK506) ameliorates skilled motor deficits produced by middle cerebral artery occlusion in rats. Stroke 1996;27:2282–2286.
99. Kuroda S, Siesjö BK. Postischemic administration of FK506 reduces infarct volume following transient focal brain ischemia. Neurosci Res Commun 1996;19:83–90.
100. Yoshimoto T, Siesjö BK. Posttreatment with the immunosuppressant cyclosporin A in transient focal ischemia. Brain Res 1999;839:283–291.
101. Kuroda S, Janelidze S, Siesjö BK. The immunosuppressants cyclosporin A and FK506 equally ameliorate brain damage due to 30-min middle cerebral artery occlusion in hyperglycemic rats. Brain Res 1999;835:148–153.
102. Friberg H, Ferrand-Drake M, Bengtsson F, et al. Cyclosporin A, but not FK 506, protects mitochondria and neurons against hypoglycemic damage and implicates the mitochondrial permeability transition in cell death. J Neurosci 1998;18:5151–5159.
103. Herr I, Martin-Villalba A, Kurz E, et al. FK506 prevents stroke-induced generation of ceramide and apoptosis signaling. Brain Res 1999;826:210–219.

104. Freeman EE, Grosskreutz CL. The effects of FK506 on retinal ganglion cells after optic nerve crush. Invest Ophthalmol Vis Sci 2000;41:1111–1115.
105. Sullivan PG, Thompson M, Scheff SW. Continuous infusion of cyclosporin A postinjury significantly ameliorates cortical damage following traumatic brain injury. Exp Neurol 2000;161:631–637.
106. Goldner FM, Patrick JW. Neuronal localization of the cyclophilin A protein in the adult rat brain. J Comp Neurol 1996;372:283–293.
107. Lad RP, Smith MA, Hilt DC. Molecular cloning and regional distribution of rat brain cyclophilin. Mol Brain Res 1991;9:239–244.
108. Lemasters JJ, Nieminen AL, Qian T, et al. The mitochondrial permeability transition in cell death: a common mechanism in necrosis, apoptosis and autophagy. Biochim Biophys Acta 1998;1366:177–196.
109. Lemasters JJ. The mitochondrial permeability transition: from biochemical curiosity to pathophysiological mechanism (editorial; comment). Gastroenterology 1998;115:783–786.
110. Lemasters JJ, Nieminen AL, Qian, T, et al. The mitochondrial permeability transition in toxic, hypoxic and reperfusion injury. Mol Cell Biochem 1997;174:159–165.
111. Kristal BS, Dubinsky JM. Mitochondrial permeability transition in the central nervous system: induction by calcium cycling-dependent and -independent pathways. J Neuroche. 1997;69:524–538.
112. Haworth RA, Hunter DR. Allosteric inhibition of the Ca^{2+}-activated hydrophilic channel of the mitochondrial inner membrane by nucleotides. J Membr Biol 1980;54:231–236.
113. Crompton M, Costi A. Kinetic evidence for a heart mitochondrial pore activated by Ca^{2+}, inorganic phosphate and oxidative stress: a potential mechanism for mitochondrial dysfunction during cellular Ca^{2+} overload. Eur J Biochem 1988;178:489–501.
114. Tanveer A, Virji S, Andreeva L, et al. Involvement of cyclophilin D in the activation of a mitochondrial pore by Ca^{2+} and oxidant stress. Eur J Biochem 1996;238:166–172.
115. Beal MF. Energetics in the pathogenesis of neurodegenerative diseases. Trends Neurosci 2000;23:298–304.
116. Tindall RS, Rollins JA, Phillips JT, et al. Preliminary results of a double-blind, randomized, placebo-controlled trial of cyclosporine in myasthenia gravis. N Engl J. Med 1987;316:719–724.
117. Tindall RS. Immunointervention with cyclosporin A in autoimmune neurological disorders. J Autoimmun 1992;5:301–313.
118. Zhao GJ, Li DK, Wolinsky JS, et al. Clinical and magnetic resonance imaging changes correlate in a clinical trial monitoring cyclosporine therapy for multiple sclerosis. The MS Study Group. J Neuroimaging 1997;7:1–7.
119. The Multiple Sclerosis Study Group. Efficacy and toxicity of cyclosporine in chronic progressive multiple sclerosis: a randomized, double-blinded, placebo-controlled clinical trial. Ann Neurol 1990;27:591–605.

120. Appel SH, Stewart SS, Appel V, et al. A double-blind study of the effectiveness of cyclosporine in amyotrophic lateral sclerosis. Arch Neurol 1988; 45:381–386.
121. Ryba M, Pastuszko M, Iwanska K, et al. Cyclosporine A prevents neurological deterioration of patients with SAH—a preliminary report. Acta Neurochir (Wien) 1991;112:25–27.
122. Manno EM, Gress DR, Ogilvy CS., et al. The safety and efficacy of cyclosporine A in the prevention of vasospasm in patients with Fisher grade 3 subarachnoid hemorrhages: a pilot study. Neurosurgery 1997;40:289–293.
123. Longa EZ, Weinstein PR, Carlson S, Cummins R. Reversible middle cerebral artery occlusion without craniotomy in rats. Stroke 1989;20:84–91.
124. Shiga Y, Onodera H, Matsuo Y, Kogure, K. Cyclosporin A protects against ischemia-reperfusion injury in the brain. Brain Res 1992;95:145–148.
125. Ogawa N, Tanaka K, Kondo Y, et al. The preventive effect of cyclosporin A, an immunosuppressant, on the late onset reduction of muscarinic acetylcholine receptors in gerbil hippocampus after transient forebrain ischemia. Neurosci Lett 1993;152:173–176.
126. Kondo Y, Ogawa N, Asanuma M, et al. Cyclosporin A prevents ischemia-induced reduction of muscarinic acetylcholine receptors with suppression of microglial activation in gerbil hippocampus. Neurosci Res 1995;22: 123–127.
127. Kondo Y, Asanuma M, Iwata E, et al. Early treatment with cyclosporin A ameliorates the reduction of muscarinic acetylcholine receptors in gerbil hippocampus after transient forebrain ischemia. Neurochem Res 1999;24:9–13.
128. Wakita H, Tomimoto H, Akiguchi I, Kimura J. Protective effect of cyclosporin A on white matter changes in the rat brain after chronic cerebral hypoperfusion. Stroke 1995;26:1415–1422.
129. Lindvall O, Rehncrona S, Brundin P, et al. Human fetal dopamine neurons grafted into the striatum in two patients with severe Parkinson's disease: a detailed account of methodology and a 6-month follow-up. Arch. Neurol. 1989;46:615–631.
130. Lindvall O, Kokaia Z, Bengzon J, et al. Neurotrophins and brain insults. Trends Neurosci 1994;17:490–496.
131. Keep MF, Elmér ME, Kokaia M, et al. Treatment of cerebral ischemia and cerebral damage with neuroprotective agents, US Patent and Trademark Office, (1999), Patent: 5,972,924, Maas BiolAB, LLC. Honolulu, HI.
132. Siesjö BK, Elmér E, Janelidze S, et al. Role and mechanism of secondary mitochondrial failure. Acta Neurochir Suppl (Wien) 1999;73:7–13.
133. Li PA, Kristian T, He QP, Siesjö BK. Cyclosporin A enhances survival, ameliorates brain damage, and prevents secondary mitochondrial dysfunction after a 30-minute period of transient cerebral ischemia. Exp Neurol 2000; 165:153–163.

134. Lemaire M, Bruelisauer A, Guntz P, Sato H. Dose-dependent brain penetration of SDZ PSC 833, a novel multidrug resistance-reversing cyclosporin, in rats. Cancer Chemother Pharmacol 1996;38:481–486.
135. Scheff SW, Sullivan PG. Cyclosporin A significantly ameliorates cortical damage following experimental traumatic brain injury in rodents. J Neurotrauma 1999;16:783–792.
136. Bochelen D, Rudin M, Sauter A. Calcineurin inhibitors FK506 and SDZ ASM 981 alleviate the outcome of focal cerebral ischemic/reperfusion injury. J Pharmacol Exp Ther 1999;288:653–659.
137. Okonkwo DO, Povlishock JT. An intrathecal bolus of cyclosporin A before injury preserves mitochondrial integrity and attenuates axonal disruption in traumatic brain injury. J Cereb Blood Flow Metab 1999;19:443–451.
138. Okonkwo DO, Buki A, Siman R, Povlishock JT. Cyclosporin A limits calcium-induced axonal damage following traumatic brain injury. NeuroReport 1999;10:353–358.
139. Buki A, Okonkwo DO, Povlishock JT. Postinjury cyclosporin A administration limits axonal damage and disconnection in traumatic brain injury. J Neurotrauma 1999;16:511–521.
140. Sullivan PG, Thompson MB, Scheff SW. Cyclosporin A attenuates acute mitochondrial dysfunction following traumatic brain injury. Exp Neurol 1999;160:226–234.
141. Albensi BC, Sullivan PG, Thompson MB, et al. Cyclosporin ameliorates traumatic brain-injury-induced alterations of hippocampal synaptic plasticity. Exp Neurol 2000;162:385–389.
142. Gogarten W, Van Aken H, Moskopp D, et al. A case of severe cerebral trauma in a patient under chronic treatment with cyclosporine A. J Neurosurg Anesthesiol 1998;10:101–105.
143. Tatton WG, Chalmers-Redman RM. Mitochondria in neurodegenerative apoptosis: an opportunity for therapy? Ann Neurol 1998;44:S134–141.
144. Schapira AH, Cooper JM, Dexter D, et al. Mitochondrial complex I deficiency in Parkinson's disease. J Neurochem 1990;54:823–827.
145. The Huntington's Disease Collaborative Research Group. A novel gene containing a trinucleotide repeat that is expanded and unstable on Huntington's disease chromosomes. Cell 1993;72:971–983.
146. Browne SE, Bowling AC, MacGarvey U, et al. Oxidative damage and metabolic dysfunction in Huntington's disease: selective vulnerability of the basal ganglia. Ann Neurol 1997;41:646–653.
147. Kong J, Xu, Z. Massive mitochondrial degeneration in motor neurons triggers the onset of amyotrophic lateral sclerosis in mice expressing a mutant SOD1. J Neurosci 1998;18:3241–3250.
148. Radisky DC, Babcock MC, Kaplan J. The yeast frataxin homologue mediates mitochondrial iron efflux. Evidence for a mitochondrial iron cycle. J Biol Chem 1999;274:4497–4499.
149. Lutsenko S, Cooper MJ. Localization of the Wilson's disease protein product to mitochondria. Proc Natl Acad Sci USA 1998;95:6004–6009.

150. Ruiz F, Alvarez G, Ramos M, et al. Cyclosporin A targets involved in protection against glutamate excitotoxicity. Eur J Pharmacol 2000;404:29–39.
151. Keller JN, Guo Q, Holtsberg FW, et al. Increased sensitivity to mitochondrial toxin-induced apoptosis in neural cells expressing mutant presenilin-1 is linked to perturbed calcium homeostasis and enhanced oxyradical production. J Neurosci 1998;18:4439–4450.
152. Cassarino DS. Swerdlow RH, Parks JK, et al. (1998) Cyclosporin A increases resting mitochondrial membrane potential in SY5Y cells and reverses the depressed mitochondrial membrane potential of Alzheimer's disease cybrids. Biochem Biophys Res Commun 1998;248:168–173.
153. Borlongan CV, Stahl CE, Keep MF, et al. Cyclosporine-A enhances choline acetyltransferase immunoreactivity in the septal region of adult rats. Neurosci Lett 2000;279:73–76.
154. Schuchmann S, Muller W, Heinemann U. Altered Ca^{2+} signaling and mitochondrial deficiencies in hippocampal neurons of trisomy 16 mice: a model of Down's syndrome. J Neurosci 1998;18: 7216–7231.
155. Hagihara M, Fujishiro K, Takahashi A, et al. Cyclosporin A, an immune suppressor, enhanced neurotoxicity of N-methyl-4-phenyl-1,2,3,6-tetrahydrodropyridine (MPTP) in mice. Neurochem Int 1989;15:249–254.
156. Chalmers-Redman RM, Fraser AD, Carlile GW, et al. Glucose protection from MPP+-induced apoptosis depends on mitochondrial membrane potential and ATP synthase. Biochem Biophys Res Commun 1999;257:440–447.
157. Cassarino DS, Parks JK, Parker WD Jr, Bennett JP Jr. The parkinsonian neurotoxin MPP+ opens the mitochondrial permeability transition pore and releases cytochrome c in isolated mitochondria via an oxidative mechanism. Biochim Biophys Acta 1999;1453:49–62.
158. Seaton, T. A., Cooper, J. M. and Schapira, A. H. (1998) Cyclosporin inhibition of apoptosis induced by mitochondrial complex I toxins. Brain Res. 809, 12–17.
159. Matsuura K, Kabuto H, Makino H, Ogawa N. Cyclosporin A attenuates degeneration of dopaminergic neurons induced by 6-hydroxydopamine in the mouse brain. Brain Res 1996;733:101–104.
160. Matsuura K, Makino H, Ogawa N. Cyclosporin A attenuates the decrease in tyrosine hydroxylase immunoreactivity in nigrostriatal dopaminergic neurons and in striatal dopamine content in rats with intrastriatal injection of 6-hydroxydopamine. Exp Neurol 1997;146:526–535.
161. Borlongan CV, Stahl CE, Fujisaki T, et al. Cyclosporine A-induced hyperactivity in rats: is it mediated by immunosuppression, neurotrophism, or both? Cell Transplant 1999;8:153–159.
162. Borlongan CV, Freeman TB, Scorcia TA, et al. Cyclosporine-A increases spontaneous and dopamine agonist-induced locomotor behavior in normal rats. Cell Transplant 1995;4:65–73.
163. Borlongan CV, Freeman TB, Hauser RA, et al. Cyclosporine-A increases locomotor activity in rats with 6-hydroxydopamine-induced hemiparkinsonism: relevance to neural transplantation. Surg Neurol 1996;46:384–388.
164. Schapira AH. Mitochondrial dysfunction in neurodegenerative disorders. Biochim Biophys Acta 1998;1366:225–233.

165. Beal MF. Mitochondrial dysfunction in neurodegenerative diseases. Biochim Biophys Acta 1998;1366:211–223.

166. Petersen A, Castilho RF, Hansson O, et al. Oxidative stress, mitochondrial permeability transition and activation of caspases in calcium ionophore A23187-induced death of cultured striatal neurons. Brain Res 2000;857: 20–29.

167. Leventhal L, Sortwell CE, Hanbury R, et al. Cyclosporin A protects striatal neurons in vitro and in vivo from 3-nitropropionic acid toxicity. J Comp Neurol 2000;425:471–478.

168. Alexi T, Borlongan CV, Faull RL, et al. Neuroprotective strategies for basal ganglia degeneration: Parkinson's and Huntington's diseases. Prog Neurobiol 2000;60:409–470.

169. Castilho RF, Hansson O, Brundin P. FK506 and cyclosporin A enhance the survival of cultured and grafted rat embryonic dopamine neurons. Exp Neurol 2000;164:94–101.

170. Lindvall O, Brundin P, Widner H, et al. Grafts of fetal dopamine neurons survive and improve motor function in Parkinson's disease. Science 1990;247:574–577.

171. Lindvall O, Widner H, Rehncrona S., et al. Transplantation of fetal dopamine neurons in Parkinson's disease: one-year clinical and neurophysiological observations in two patients with putaminal implants. Ann Neurol 1992; 31:155–165.

172. Lindvall O. Clinical application of neuronal grafts in Parkinson's disease. J Neurol 1994;242:S54–S56.

173. Lindvall O. Update on fetal transplantation: the Swedish experience. Mov Disord 1998;13:83–87.

174. Kordower JH, Freeman TB, Snow BJ, et al. Neuropathological evidence of graft survival and striatal reinnervation after the transplantation of fetal mesencephalic tissue in a patient with Parkinson's disease. N Engl J Med 1995;332:1118–1124.

175. Kordower JH, Rosenstein JM, Collier TJ, et al. Functional fetal nigral grafts in a patient with Parkinson's disease: chemoanatomic, ultrastructural, and metabolic studies. J Comp Neurol 1996;370:203–230.

176. Kordower JH, Freeman TB, Chen EY, et al. Fetal nigral grafts survive and mediate clinical benefit in a patient with Parkinson's disease. Mov Disord 1998;13:383–393.

177. Shannon KM, Kordower JH. Neural transplantation for Huntington's disease: experimental rationale and recommendations for clinical trials. Cell Transplant 1996;5:339–352.

178. Kopyov OV, Jacques S, Lieberman A, et al. Safety of intrastriatal neurotransplantation for Huntington's disease patients. Exp Neurol 1998;149:97–108.

179. Bachoud-Levi A, Bourdet C, Brugieres P, et al. Safety and tolerability assessment of intrastriatal neural allografts in five patients with Huntington's disease. Exp Neurol 2000;161:194–202.

180. Watts C, Dunnett SB. Towards a protocol for the preparation and delivery of striatal tissue for clinical trials of transplantation in Huntington's disease. Cell Transplant 2000;9:223–234.

181. Fink JS, Schumacher JM, Ellias SL, et al. Porcine xenografts in Parkinson's disease and Huntington's disease patients: preliminary results. Cell Transplant 2000;9:273–278.

182. Kondziolka D, Wechsler L, Goldstein S, et al. Transplantation of cultured human neuronal cells for patients with stroke. Neurology 2000;55:565–569.

II

Immunosuppressants and Parkinson's Disease

2

Cyclosporin-Mediated Amelioration of Degeneration of Dopaminergic Neurons in Experimental Models of Parkinsonism

Norio Ogawa and Ken-ichi Tanaka

INTRODUCTION

Parkinson's disease (PD) is a slowly progressive neurodegenerative disease, the principal pathological feature of which is the progressive degeneration of dopaminergic neurons in the nigrostriatal system. This degeneration of the nigrostriatal system results in a deficiency in dopamine (DA) content both in the striatum and substantia nigra, which causes the characteristic symptoms of PD, that is, resting tremor, rigidity, and bradykinesia or akinesia. There are several strategies for the treatment of PD, such as supplying DA by providing the precursor levodopa, activating the DA receptor with DA agonists, or grafting with DA-producing tissues. Levodopa treatment, which was developed based on the observation of a decrease in striatal DA levels, has been the most successful of these strategies. Levodopa is the gold standard for the treatment of PD and is widely used because of its outstanding clinical efficacy. However, long-term levodopa treatment causes severe clinical complications, including the wearing-off phenomenon, on–off phenomenon, dyskinesia, and psychiatric symptoms *(1–3)*. Moreover, since degeneration of dopaminergic neurons continues even during levodopa treatment, recent efforts in the treatment of PD have focused on the development of agents and strategies that suppress or delay disease progression. These include free-radical scavengers *(4)*, antioxidants *(5)*, the iron-chelator desferrioxamine *(6)*, excitatory amino acid receptor antagonists *(4,7)*, and neurotrophic factors such as glial cell-derived neurotrophic factor (GDNF) *(8,9)* and brain-derived neurotrophic factor (BDNF) *(10–13)*.

It has also been suggested that immunological reactions play an important role in PD, Alzheimer's disease, and cerebrovascular disease *(14–17)*.

From: *Immunosuppressant Analogs in Neuroprotection*
Edited by: C. V. Borlongan, O. Isacson, and P. R. Sanberg © Humana Press Inc., Totowa, NJ

Cyclosporin A (CsA) is a potent immunosuppressant widely used to inhibit rejection after transplantation and to treat autoimmune diseases, and protective effects of CsA against ischemia–reperfusion injury in rat and gerbil models of transient ischemia *(15,16,18)*, and against 1-methyl-4-phenyl-1,2,3,6-tetrahydropyridine (MPTP)-induced striatal DA depletion in mice *(19)* have been reported. In this chapter, we summarize the effects of CsA on the depletion and degeneration of dopaminergic neurons in experimental animal models of parkinsonism.

EFFECTS OF CYCLOSPORIN A ON THE DEGENERATION OF DOPAMINERGIC NEURONS IN EXPERIMENTAL ANIMAL MODELS OF PARKINSONISM

Several animal models of parkinsonism have been established that employ intracerebroventricular, intranigral, or intraforebrain bundle injections of 6-hydroxydopamine (6-OHDA), or systemic injections of MPTP to induce rapid and selective lesioning of nigrostriatal dopaminergic neurons. However, these models have faster time courses than PD, the slow progression of which is due to a sustained loss of nigrostriatal dopaminergic neurons. Furthermore, the MPTP model can show spontaneous improvement in indices of dopaminergic function *(20–22)*. We have previously used two experimental animal models of parkinsonism: acute degeneration of dopaminergic neurons induced by intracerebroventricular injection of 6-OHDA in mice, and slowly progressive degeneration of dopaminergic neurons induced by intrastriatal injection of 6-OHDA in rats.

6-Hydroxydopamine-Induced Parkinsonism in Mice

In the first study, we investigated the protective effects of the immuno-suppressant CsA against 6-OHDA-induced injury of nigrostriatal dopaminergic neurons in male ICR mice *(23)*. Intracerebroventricular (icv) injections of 6-OHDA (80 µg) or physiological saline containing ascorbic acid (SA) as a control were performed under light ether anesthesia 30 min after injection of desipramine (25 mg/kg ip), which prevents the uptake of 6-OHDA by noradrenergic neurons. CsA or the same volume of vehicle (V; 0.2% castor oil) was injected subcutaneously 24 h and 30 min before, 5 h after, and once daily from d 1 to d 6 after 6-OHDA injection. At 7 d after the injection of 6-OHDA, the concentrations of DA and its metabolites dihydroxyphenyl-acetic acid (DOPAC) and homovanillic acid (HVA) in the striatum and the substantia nigra were determined (Fig. 1).

Although CsA had no effect on DA or its metabolites in the substantia nigra of SA-treated control mice, it induced a slight increase in striatal HVA in such mice. At 7 d after the induction of 6-OHDA lesions, DA, DOPAC,

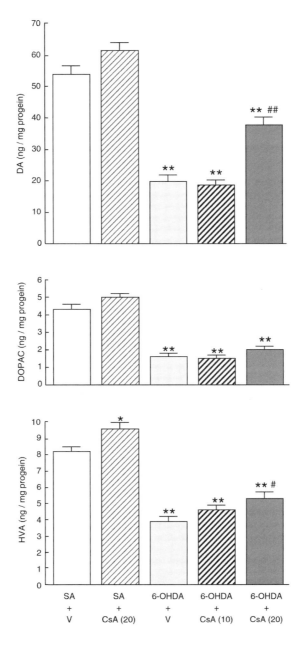

Fig. 1. Effects of CsA on the striatal DA, DOPAC, and HVA concentrations in mice at 7 d after intracerebroventricular injection of 6-OHDA. Numbers in parentheses are the daily dose of CsA in milligrams per kilogram. Each value is the mean ±SEM for 30–35 mice. *$p < .05$, **$p < .01$ vs SA (i.c.v.) + V (vehicle)-injected group; #$p < .05$, ##$p < .01$ vs 6-OHDA (i.c.v.) + V-injected group.

and HVA in the striatum were depleted by 63%, 63%, and 52%, respectively (Fig. 1). However, striatal DA and HVA in the 6-OHDA+CsA (20 mg/kg)-treated group were significantly higher than in the 6-OHDA+ V-treated group, indicating that CsA (20 mg/kg) elevated both striatal DA and striatal HVA in the 6-OHDA-lesioned mice. Although HVA and DOPAC in the substantia nigra were depleted by 40% in 6-OHDA-lesioned mice, CsA significantly increased both HVA and DOPAC (data not shown in Fig. 1). Thus, CsA is beneficial in reducing 6-OHDA-induced injury of nigrostriatal DA neurons in mice, indicating its therapeutic potential in the treatment of PD. Similar protective effects were obtained by another immunosuppressant, FK506, and the nonimmunosuppressive analogue GPI1046 (data not shown in Fig. 1).

Slowly Progressive Dopaminergic Neurodegeneration Model in Rats

In the second study, we investigated the effects of CsA on the degeneration of dopaminergic neurons in a rat model of slowly progressive dopaminergic neurodegeneration after intrastriatal injections of 6-OHDA *(24)*. In this animal model, intrastriatal injection of 6-OHDA induces slowly progressive degeneration of dopaminergic neurons, and neurotrophins or other factors can be tested for their effects on the residual dopaminergic neurons *(5,11)*. Under sodium pentobarbital anesthesia (35 mg/kg, ip), rats were intrastriatally injected with 6-OHDA (5 µg at four sites) or SA as a control. CsA or the same volume of vehicle (V; 0.2% castor oil) was injected subcutaneously (s.c.) 24 h and 30 min before, 5 h after, and once daily on d 1 to d 6 after 6-OHDA (or SA) injection. Rats were sacrificed 1 or 4 wk after 6-OHDA injection and were divided into two groups: one for neurochemical analysis and the other for histological analysis.

At 1 and 4 wk after 6-OHDA injection, DA, DOPAC, and HVA in the striatum and the substantia nigra were measured (Fig. 2). At 1 wk after 6-OHDA injection, there was no difference in DA levels in the striatum or substantia nigra between SA+V- and SA+CsA-treated groups, although DA levels of 6-OHDA+V- and 6-OHDA+CsA-treated groups were significantly lower than those of control (SA+V-treated) rats in the striatum (Fig. 2). At 4 wk after 6-OHDA injection, however, the striatal DA level in the CsA-treated group was significantly higher than in the V-treated group, indicating that CsA significantly attenuated the toxic effects of 6-OHDA on dopaminergic neurons (Fig. 2). Nigral DA level in the 6-OHDA+V-treated group was significantly lower than that in the SA+V treated group, but there was no significant difference in DA levels between SA+V-treated rats and 6-OHDA+CsA-treated rats at 4 wk after 6-OHDA injection, indicating that the CsA also had an effect on nigral DA depletion (Fig. 2).

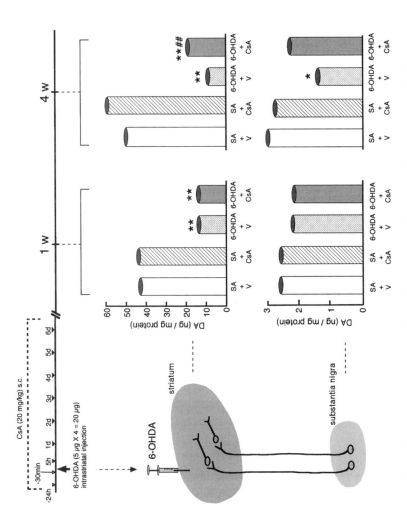

Fig. 2. Effects of CsA on DA concentrations in the striatum and substantia nigra of rats at 1 wk and 4 wk after intrastriatal injections of 6-OHDA. Data are expressed as the mean of 6 animals. $*p < .05$, $**p < .01$ vs SA (intrastriatal) + V (vehicle)-injected group; $\#\#p < .01$ vs 6-OHDA (intrastriatal) + V-injected group.

Previous studies have given contradictory results on neurochemical changes in the striatum of intrastriatal 6-OHDA-lesioned rats. Although Altar and colleagues *(25)* found that the levels of DA and its metabolites partially recovered between 1 and 4 wk after striatal injection of 6-OHDA, Venero and colleagues *(26)* observed no recovery in the levels of striatal DA and its metabolites between 2 d and 4 wk after striatal injection of 6-OHDA. In the present study, we also observed no spontaneous recovery of nigrostriatal DA content (Fig. 2). There was no significant difference in striatal DA levels between 1 and 4 wk after 6-OHDA injection in the SA-treated group. Further, although the nigral DA level in this group was not significantly different from the level in controls at 1 wk after injection, it was significantly decreased at 4 wk (Fig. 2), indicating that progressive degeneration of dopaminergic neurons occurred in this rat model.

In a previous histological study, tyrosine hydroxylase (TH) immunoreactivity (TH-IR) of nigral cell bodies and dendrites in the substantia nigra ipsilateral to injection was lower than that on the contralateral side at 4 wk after 6-OHDA injection *(24)*. The number of TH-positive neurons in the substantia nigra pars compacta on the 6-OHDA-injected side was decreased by 36% in the V-treated group and by 13% in the CsA-treated group. The loss of TH-IR was therefore significantly less in the CsA-treated group, indicating that CsA attenuated damage to the dopaminergic neurons. Without 6-OHDA injection, there was no decrease in the number of TH-immunoreactive neurons in the V-treated group or CsA-treated group, indicating that neither SA nor CsA by itself had any effect on the number of TH-immunoreactive neurons in the substantia nigra.

TH-IR is a good and sufficient marker for evaluating the depletion of tissue DA levels in the nigrostriatal system *(27)*, and changes in nigral TH-IR can be detected from 2 wk after 6-OHDA injection *(27)*. Thus, CsA treatment for 7 d significantly attenuated the decrease in TH-IR in the substantia nigra at 4 wk postinjection. These data again indicate that there is progressive degeneration of dopaminergic neurons in the present rat model, as in PD, and that CsA treatment significantly attenuated this degeneration.

MECHANISM OF ACTION OF CYCLOSPORIN A

The major findings of the above-mentioned two studies are that CsA elevated striatal DA levels in 6-OHDA-lesioned mice and rats. In the mouse model study, DA in the striatum was depleted by 63% at 7 d after intracerebroventricular injection of 6-OHDA, and repeated high-dose CsA (20 mg/kg) treatment significantly protected against this DA depletion *(23)*. Intrastriatal injection of 6-OHDA in the rat can cause a slowly progressive degeneration of dopaminergic neurons *(5,10,25,27–29)*. High-dose CsA daily for 7 d significantly attenuated the decrease in DA on the lesioned side of the striatum, and the number of TH-immunoreactive neurons in the substantia nigra at 4 wk after 6-OHDA lesions. Because tissue DA levels are known to be a good index of the degree of striatal dopaminergic denervation after the administration of 6-OHDA *(30)*, the present findings indicate that CsA may inhibit degeneration and/or promote regeneration of dopaminergic neurons. This is in agreement with earlier studies in which CsA was found to protect against MPTP-induced DA depletion in the striatum of mice *(19)*.

There have been a number of reports on the neuroprotective effects of various substances on damaged dopaminergic neurons in vivo *(4)*. We have provided the first evidence that CsA has a neuroprotective effect on dopaminergic neurons in experimental animal models of parkinsonism *(23,24)*.

One might not expect CsA to cross the blood–brain barrier. However, when brain lesions appear, the barrier is impaired, and CsA is able to cross it *(15,17,23)*; for this reason, long-term administration of CsA produces various central nervous system (CNS) side effects *(31)*, indicating that peripherally administered CsA can affect the CNS.

Immunosuppressive Effects via Calcineurin

It is known that glial cells accumulate at sites surrounding lesioned regions in PD, Alzheimer's disease, cerebrovascular disease, and in animal models of these diseases *(14–16,32)*. Several studies have reported that CsA particularly suppresses the ischemia-induced accumulation of reactive glial cells in the brain *(15,16,18)*. Thus, it is possible that CsA protects dopaminergic neurons by suppressing microglial cytotoxicity, which can occur via mechanisms such as the production of reactive oxygen intermediates, proteinases, and cytokines *(32,33)*.

CsA achieves immunosuppression mainly by inhibiting production of interleukin (IL)-2, which activates T cells. Foreign antigens displayed on the surface of antigen-presenting cells activate the T-cell receptor to initiate signal pathways that lead to increases in intracellular Ca^{2+}. Ca^{2+} binds to calmodulin and calcineurin B, which activate the phosphatase activity of the catalytic subunit (calcineurin A) of calcineurin. The phosphatase dephosphorylates the nuclear factor of activated T-cell (NFAT), allowing it to enter the nucleus and activate the transcription of IL-2 and IL-2 receptor *(34)*. CsA forms a complex with cyclophilin, an immunophilin. The CsA–cyclophilin complex binds to and inhibits calcineurin, preventing NFAT dephosphorylation and its subsequent transcription to the nucleus, leading to inhibition of T-cell activation *(35,36)*. Since calcineurin has been reported to dephosphorylate DARPP-32 (a dopamine-regulated neuronal phosphop-rotein) and to be richly distributed in the caudate putamen, substantia nigra, and striatonigral pathway, calcineurin may play a role in the function of dopaminergic neurons *(37–40)*. Thus, it might be assumed that CsA protects striatal DA and elevates nigral TH-IR–striatal DA levels by inhibiting calcineurin activity.

Neuroprotective and Neurorestorative Effects Independent of Immunosuppressive Properties

The intrastriatal 6-OHDA injection model is advantageous for studies of the microglial and astrocytic response because there is no mechanical dam-age to the substantia nigra. In the rat model *(24)*, a strong microglial reac-tion was observed in the substantia nigra after injection of either SA or 6-OHDA, although the 6-OHDA injection induced a more lasting reaction than did the SA. This reaction occurred during the initial neuronal degenera-tion stage but declined after about 4 wk, even though neuronal degeneration was still progressing in the 6-OHDA injection group *(27,41)*. It might be expected that CsA protects dopaminergic neurons by suppressing micro-glial cytotoxicity, which occurs via mechanisms such as the production of reactive oxygen intermediates, proteinases, and cytokines *(32,33)*. In our study, however, microglial activation in the substantia nigra was not affected by CsA treatment, and no significant change in GFAP staining was observed in the substantia nigra *(24)*. This suggests that CsA acts directly on neurons of the damaged dopaminergic system, rather than indirectly through immu-nosuppression. This is further supported by the finding that short-term CsA treatment during only the initial stages of neuronal damage either prevented degeneration or accelerated regeneration of the nigrostriatal dopaminergic neurons *(24)*. We have also shown that, in the mouse intracerebroventricular 6-OHDA injection model, both the initial CsA treatment *(42)* and continuous daily administration of CsA *(23)* promote the recovery of striatal DA levels.

Activated microglia generate free radicals. It is believed that ithis activ-ity can be inhibited by the administration of immunosuppressants, which involves binding of the CsA–cyclophilin complex with calcineurin to inhibit the dephosphorylating effect of calcineurin. However, cyclophilin has been identified with peptidylprolyl-*cis-trans*-isomerase (rotamase), an enzyme related to folding of proteins *(43,44)*, and CsA specifically sup-presses the rotamase activity of cyclophilin. Futhermore, long-term con-tinuous administration of CsA is not always necessary for neuroprotective action. In experiments using animal models of transient cerebral ischemia *(45)* and PD *(23,24)*, we have found that administration only in the initial stage after injury was sufficient. This raises the possibility that the neuroprotective and neurorestorative mechanisms of CsA differ from the immunosuppressive mechanisms.

Recently, it has been reported that agents that bind to immunophilins but have no immnunosuppressive effect show neurotrophiclike activity *(46,47)*. These agents (nonimnunosuppressive immunophilin ligands) are attracting attention as new candidates for neuroprotection and neurorestoration because they are not expected to have the adverse effects of immunosuppressants. Thus, the neuroprotective effects of CsA and other immunophilin ligands do not parallel their calcineurin-inhibitory effects, but are in parallel with the inhibitory effect on rotamase activity *(47)*; furthermore, the neuroprotective effects are not related to the inhibition of calcineurin, as was assumed in the past *(47)*.

POSSIBLE RESTORATIVE EFFECTS OF CYCLOSPORIN A ON DOPAMINERGIC NEURONS

In addition to its protective effects, CsA may also promote dopaminergic neurons. In the iminodipropionitrile (IDPN)-induced rat model of dyskinesia, the addition of CsA treatment exacerbated IDPN-induced dyskinesia *(48)*. The injection of both CsA and IDPN increased the concentration of DA and the binding activities of transcription factors to the TPA (12-*O*-tetradecanoylphorbol-13-acetate)-responsive element (TRE) and to the cAMP response element (CRE) in the striatum, compared with those in rats treated with IDPN alone (Fig. 3). Since the 5' upstream region of the rat tyrosine hydroxylase (TH) gene contains both TRE and CRE *(49)*, increased DA levels in the basal ganglia of the CsA + IDPN group may be partly due to transcriptional activation of the TH gene by increases in the DNA-binding activity of both TRE and CREB. In the present study, the levels of D1-receptor mRNA, but not D2-receptor mRNA, in the striatum were significantly decreased in the IDPN-treated rats but were at the control level in the rats given CsA + IDPN (Fig. 3). Since the rat D1-receptor gene posseses both TRE and CRE in the promoter region *(50)*, while the rat D2-receptor gene has only TRE *(51)*, increases in the activity of these transcription factors in the striatum of CsA + IDPN-treated rats may lead to the increases in the striatal D1-receptor mRNA. These findings suggest that the behavioral aggravation of the IDPN-induced dyskinesia caused by CsA administration may be due to the acceleration of the pre- and postsynaptic dopaminergic systems via activation of transcription factors that bind upstream to TH- and D1-receptor genes. Thus, CsA both restores and protects dopaminergic neurons, and, further, the restorative-neurotrophic effects of immunophilin ligands are restricted to damaged neurons *(46–48)*.

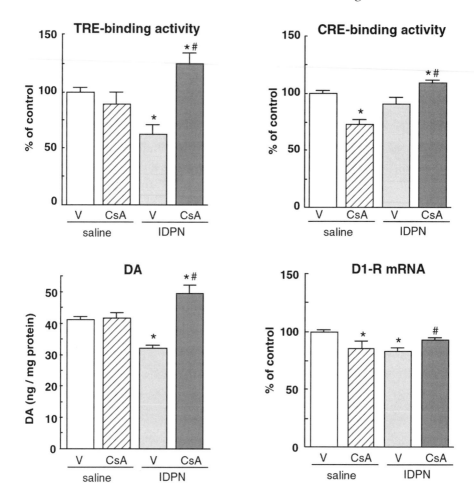

Fig. 3. Effects of CsA and IDPN, alone or togather, on TRE-binding activity, CRE-binding activity, DA concentrations, and D1-R mRNA levels in the rat striatum. Data are the mean ±SEM (n = 4–6). *p < .05 vs V (vehicle) + saline-injected group; [#] p < .05 vs V + IDPN-injected group.

These findings indicate that CsA should be advantageous for therapeutic use for PD.

CONCLUDING REMARKS

The pathogenesis of various important neurodegenerative diseases appears to be related to structural abnormalities, inactivation, or deposition of proteins such as β-amyloid, α-synuclein, polyglutamine, or prions (52). CsA has a neuroprotective effect against degeneration of dopaminergic neurons and shows neurotrophiclike activity. Through its interaction with cyclophilins, which are a highly conserved family of protein chaperones showing prolyl isomerase (rotamase) activity, CsA is deeply involved in the modulation of protein conformation. Therefore, it is possible that the neuroprotective action of immunophilin ligands can be applied to the treatment of conformational diseases. Cyclophilin is one of the immunophilins and is a highly efficient catalyst for the delayed refolding of damaged proteins *(53)*, but it shows almost no catalytic effect on delayed refolding of intact proteins *(54)*. Because immunophilin ligands act mainly on damaged proteins *(46–48)*, they are unlikely to have much effect on normal tissues, and should cause few adverse reactions. Thus, immunophilin ligands that were initially considered to be immunosuppressants are now expected to be useful in the treatment of neurodegenerative diseases via modulation of protein structures.

In conclusion, CsA showed protective and restorative effects against dopaminergic neuronal damage in experimental animal models, and these results suggest that CsA might offer a new approach to the treatment of PD and other neurodegenerative diseases.

ACKNOWLEDGMENTS

This work was supported in part by grants from Research on Brain Science and the Research Committee on the Neurodegenerative Diseases from the Japanese Ministry of Health and Welfare, and Grants-in-Aid for Scientific Research on Priority Areas and Scientific Research (C) from the Japanese Ministry of Education, Science, Sports and Culture.

REFERENCES

1. Pantelatos A, Fornadi, F. Clinical features and medical treatment of Parkinson's disease in patient groups selected in accordance with age at onset. Adv Neurol 1993;60:690–697.
2. Ogawa N. Levodopa and dopamine agonists in the treatment of Parkinson's disease: advantages and disadvantages. Eur Neurol 1994;34(Suppl. 3):20–28.
3. Ogawa N. Factors affecting levodopa effects in Parkinson's disease. Acta Med Okayama 2000;54:95–101.
4. Ogawa N. Possible neuroprotective therapy for Parkinson's disease. Acta Med Okayama 1995;49:179–185.
5. Cadet JL, Katz M, Jackson LV, Fahn S. Vitamin E attenuates the toxic effects of intrastriatal injection of 6-hydroxydopamine (6-OHDA) in rats: behavioral and biochemical evidence. Brain Res 1989;476:10–15.
6. Ben SD, Eshel G, Finberg JP, Youdim MB. The iron chelator desferrioxamine (Desferal) retards 6-hydroxydopamine-induced degeneration of nigrostriatal dopamine neurons. J Neurochem 1991;56:1441–1444.

7. Lange KW, Riederer P. Glutamatergic drugs in Parkinson's disease. Life Sci 1994;55:2067–2075.

8. Tomac A, Lindqvist E, Lin LF, et al. Protection and repair of the nigrostriatal dopaminergic system by GDNF in vivo. Nature 1995;373:335–339.

9. Bowenkamp KE, Hoffman AF, Gerhardt GA, et al. Glial cell line-derived neurotrophic factor supports survival of injured midbrain dopaminergic neurons. J Comp Neurol 1995;355:479–489.

10. Altar CA, Boylan CB, Jackson C, et al. Brain-derived neurotrophic factor augments rotational behavior and nigrostriatal dopamine turnover in vivo. Proc Natl Acad Sci USA 1992;89:11,347–11,351.

11. Altar CA, Boylan CB, Fritsche M, et al. Efficacy of brain-derived neurotrophic factor and neurotrophin-3 on neurochemical and behavioral deficits associated with partial nigrostriatal dopamine lesions. J Neurochem 1994;63:1021–1032.

12. Spina MB, Squinto SP, Miller J, et al. Brain-derived neurotrophic factor protects dopamine neurons against 6-hydroxydopamine and N-methyl-4-phenylpyridinium ion toxicity: Involvement of the glutathione system. J Neurochem 1992;59:99–106.

13. Martin-Iverson MT, Todd KG, Altar CA. Brain-derived neurotrophic factor and neurotrophin-3 activates striatal dopamine and serotonin metabolism and related behaviors: interactions with amphetamine. J Neurosci 1994; 14:1262–1270.

14. McGeer PL, Itagaki S, Boyes BE, McGeer EG. Reactive microglia are positive for HLA-DR in the substantia nigra of Parkinson's and Alzheimer's disease brains. Neurology 1988;38:1285–1291.

15. Ogawa N, Tanaka K, Kondo Y, et al. The preventive effect of cyclosporin A, an immunosuppressant,on the late onset reduction of muscarinic acetylcholine receptors in gerbil hippocampus after transient forebrain ischemia. Neurosci Lett 1993;152:173–176.

16. Shiga Y, Onodera H, Matsuo Y, Kogure K. Cyclosporin A protects against ischemia-reperfusion injury in the brain. Brain Res 1992;595:145–148.

17. Wakita H, Tomimoto H, Akiguchi I, Kimura J. Protective effect of cyclosporin A on white matter changes in the rat brain after chronic cerebral hypoperfusion. Stroke 1995;26:1415–1422.

18. Kondo Y, Ogawa N, Asanuma M, Niet al. Cyclosporin A prevents ischemia-induced reduction of muscarinic acetylcholine receptors with suppression of microglial activation in gerbil hippocampus. Neurosci Res 1995;22:123–127.

19. Kitamura Y, Itano Y, Kubo T, Nomura Y. Suppressive effect of FK506, a novel immunosuppressant, against MPTP-induced dopamine depletion in the striatum of young C57BL/6 mice. J Neuroimmunol 1994;50:221–224.

20. Espino A, Cutillas B, Tortosa A, et al. Chronic effects of single intrastriatal injections of 6-hydroxydopamine or 1-methyl-4-phenylpyridinium studied by microdialysis in freely moving rats. Brain Res 1995;695:151–157.

21. Ricaurte GA, DeLanney LE, Irwin I, Langston JW. Older dopminergic neurons do not recover from the effects of MPTP. Neuropharmacology 1987; 26:97–99.

22. Schneider JS. Effects of age on GM1 ganglioside-induced recovery of concentrations of dopamine in the striatum in 1-methyl-4-phenyl-1,2,3,6-tetrahydropyridine-treated mice. Neuropharmacology 1992;31:185–192.

23. Matsuura K, Kabuto H, Makino H, Ogawa N. Cyclosporin A attenuates degeneration of dopaminergic neurons induced by 6-hydroxydopamine in the mouse brain. Brain Res 1996;733:101–104.

24. Matsuura K, Makino H, Ogawa N. Cyclosporin A attenuates the decrease in tyrosine hydroxylase immunoreactivity in nigrostriatal dopaminergic neurons and in striatal dopamine content in rats with intrastriatal injection of 6-hydroxydopamine. Exp Neurol 1997;146:526–535.

25. Altar CA, Jakeman LB, Acworth IN, et al. Regionally restricted loss and partial recovery of nigrostriatal dopamine input following intrastriatal 6-hydroxydopamine. Neurodegeneration 1992;1:123–133.

26. Venero JL, Romero RM, Revuelta M, et al. Intrastriatal quinolinic acid injections protect against 6-hydroxydopamine-induced lesions of the dopaminergic nigrostriatal system. Brain Res 1995;672:153–158.

27. Ichitani Y, Okamura H, Nakahara D, et al. Biochemical and immunocytochemical changes induced by intrastriatal 6-hydroxydopamine injection in the rat nigrostriatal dopamine neuron system: evidence for cell death in the substantia nigra. Exp Neurol 1994;130:269–278.

28. Berger K, Przedborski S, Cadet JL. Retrograde degeneration of nigrostriatal neurons induced by intrastriatal 6-hydroxydopamine injection in rats. Brain Res Bullet 1991;26:301–307.

29. Jones BE, Boylan CB, Fritsche M, et al. A continuous striatal infusion of 6-hydroxydopamine produces a terminal axotomy and delayed behavioral effects. Brain Res 1996;709:275–284.

30. Altar CA, Marien MR, Marshall JF. Time course of adaptations in dopamine biosynthesis, metabolism, and release following nigrostriatal lesions: implications for behavioral recovery from brain injury. J Neurochem 1989;48:390–399.

31. Berden JHM, Hottsuma AJ, Merx JL, Keyser A. Severe central-nervous-system toxicity associated with cyclosporin. Lancet 1985;1:219–220.

32. Banati RB, Gehrmann J, Schubert P, et al. Cytotoxicity of microglia. Glia 1993;7:111–118.

33. Slivka A, Cohen G. Hydroxyl radical attack on dopamine. J Biol Chem 1985;15:15,466–15,472.

34. Shaw JP, Utz PJ, Durand, DB, et al. Identification of a putative regulator of early T cell activation genes. Science 1988;241:202–205.

35. Emmel EA, Verweij CL, Durand, D. B., et al. Cyclosporin A specifically inhibits function of nuclear proteins involved in T cell activation. Science 1989;246:1617–1620.

36. Mattila PS, Ullman KS, Fiering S, et al. The actions of cyclosporin A and FK506 suggest a novel step in the activation of T lymphocytes. EMBO J 1990;9:4425–4433.

37. Goto S, Matsykado Y, Mihara Y, et al. The distribution of calcineurin in rat brain by light and electron microscopic immunohistochemistry and enzyme-immunoassay. Brain Res 1986;397:161–172.

38. Steiner JP, Dawson TM, Fotuhi M, et al. High brain densities of the immunophilin FKBP colocalized with calcineurin. Nature 1992;358:584–587.
39. Walaas SI, Aswad DW, Greengard P. A dopamine- and cyclic AMP-regulated phosphoprotein enriched in dopamine innervated brain regions. Nature 1983;301:69–71.
40. Wera S, Neyts J. Calcineurin as a possible new target for treatment of Parkinson's disease. Med Hypotheses 1994;43:132–134.
41. Sauer H, Oertel WH. Progressive degeneration of nigrostriatal dopamine neurons following intrastriatal terminal lesions with 6-hydroxydopamine: a combined retrograde tracing and immunocytochemical study in the rat. Neuroscience 1994;59:401–415.
42. Matsuura K, Kabuto H, Makino H, Ogawa N. Initial cyclosporin A but not glucocorticaoid treatment promotes recovery of striatal dopamine concentration in 6-hydroxydopamine lesioned mice. Neurosci Lett 1997;230:191–194.
43. Takahashi N, Hayano T, Suzuki M. Peptidyl-prolyl cis-trans isomerase is the cyclosporin A-binding protein cyclophilin. Nature 1989;337:473–475.
44. Fischer G, Wittmann-Liebold B, Lang K, et al. Cyclophilin and peptidyl-prolyl cis-trans isomerase are probably identical proteins. Nature 1989;337:476–478.
45. Kondo Y, Asanuma M, Iwata E, et al. Early treatment with cyclosporin A ameliorates the reduction of muscarinic acetylcholine receptors in gerbil hippocampus after transient forebrain ischemia. Neurochem Res 1999;24:9–13.
46. Snyder SH, Sabatini DM, Lai MM, et al. Neural actions of immunophilin ligands. Trends Pharmacol Sci 1998;19:21–26.
47. Steiner JP, Hamilton GS, Ross DT, et al. Neurotrophic immunophilin ligands stimulate stracural and functional recovery in neurodegenerative animal models. Proc Natl Acad Sci USA 1997;94:2019–2024.
48. Iida K, Iwata E, Asanuma M, et al. Effects of repeated cyclosporin A administration on iminodipropionitrile-induced dyskinasia and TRE-/CRE-binding activities in rat brain. Neurosci Res 1998;30:185–193.
49. Cambi F, Fung B, Chikaraishi D. 5' Flanking DNA sequences direct cell-specific expression of rat tyrosine hydroxylase. J Neurochem 1989;53:1656–1659.
50. Zhou Q-Y, Li C, Civelli O. Characterization of gene organization and promoter region of the rat dopamine D1 receptor gene. J Neurochem 1992; 59:1875–1883.
51. Minowa T, Minowa MT, Mouradian MM. Analysis of the promoter region of the rat D2 dopamine receptor gene. Biochemistry 1992;31:8389–8396.
52. Carrell RW, Lomas DA. Conformational disease. Lancet 1997;350:134–138.
53. Lang K, Scmid FX, Fischer G. Catalysis of protein folding by prolyl isomerase. Nature 1987;329:268–272.
54. Fischer G, Bang H. The folding of urea denatured ribonuclease A is catalysed by peptidyl prolyl cis-trans isomerase. Biochim Biophys Acta 1985;828:39–45.

3

Immunophilin Ligands and Dopamine Neurons

Specific Effects in Culture and In Vivo

Lauren C. Costantini and Ole Isacson

INTRODUCTION

The search for compounds that can alter the development and health of a neuron has been the focus of a growing field of research. Several neurotrophic factors have shown impressive growth-inducing effects during development and protective effects in animal models of neurodegeneration, including brain-derived neurotrophic factor (BDNF) *(1–3)*, glial-derived neurotrophic factor (GDNF) *(4–8)*, transforming growth factor (TGF)-beta *(9,10)*, and basic fibroblast growth factor (bFGF) *(11)*. Identification of these factors helped pave the way for detection and analyses of the effects of other molecules and compounds with specific trophic and tropic effects on subsets of neuronal populations. Effects have also been shown with a variety of antioxidants *(12,13)*, glutamate antagonists *(14)*, caspase inhibitors *(15)*, and antiapoptotic agents *(16,17)*.

However the translation of these positive effects into the clinical setting has been cumbersome or largely negative due to difficulties in routes of administration and dosing parameters *(18,19)*. Systemic delivery of a trophic compound would provide an ideal strategy for clinical utilization.

IMMUNOSUPPRESSIVE IMMUNOPHILIN LIGANDS

Initial findings that the systemically administered immunosuppressive immunophilin ligand FK506 promotes neurite outgrowth in cell lines *(20)*, protects against glutamate toxicity in vitro *(21)*, and protects against focal ischemia in vivo *(22–24)*, stimulated interest in this family of compounds. Already utilized in the clinic for organ transplant recipients, the extension of their effects to a neuroprotective or neuroregenerative indication was an attractive possibility. Further animal studies show that FK506 protects

From: *Immunosuppressant Analogs in Neuroprotection*
Edited by: C. V. Borlongan, O. Isacson, and P. R. Sanberg © Humana Press Inc., Totowa, NJ

against kainate-induced neuronal death *(25)* and medial forebrain bundle transection *(26)*, increases regeneration after sciatic-nerve crush injury (reviewed in ref. *27)*, improves morphological and functional recovery after spinal cord injury *(28–30)*, and protects retinal ganglion cells after optic nerve crush *(31)*.

Animal studies have shown similar trophic and protective effects with the immunosuppressive drug CsA, including attenuation of neuronal degeneration in PD models *(32–34)* and Huntington's disease models *(35)*, and reduced area of injury after both ischemia *(36–40)* and traumatic brain injury *(41–43)*.

However the immunosuppressive and associated adverse effects of these drugs make them unsuitable for long-term treatment for neurological disorders. Long-term CsA induces neurological side effects in up to 40% of patients, including encephalopathy, peripheral neuropathy, and seizures *(44–47)*. In addition, owing to the inability of CsA to effectively cross the blood–brain barrier, treatment in neurodegenerative models requires an intrastriatal saline injection, lesion, or intravenous bradykinin receptor agonist *(35,38,48)* to disrupt the blood–brain barrier.

The neurotrophic activities of these immunophilin ligands can be separated from the immunosuppressive pathway. The neurotrophic effects of FK506 are due, in part, to its complexing with FKBP12, one of several immunophilins, which is highly concentrated in the brain and localized almost exclusively to neurons *(49)*. The immunosuppressive properties of FK506 are a consequence of the subsequent inhibition of the phosphatase calcineurin by the FK506/FKBP12 complex *(50)*. Inhibition of calcineurin augments phosphorylation of several substrates, leading to cytokine synthesis *(51)* and immunosuppression.

NONIMMUNOSUPPRESSIVE IMMUNOPHILIN LIGANDS

It has been postulated that FKBP12 plays a role in neuronal regeneration, since facial and sciatic nerve crush augments neuronal expression of FKBP12 mRNA, which parallels increases in GAP43 mRNA *(52)*. Based on the FKBP/FK506 complex structure, several novel small-molecule immunophilin ligands have been designed that bind the immunophilin FKBP12 yet do not interact with calcineurin, and are thus devoid of immunosuppressive activity. These *nonimmunosuppressive* immunophilin ligands demonstrate neurotrophic activity analogous to that obtained with FK506. Studies in culture illustrate the potent growth-stimulating effects of these compounds: while the extension of neurites from SH-SY5Y and PC12 cell lines, as well as sensory neurons in culture, occurs in the presence of NGF, the addition of nonimmunosuppressive immunophilin ligands enhances the extension of neurites in these systems *(53,54)*.

Effects of Nonimmunosuppressive Immunophilin Ligands on Developing DA Neurons in Culture

Although PC12 cell lines are catecholaminergic and secrete dopamine, they nonetheless represent a transformed cell that is not physiologically a dopamine neuron. Primary cultures of dopamine neurons from ventral mesencephalon (VM) provide a more direct analysis of the mechanisms involved in phenotypic DA survival, growth, and neurite extension. When these primary neurons were treated with nonimmunosuppressive immunophilin ligands, significant increases in neurite outgrowth were observed: branching of neurites from DA neurons [expressing tyrosine hydroxylase, (TH)] was significantly increased. Treatment of these cells with immunosuppressive immunophilin ligands FK506 and CsA significantly enhanced elongation of neuritis from TH+ neurons *(55,56)*.

The specificity of these results indicates that immunophilin ligands have different mechanisms of action on dopamine neurons, and elongation is dependent on the maintained phosphorylation of cell substrates (FK506 and CsA inhibit the phosphatase calcineurin), while branching does not require this pathway (nonimmunosuppressive immunophilin ligands do not inhibit calcineurin). The inhibition of calcineurin not only increases the phosphorylation of nuclear factor of activated T cells, thereby inhibiting subsequent interleuki (IL)-2 production, but it also increases the phosphorylation of other proteins, such as protein kinase C substrates *(57)*, Na^+/K^+-ATPase *(58)*, nitric oxide synthase (NOS) *(21)*, and GAP43 *(59)*. The mechanism underlying these effects may explain the contrasting effects observed here.

To determine whether this mechanism was a calcineurin-dependent phenomenon and not an immunosuppressive effect, we treated these cells with rapamycin (an immunosuppressive drug that does not inhibit calcineurin) and observed enhanced branching. Cell-type specificity was also observed, since there were no effects on growth of the γ-aminobutyric acid (GABA) neurons that are also included in primary VM cultures. No effects on total cell survival or TH+ cells were observed *(55,56)*.

The distinction between branching and elongation of DA neurites was made evident when DA neurons formed in the presence of growth factors *(60–62)* and their target striatal cells *(63)*. For instance, exposure of DA neurons to conditioned medium from VM induces the growth of dendritelike neurites (short, with a large number of branches), while growth in a medium conditioned with target striatal tissue stimulates the growth of axonlike neurites (long, with few branches) *(64)*. These factors may differentially modify subsets of cytoskeletal proteins, cell adhesion molecules, or extracellular matrix components *(65)*. The actions of immunophilin ligands may also involve these modifications, specifically at the growth cone, which has been shown to serve a stabilizing function in outgrowth *(66)*.

Effects of Nonimmunosuppressive Immunophilin Ligands Degenerating DA Neurons

When such robust effects of a trophic compound are observed on DA neurons in culture, the next step often moves toward one of many animal models of PD with the anticipation of therapeutic potential. The debilitating rigidity, tremor, bradykinesia, and postural instability experienced by PD patients eventually destroy their capability for physical movement and coordination, leaving them incapable of caring for themselves. These impairments that accompany the loss of dopamine neurons within the substantia nigra (SN) are only the first in a series of motor disabilities brought on by the disease as well as its treatments. The most common therapies for PD revolve around pharmaceutical substitutes for DA; however, as DA neurons continue their progressive degeneration; the effectiveness of these substitutes decreases, and eventually dyskinesias and motor fluctuations outweigh the benefits of drugs such as L-dopa *(67,68)*.

The development of drugs that enhance or prolong the effectiveness of L-dopa have had impressive results for a limited period of time. Alleviation of some symptoms has been obtained with surgical procedures such as pallidotomy ("short circuiting" the overactive pallidum and reducing dyskinesias), thalamotomy (lesioning the ventral intermediate nucleus for tremor reduction), and deep brain stimulation (inhibiting directly or stimulating inhibitory pathways in underactive regions of the basal ganglia) *(69–71)*. "Restoration by reconstruction" through the transplantation of DA-producing cells to the putamen has shown success *(72–75)*, although strategies to increase the survival and reinnervation capacity of the transplanted cells remain a top priority in preclinical studies of this field (discussed below). A variety of strategies are highly effective in treating the symptoms of the disease, but they do not alter the progression of the disease in order to continue to minimize symptoms effectively. This is the next challenge: to alter the underlying progression of the disease. Although the decreased DA transmission in PD impacts on a series of neuronal populations (motor symptoms of PD occur after 80% of DA neurons are lost), the protection or reestablishment of DA transmission may be the most efficient therapeutic strategy.

MPTP Mice

Several animal models of PD exist, each with its own "pros and cons." The MPTP (1-methyl-4-phenyl-1,2,3,6-tetrahydropyridine) mouse model of PD produces a specific degeneration of the nigrostriatal DA system *(11,76,77)* and has been extensively used to the illustrate the protective effects of peptidergic factors after various routes of intracranial administration *(78–81)*. To test the protective and regenerative capacity of nonimmunosuppressive immunophilin ligands, subcutaneous *(53)* and oral *(55)* immunophilin ligands were administered to MPTP-exposed mice. Oral administration for 10 d completely protected against the loss of striatal DA fibers when given concurrently with MPTP *(55,82)*. Regenerative effects were also observed when nonimmunosuppressive immunophilin ligand was administered *after* MPTP lesion, although a 5-d extension after treatment was required owing to the smaller pool of spared axons present for the immunophilin ligand to act upon. The protective effect after oral administration was more pronounced than that obtained by using subcutaneous delivery of a nonimmunosuppressive immunophilin ligand *(53)*. It is possible that oral administration may have a preferable pharmacokinetic profile compared to subcutaneous delivery; in fact, we found the neuroprotective effects of immunophilin ligands were significantly greater with oral administration when compared with subcutaneous delivery in our animal model (L. C. Costantini, unpublished observations). Nonetheless, it is reasonable to assume that even an incomplete restoration of DA innervation may provide therapeutic relief for parkinsonian patients, in which 60–80% depletion of striatal DA is endured before symptoms are observed.

The protective effects in this parkinsonian model were dose-dependent *(55,82)*, demonstrating the specificity of these compounds on the degenerating DA system. The effects have also been observed with several different novel nonimmunosuppressive immunophilin ligands but not with the immunosuppressive immunophilin ligand FK506. The observed protection and regeneration of striatal DA innervation in the MPTP-treated mouse model may be obtained through enhanced neuronal survival, metabolism, and/or neurite outgrowth, and can be interpreted in the context of our in vitro data, which showed growth-promoting effects on DA neurites in primary culture that were distinct from the neurite-elongating effects obtained with FK506. Alternatively, the loss of striatal TH+ innervation after MPTP-induced neurotoxicity may be an injury response by downregulation of TH levels, since we do not observe a loss of DA neurons in the SN after MPTP (L. C. Costantini, unpublished observations). Recovery of TH expression would nonetheless enhance functional DA transmission in spared neurons.

A structurally similar nonimmunosuppressive immunophilin ligand that does not interact with FKBP12 also confers complete protection against MPTP-induced toxicity *(82)*, indicating a mechanism independent of FKBP12 inhibition for these effects.

6-OHDA Rats

Another extensively used animal model of PD is the 6-hydroxydopamine (6-OHDA) rat model. The dose and site of administration of the toxin determine the severity and time course of dopamine degeneration. For instance, a lesion of the SN or transection of the medial forebrain bundle produces an immediate loss of DA fibers within the striatum and loss of DA cell bodies within the SN. Unilaterally lesioned rats rotate ipsilateral to the lesioned hemisphere when injected with the DA-releasing drug amphetamine, thus a decrease in this rotation after treatment indicates a degree of functional DA recovery.

Subcutaneous delivery of a nonimmunosuppressive immunophilin ligand increased striatal TH+ fiber density when administered after an *acute* lesion of the rat nigrostriatal system (intranigral 6-OHDA), and decreased the rate of amphetamine-induced rotations; analysis of SN DA cell number was not presented *(53)*. In a separate study using the same compound in the acute intranigral 6-OHDA model, Harper and colleagues observed no sparing effect on striatal TH+ fibers or DA neurons after subcutaneous delivery *(82a)*. No functional effects were observed in animals treated with this compound. Harper and colleagues also showed that this compound is cleaved after subcutaneous delivery to a free acid that shows no trophic activity. Utilizing a medial forebrain bundle transection model, Winter and colleagues *(26)* also showed that this particular nonimmunosuppressive immunophilin ligand was ineffective in protecting DA neurons.

Intrastriatal injection of low doses of the 6-OHDA lesion more closely represents the degeneration seen in PD, with DA terminal degeneration and subsequent retrograde atrophy and partial cell death of DA cell bodies occurring over several weeks *(83)*. There is long-term atrophy of SN DA neurons, and TH downregulation 1–4 wk after the lesion. The incomplete loss of DA neurons and partial remaining striatal TH+ fibers resemble the early stages of PD, leaving part of the nigrostriatal system intact as a potential substrate for sprouting and functional recovery after administration of growth-promoting factors *(84)*. When nonimmunosuppressive immunophilin ligands were orally administered for 21 d after the lesion, protection of the DA system at both the striatal and SN levels was observed *(82)*. Specifically, the area of the striatum that was depleted of DA terminals by lesion was significantly smaller in animals orally treated with the compound, and close microscopic analyses revealed DA fibers extending into the lesion area, reflecting a sprouting of the spared fibers. A trend toward decreased rotations in response to amphetamine indicated a recovery of DA function in this unilateral lesion model *(82)*.

The effects observed in this model are similar in magnitude to those obtained with peptide growth factors (where the route of administration has been a recurring problem). For example, protection of TH+ neurons was obtained (but no protection of striatal DA innervation) with GDNF, but only after repeated intranigral injections *(5,85)*. Intranigral infusion of GDNF after acute lesion of the nigrostriatal pathway, either prior to lesion *(86)* or 2 wk after lesion *(87)*, also showed sparing of TH+ cells but had no effect on striatal innervation or lesion-induced decreases in TH levels.

Protection at both the striatal and SN levels can be obtained, but only after intrastriatal injection of GDNF *(4,88)*. Neurturin partially protects TH+ neurons only after intrastriatal administration, but shows no effect after ICV injection *(89)*. This illustrates the problematic diffusion kinetics of peptidergic factors after intracranial administration, resulting in limited diffusion and hence incomplete protection of damaged areas. By contrast, as described here, immunophilin ligands exert growth-promoting effects on both spared and damaged axons as well as DA neurons in the lesioned adult nigrostriatal DA system after oral administration. Although protection was not complete, the maintenance of almost 60% of striatal DA innervation and almost 50% of DA neurons could potentially overcome the threshold for parkinsonian symptoms.

Effects of Nonimmunosuppressive Immunophilin Ligands on DA Neuron Transplants

In addition to pharmacological and surgical lesion–stimulator treatments for PD, the transplantation of DA-producing cells has shown promising results *(72–75)*. Long-term studies have proven the continued survival and maintained (and even enhanced) functional benefits that transplanted fetal cells can bring to PD patients. However, not all parkinsonian signs and motor deficits are relieved. Postmortem studies have shown low survival of transplanted DA fetal cells (approx 5–10%), and only partial reinnervation of the host striatum. Although the survival of transplanted DA neurons is critical for this therapy, and several strategies have been used to enhance the survival of transplanted cells *(83,90–96)*, the reinnervation and synaptic integration of the transplanted neurons plays a crucial role in complete and sustained symptomatic relief.

Based on the significant effects on the DA system in primary DA cultures and several in vivo models, we asked whether fetal DA neurons maintain their responsiveness to nonimmunosuppressive immunophilin ligands after transplantation to adult brain. Rats with unilateral 6-OHDA lesions of the nigrostriatal dopamine system were transplanted into the striatum with rat embryonic d 14 ventral mesencephalon, then treated orally with non-immunosuppressive immunophilin ligand for 14 d. All transplanted animals regained complete DA function over 10 wk (indicated by decrease and reversal of amphetamine-induced rotation); however, nonimmuno-suppressive immunophilin ligand-treated animals showed a more pronounced motor response during the first 10 min after amphetamine injection. This enhanced motor response correlated morphologically with significantly higher density of DA fibers reinnervating the lesioned striatum, both immediately surrounding the transplant and at a distance from the transplant–host interface *(97)*.

With regard to DA cell survival, the number of TH+ cells within the transplants was not increased in animals treated with nonimmuno-suppressive immunophilin ligand, indicating enhancement of growth and function of the same number of transplanted cells. Although survival of transplanted cells is critical for behavioral recovery, reinnervation of the DA-depleted striatum has been difficult to improve. This increased DA fiber density observed with oral nonimmunosuppressive immunophilin ligand treatment could indicate a higher number of fibers extended by the transplanted DA neurons, which is consistent with our previous findings in culture: immunophilin ligands enhanced neurite outgrowth from fetal DA neurons without increasing the number of surviving DA neurons *(55,56)*. This augmented outgrowth may increase synaptic contacts in functionally relevant regions of the striatum, thus enhancing and sustaining the function of DA transplants.

The plateau in *overall* amphetamine-induced rotation in both non-immunosuppressive immunophilin ligand- and vehicle-treated groups may reflect a threshold effect. Studies showing morphologically enhanced DA cell transplants often observe significant decreases in rotational behavior in both treated and untreated groups, with no differences between groups *(95,98–101)*. This reflects a threshold of functional effects in this behavioral test even in the presence of morphological enhancement. Behavioral compensation plateaus at a threshold number of TH+ cells [ranging from 300–2500 rat TH+ cells *(102–105)* to 850–1000 pig TH+ cells *(106,107)*]. Therefore, even in the presence of nonimmunosuppressive immunophilin ligand-induced enhancement, animals may reach the maximum level of com-pensation in the amphetamine test, or due to threshold levels of amphet-amine-induced DA release and autoregulation with the level of reinnervation reached in both groups *(108)*.

MECHANISMS

Studies with these nonimmunosuppressive immunophilin ligands in other animal models extended these positive results, enhancing nerve regeneration and functional recovery after sciatic nerve crush *(54,109,110)* and reversing spatial memory impairment and cholinergic cell atrophy in aged animals *(111)*. The effects of these compounds in such a variety of models is likely to be mediated by their binding with FKBPs and subsequent effects on Ca^+ homeostasis, consistent with the understanding that an optimal Ca^+ concentration is involved in neurotrophic effects *(112)*. FKBPs complex with several Ca^+ channels *(113–115)*, and transient changes in intracellular Ca^+ can alter structural proteins, neurotransmitter release, synaptic transmission, excitotoxic cell death, and gene expression *(116)*. Intracellular Ca^+ concentrations can be altered by flux from internal stores, and distinct Ca^+ channels in subcellular regions of the neuron generate highly compartmentalized Ca^+ signaling *(117)*.

The bell-shaped dose-response curves observed in several studies using nonimmunosuppressive immunophilin ligands and growth factors suggest an optimal concentration for maximal trophic effects. Such effects have previously been explained by the "set-point hypothesis" of both growth factors and Ca^+ levels *(112)*, with a midlevel of intracellular Ca^+ producing optimal trophic effects versus a suboptimal low level and a high level, that is toxic to neurons. Additionally, the intrinsic protein-folding rotamase activity of FKBPs is inhibited by the immunophilin ligands *(118)* and may also contribute to the effects observed. It is reasonable to assume that inhibition of rotamase activity may affect the conformation of membrane proteins such as ion channels or receptors *(119)*.

Finally, other FKBPs that immunophilin ligands may associate with include: FKBP13, which possesses a target sequence for the lumen of the endoplasmic reticulum; FKBP25, which is concentrated in the nucleus and associates with nucleolin and kinases, yet has a low affinity for FK506; FKBP52, which is a component of glucocorticoid–receptor complex via hsp90 and is expressed in the brain *(120)*.

In these studies, the neurotrophic effects of nonimmunosuppressive immunophilin ligands were comparable to those obtained with other compounds in similar models *(1–8,10,106)*; however, the necessity for intracerebral administration of these compounds has hampered their clinical application, although systemic-delivery methods, such as conjugation of the trophic factor to a transferrin receptor antibody *(121)*, have shown some success. Since the nonimmunosuppressive immunophilin ligands have biological activity in the CNS after oral administration, and with a once-per-day dosing, they could provide a more practical agent for the treatment of PD.

ACKNOWLEDGMENTS

These studies were supported by research funds at McLean Hospital, NINDS Morris K. Udall Parkinson's Disease Center of Excellence P50NS39793 (OI), NINDS NS41263 (OI), the Century Foundation, Sarasota, FL and the Parkinson Alliance.

REFERENCES

1. Altar CA, Boylan CB, Fritsche M, et al. Efficacy of brain-derived neurotrophic factor and neurotrophin-3 on neurochemical and behavioral deficits associated with partial nigrostriatal dopamine lesions. J Neurochem 1994;63:1021–1032.
2. Galpern WR, Frim DM, Tatter SB, et al. Cell-mediated delivery of brain-derived neurotrophic factor enhances dopamine levels in an MPP+ rat model of substantia nigra degeneration. Cell Transplant 1996;5:225–232.
3. Frim DM, Uhler TA, Galpern WR, et al. Implanted fibroblasts genetically engineered to produce brain-derived neurotrophic factor prevent 1-methyl-4-phenylpyridinium toxicity to dopaminergic neurons in rat. Proc Nat Acad Sci USA 1994;91:5104–5108.
4. Tomac A, Lindquist E, Lin LF, et al. Protection and repair of the nigrostriatal dopaminergic system by GDNF in vivo. Nature 1995;373:335–339.
5. Kearns CM, Gash DM, GDNF protects nigral dopamine neurons against 6-hydroxydopamine in vivo. Brain Res 1995;672:104–111.
6. Hoffer BJ, Hoffman A, Bowenkamp K, et al. Glial cell-line derived neurotrophic factor reverses toxin-induced injury to midbrain dopaminergic neurons in vivo. Neurosci Lett 1994;82:107–111.
7. Hou JG, Lin LH, Mytilineou C, Glial cell-line derived neurotrophic factor exerts neurotrophic effects on dopaminergic neurons in vitro and promotes their survival and regrowth after damage by 1-methyl-4-phenylpyridinium. J Neurochem 1996;66:74–82.
8. Sauer H, Rosenblad C, Bjorklund A. Glial cell-line derived neurotrophic factor but not transforming growth factor B3 prevents delayed degeneration of nigral dopaminergic neurons following striatal 6-hydroxydopamine lesion. Proc Nat Acad Sci USA 1995;92:8935–8939.
9. Krieglstein K, Unsicker, K. Transforming growth factor-B promotes survival of midbrain dopaminergic neurons and protects them against N-methyl-4-phenylpiridinium ion toxicity. Neuroscience 1994;63:1189–1196.
10. Kreiglstein K, Suter-Crazzolara C, Fischer WH, Unsicker K. TGF-beta superfamily members promote survival of midbrain dopaminergic neurons and protect them against MPP+ toxicity. EMBO J 1995;14:736–742.
11. Date I, Yoshimoto Y, Imaoko T, et al. Enhanced recovery of the nigrostriatal dopaminergic system in MPTP-treated mice following intrastriatal injection of basic fibroblast growth factor in relation to aging. Brain Res 1993;621:150–154.
12. Beal M. Coenzyme Q10 administration and its potential for treatment of neurodegenerative diseases. Biofactors 1999;9:261–266.

13. Ebadi M, Srinivasan S, Baxi M. Oxidative stress and antioxidant therapy in Parkinson's disease. Prog Neurobiol 1996;48:1–19.
14. Rodriguez M, Obeso J, Olanow W. Subthalamic nucleus-mediated excitotoxicity in Parkinson's disease: a target for neuroprotection. Ann Neurol 1998;44(Suppl):S175–S188.
15. Boonman A, Isacson O. Apoptosis in neuronal development and transplantation: role of caspases and trophic factors. Exp Neurol 1999;156:1–15.
16. Koller W. Neuroprotection for Parkinson's disease. Ann Neurol 1998; 44(Suppl):S155–S159.
17. Olanow W, Jenner P, Brooks D. Dopamine agonists and neuroprotection in Parkinson's disease. Ann Neurol 1998;44(Suppl):S167–S174.
18. Shoulson I. Mortality in DATATOP: a multicenter trial in early Parkinson's disease. Ann Neurol 1998;43:318–325.
19. Palfi S. Clinical and pathological evaluation of patient with Parkinson's disease (PD) following intracerebroventricular (icv) GDNF. Soc Neurosci Abstr 1998;24:42.
20. Lyons WE, George EB, Dawson TM, et al. Immunosuppressant FK506 promotes neurite outgrowth in cultures of PC12 cells and sensory ganglia. Proc Nat Acad Sci USA 1994;91:3191–3195.
21. Dawson TM, Steiner JP, Dawson VL, et al. Immunosuppressant FK506 enhances phosphorylation of nitric oxide synthase and protects against glutamate toxicity. Proc Nat Acad Sci USA 1993;90:9808–9812.
22. Sharkey J, Butcher SP. Immunophilins mediate the neuroprotective effects of FK506 in focal cerebral ischaemia. Nature 1994;371:336–339.
23. Butcher SP, Henshall DC, Teramura Y, et al. Neuroprotective actions of FK506 in experimental stroke: in vivo evidence against an antiexcitotoxic mechanism. J Neurosci 1997;17:6939–6946.
24. Nakai A, Kuroda S, Kristian T, Siesjo BK. The immunosuppressant drug FK506 ameliorates secondary mitochondrial dysfunction following transient focal cerebral ischemia in the rat. Neurobiol Dis 1997;4:288–300.
25. Moriwaki A, Lu Y, Tomizawa K, Matsui H. An immunosuppressant, FK506, protects agianst neuronal dysfunction and death but has no effect on electrographic and behavioral activities induced by systemic kainate. Neuroscience 1998;86:855–865.
26. Winter C, Schenkel J, Burger E, et al. The immunophilin ligand FK506, but not GPI-1046, protects against neuronal death and inhibits c-Jun expression in the substantia nigra pars compacta following transection of the rat medial forebrain bundle. Neuroscience 2000;95:753–762.
27. Gold BG. FK506 and the role of immunophilins in nerve regeneration. Mol Neurobiol 1997; 285–306.
28. Madsen JR, MacDonald P, Irwin N, et al. Tacrolimus (FK506) increases neuronal expression of GAP-43 and improves functional recovery after spinal cord injury in rats. Exp Neurol 1998;154:673–683.
29. Bavetta S, Hamlyn PJ, Burnstock G, et al. The effects of FK506 on dorsal column axons following spinal cord injury in adult rats: neuroprotection and local regeneration. Exp Neurol 1999;158:382–393.

30. Wang MS, Zeleny-Pooley M, Gold, BG. Comparative dose-dependence study of FK506 and cyclosporin A on the rate of axonal regeneration in the rat sciatic nerve. J Pharmacol Exp Ther 1997;282:1084–1093.

31. Freeman EE, Grosskreutz, CL. The effects of FK506 on retinal ganglion cells after optic nerve crush. Invest Ophthalmol Vis Sci 2000;41:1111–1115.

32. Matsuura K, Makino H, Ogawa H, Cyclosporin N. A attenuates degeneration of dopaminergic neurons induced by 6-hydroxydopamine in the mouse brain. Brain Res 1996;733:101–104.

33. Kitamura Y, Itano Y, Kubo T, Nomura, Y. Suppressive effect of FK506, a novel immunosuppressant, against MPTP-induced dopamine depletion in the striatum of young C57BL6 mice. J Neuroimmunol 1994;50:221–224.

34. Matsuura K, Makino H, Ogawa, N. Cyclosporin A attenuates the decrease in tyrosine hydroxylase immunoreactivity in nigrostriatal dopaminergic neurons and in striatal dopamine content in rats with intrastriatal injection of 6-hydroxydopamine. Exp Neurol 1997;146:526–535.

35. Leventhal L, Sortwell CE, Hanbury R, et al. Cyclosporin A protects striatal neurons in vitro and in vivo from 3-nitropropionic acid toxicity. J Comp Neurol 2000;425:471–478.

36. Uchino H, Elmer E, Uchino K, et al. Amelioration by cyclosporin A of brain damage in transient forebrain ischemia in the rat. Brain Res 1998;812: 216–226.

37. Li J, Samulski RJ, Xiao X. Role for highly regulated rep gene expression in adeno-associated virus vector production. J Virol 1997;71:5236–5243.

38. Li PA, Kristian T, He QP, Siesjo, BK. Cyclosporin A enhances survival, ameliorates brain damage, and prevents secondary mitochondrial dysfunction after a 30-minute period of transient cerebral ischemia. Exp Neurol 2000;165:153–163.

39. Friberg H, Ferrand-Drake M, Bengtsson F, et al. Cyclosporin A, but not FK 506, protects mitochondria and neurons against hypoglycemic damage and implicates the mitochondrial permeability transition in cell death. J Neurosci 1998;1814:5151–5159.

40. Yoshimoto T, Siesjo, BK. Posttreatment with the immunosuppressant cyclosporin A in transient focal ischemia. Brain Res 1999;8392:283–291.

41. Sullivan PG, Thompson M, Scheff, S.W. Continuous infusion of cyclosporin A postinjury significantly ameliorates cortical damage following traumatic brain injury. Exp Neurol 2000;1612: 631–637.

42. Scheff SW, Sullivan PG, Cyclosporin A significantly ameliorates cortical damage following experimental traumatic brain injury in rodents. J Neurotrauma 1999;169:783–792.

43. Buki A, Okonkwo DO, Povlishock, JT. Postinjury cyclosporin A administration limits axonal damage and disconnection in traumatic brain injury. J Neurotrauma, 1999. 16(6): pp. 511–521.

44. Shah AK. Cyclosporine A neurotoxicity among bone marrow transplant recipients. Clin Neuropharmacol 1999;22:67–73.

45. Gijtenbeek JM, van den Bent MJ, Vecht, CJ. Cyclosporine neurotoxicity: a review. J Neurol 1999;246:339–346.

46. Uoshima N, Karasuno T, Yagi T, et al. Late onset cyclosporine-induced cerebral blindness with abnormal SPECT imagings in a patient undergoing unrelated bone marrow transplantation. Bone Marrow Transplant 2000; 26:105–108.

47. Wong M, Yamada, KA. Cyclosporine induces epileptiform activity in an in vitro seizure model. Epilepsia 2000;41:271–276.

48. Borlongan, CV, Emerich DF, Hoffer BJ, Bartus, RT. Transient blood-brain barrier opening via the intravenous injection of bradykinin receptor agonist, cereport, facilitates low dose cyclosporine-A-induced protection against 6-Hydroxydopamine neurotoxicity. Society for Neuroscience 2000, http:// stn.scholarone.com/itin2000/Prog # 798-4.

49. Steiner JP, Dawson TM, Fotuhi M, et al. High brain densities of the immunophilin FKBP colocalized with calcineurin. Nature 1992;358:584–586.

50. O'Keefe SJ, Tamura J, Kincaid RL, et al. FK506- and CsA-sensitive activation of the interleukin-2 promoter by calcineurin. Nature 1992;357:692–694.

51. Liu J, Wandless TJ, Alberg DG, et al. Inhibition of T cell signalling by immunophilin-ligand complexes correlates with loss of calcineurin phosphatase activity. Biochemistry 1992;31:3896–3901.

52. Lyons WE, Steiner JP, Snyder SH, Dawson, TM. Neuronal regeneration enhances the expression of the immunophilin FKBP-12. J Neurosci 1995; 15:2985–2994.

53. Steiner JP, Connelly MA, Valentine HL, et al. Neurotrophic actions of nonimmunosuppressive analogues of immunosuppressive drugs FK506, rapamycin, and cyclosporin A. Nat Med 1997;3:421–428.

54. Gold BG, Zeleny-Pooley M, Wang MS, et al. A non-immunosuppressive FKBP-12 ligand increases nerve regeneration. Exp Neurol 1997;147:269–278.

55. Costantini L, Chaturvedi P, Armistead D, et al. A novel immunophilin ligand: distinct branching effects on dopaminergic neurons in culture and neurotrophic actions after oral administration in an animal model of Parkinson's disease. Neurobiol Dis 1998;5:97–106.

56. Costantini LC, Isacson O. Immuophilin ligands and GDNF enhance neurite branching or elongation from developing dopamine neurons. Exp Neurol 2000;164:60–70.

57. Seki K, Chen HC, Huang KP. Dephosphorylation of protein kinase C substrates, neurogranin, neuromodulin, and MARCKS, by calcineurin and protein phosphatases 1 and 2A. Arch Biochem Biophys 1995;316:673–679.

58. Marcaida G, Kosenko E, Minana MD, et al. Glutamate induces calcineurin-mediated dephosphorylation of Na+, K(+)-ATPase that results in its activation in cerebellar neurons in culture. J Neurochem 1996;66:99–104.

59. Snyder SH, Sabatini DM. Immunophilins and the nervous system. Nat Med 1995;1:32–37.

60. Aoyagi A, Nishikawa K, Saito H, Abe K. Characterization of basic fibroblast growth factor-mediated acceleration of axonal branching in cultured rat hippocampal neurons. Brain Res 1994;661:117–126.

61. Beck KD, Knusel B, Hefti F. The nature of the trophic action of brain-derived neurotrophic factor, sed(1-3)-insulin-like growth factor-1, and basic fibroblast

growth factor on mesencephalic dopaminergic neurons developing in culture. Neuroscience 1993;52:855–866.

62. Studer L, Spenger C, Seiler RW, et al. Comparison of the effects of the neurotrophins on the morphological structure of dopaminergic neurons in cultures of rat substantia nigra. European J Neurosci 1995;7:223–233.

63. Hemmendinger LM, Garber BB, Hoffmann PC, Heller A. Target neuron-specific process formation by embryonic mesencephalic dopamine neurons in vitro. Proc Nat Acad Sci USA 1981;78:1264–1268.

64. Rousselet A, Felter L, Chamak B, Prochiantz A. Rat mesencephalic neurons in culture exhibit different morphological traits in the presence of media conditioned on mesencephalic or striatal astroglia. Dev Biol 1988;129:495–504.

65. Bixby JL, Jhabvala P. Extracellular matrix molecules and cell adhesion molecules induce neurites through different mechanisms. J Cell Biol 1990; 111:2725–2732.

66. Mattson MP, Kater SB. Calcium regulation of neurite elongation and growth cone motility. J Neurosci 1987;7:4034–4043.

67. Chase TN. Levodopa therapy: consequences of the nonphysiologic replacement of dopamine. Neurology 1998;50:S17–S25.

68. Oertel W, Quinn N. Parkinsons disease: drug therapy. Baillieres Clin Neurol 1997;6:89–108.

69. Pal PK, Samii A, Kishore A, et al. Long term outcome of unilateral pallidotomy: follow up of 15 patients for 3 years. J Neurol Neurosurg Psychiatry 2000;69:337–344.

70. Lang AE. Surgery for Parkinson disease: A critical evaluation of the state of the art. Arch Neurol 2000;57:1118–1125.

71. Fine J, Duff J, Chen R, et al. Long-term follow-up of unilateral pallidotomy in advanced Parkinson's disease. N Engl J Med, 2000. 342(23):1708–1714.

72. Piccini P, Lindvall O, Bjorklund A, et al. Delayed recovery of movement-related cortical function in Parkinson's disease after striatal dopaminergic grafts. Ann Neurol, 2000;48:689–695.

73. Hauser RA, Freeman TB, Snow BJ, et al. Long-term evaluation of bilateral fetal nigral transplantation in Parkinson disease. Arch Neurol, 1999;56:179–187.

74. Schumacher J, Ellias S, Palmer E, et al. Transplantation of embryonic porcine mesencephalic tissue in patients with Parkinson's disease. Neurology, 2000;54:1042–1050.

75. Freed CR, Breeze RE, Greene PE, et al. Double blind placebo-controlled human embryonic dopamine cell transplants in advanced Parkinson's disease-long term unblinded followup. Society for Neuroscience 2000, http://stn.scholarone.com/itin2000/Prog # 209-2.

76. Date I, Felton DL, Felton SY. Long-term effect of MPTP in the mouse brain in relation to aging: neurochemical and immunocytochemical analysis. Brain Res 1990;519:266–276.

77. Otto D, Unsicker K. FGF-2 modulates dopamine and dopamine-related striatal transmitter systems in teh intact and MPTP-lesioned mouse. Eur J Neurosci 1993;5:927–932.

78. Eberhardt O, Coelln RV, Kugler S, et al. Protection by synergistic effects of adenovirus-mediated X-chromosome-linked inhibitor of apoptosis and glial cell line-derived neurotrophic factor gene transfer in the 1-methyl-4-phenyl-1,2,3,6-tetrahydropyridine model of Parkinson's disease. J Neurosci 2000; 20:9126–9134.

79. Ferger B, Teismann P, Earl CD, et al. The protective effects of PBN against MPTP toxicity are independent of hydroxyl radical trapping. Pharmacol Biochem Behav 2000;65:425–431.

80. Grunblatt E, Mandel S, Berkuzki T, Youdim MB. Apomorphine protects against MPTP-induced neurotoxicity in mice. Mov Disord 1999;14:6 12–618.

81. Cheng FC, Ni DR, Wu MC, Kuo JS, Chia LG. Glial cell line-derived neurotrophic factor protects against 1-methyl-4-phenyl-1,2,3,6-tetrahydropyridine (MPTP)-induced neurotoxicity in C57BL/6 mice. Neurosci Lett 1998;252:87–90.

82. Costantini LC, Cole D, Chaturvedi P, Isacson O. Immunophilin ligands can prevent progressive dopaminergic degeneration in animal models of Parkinson's disease. Eur J Neurosci 2100;13:1085–1092.

82a. Harper S, Bilsland J, Young L, et al. Analysis of the neurotrophic effects of GPI-1046 on neuron survival and regeneration in culture and in vivo. Neuroscience 1999;88:257–267.

83. Bjorklund A, Rosenblad C, Winkler C, Kirik D. Studies on neuroprotective and regenerative effects of GDNF in a partial lesion model of Parkinson's disease. Neurobiol Dis 1997;4:186–200.

84. Lee C, Sauer H, Bjorklund A. Dopaminergic neuronal degeneration and motor impairments following axon terminal lesion by intrastriatal 6-hydroxydopamine in the rat. Neuroscience 1996;72:641–653.

85. Winkler C, Sauer H, Lee C, Bjorklund A. Short-term GDNF treatment provides long-term rescue of lesioned nigral DA neurons in a rat model of Parkinson's disease. J Neurosci 1996;16:7206–7215.

86. Lu X, Hagg T. Glial cell line-derived neurotrophic factor prevents death, but not reductions in tyrosine hydroxylase, of injured nigrostriatal neurons in adult rats. J Comp Neurol 1997;388:484–494.

87. Bowenkamp KE, Hoffman AF, Gerhardt GA, et al. Glial cell line-derived neurotrophic factor supports survival of injured midbrain dopaminergic neurons. J Comp Neurol 1995;355:479–489.

88. Rosenblad C, Martinez-Serrano A, Bjorklund A. Intrastriatal glial cell line-derived neurotrophic factor promotes sprouting of spared nigrostriatal dopaminergic afferents and induces recovery of function in a rat model of Parkinson's disease. Neuroscience 1998;82:129–137.

89. Rosenblad C, Kirik D, Bkorklund A. Neurturin enhances the survival of intrastriatal fetal dopaminergic transplants. Neuroreport 1999;10:1783–1787.

90. Apostilides C, Sanford E, Hong M, Mendez I. Glial cell line-derived neurotrophic factor improves intrastriatal graft survival of stored dopaminergic cells. Neuroscience 1998;83:363–372.

91. Brundin P, Isacson O, Gage F, et al. The rotating 6-hydroxydopamine-lesioned mouse as a model for assessing functional effects of neuronal grafting. Brain Re 1986;366:346–349.
92. Costantini LC, Snyder-Keller A. Co-transplantation of fetal lateral ganglionic eminence and ventral mesencephalon can augment function and development of intrastriatal transplants. Exp Neurol 1997;145:214–227.
93. Mayer E, Dunnett S, Fawcett J. Mitogenic effect of basic fibroblast growth factor on embryonic ventral mesencephalic dopaminergic neuron precursors. Dev Brain Res 1993;72:253–258.
94. Nakao N, Frodl E, Duan WM, Widner H, Brundin P. Lazaroids improve the survival of grafted embryonic dopamine neurons. Proc Nat Acad Sci USA 1994;91:12,408–12,412.
95. Rosenblad C, Kirik D, Devaux B, et al. Protection and regeneration of nigral dopaminergic neurons by neurturin or GDNF in a partial lesion model of Parkinson's disease after administration into the striatum or lateral ventricle. Eur J Neurosci 1999;11:1554–1566.
96. Yurek D, Lu W, Hipkens S, Wiegand S. BDNF enhances the functional reinnervation of the striatum by grafted fetal dopamine neurons. Exp Neurol 1996;137:105–118.
97. Costantini LC, Isacson O. Neuroimmunophilin ligand enhances neurite outgrowth and effect of fetal dopamine transplants. Neuroscience 2000; 100:515–520.
98. Granholm A, Mott J, Bowenkamp K, et al. Glial cell line-derived neurotrophic factor improves survival of ventral mesencephalic grafts to the 6-hydroxy-dopamine lesioned striatum. Exp Brain Res 1997;116:29–38.
99. Sinclair S, Svendsen C, Torres E, et al. GDNF enhances dopaminergic cell survival and fibre outgrowth in embryonic nigral grafts. Neuroreport 1996;7:2547–2552.
100. Wang Y, Tien L, Lapchak P, Hoffer B. GDNF triggers fiber outgrowth of fetal ventral mesencephalic grafts from nigra to striatum in 6-OHDA-lesioned rats. Cell Tissue Res 1996;286:225–233.
101. Wilby M, Sinclaie S, Muir E, et al. A glial cell line-derived neurotrophic factor-secreting clone of the schwann cell line SCTM41 enhances survival and fiber outgrowth from embryonic nigral neurons grafted to the striatum and to the lesioned substantia nigra. J Neurosci 1999;19:2301–2312.
102. Brundin P, Isacson O, Björklund A. Monitoring of cell viability in suspensions of embryonic CNS tissue and its use as a criterion for intracerebral graft survival. Brain Res 1985;331:251–259.
103. Haque N, Isacson O. Antisense gene therapy for neurodegenerative disease? Exp Neurol 1997;144:139–146.
104. Rioux L, Gaudin D, Bui L, et al. Correlation of functional recovery after 6-OHDA lesion with survival of grafted fetal neurons and release of dopamine in the striatum of the rat. Neuroscience 1991;40:123–131.
105. Sauer H, Frodl E, Kupsch A, et al. Cryopreservation, survival and function of intrastriatal fetal mesencephalic grafts on a rat model of Parkinson's disease. Exp Brain Res 1992;90:54–62.

106. Galpern WR, Burns LH, Deacon TW, et al. Xenotransplantation of porcine fetal ventral mesencephalon in a rat model of Parkinson's disease: functional recovery and graft morphology. Exp Neurol 1996;140:1–13.

107. Huffaker T, Boss B, Morgan A, et al. Xenografting of fetal pig ventral mesencephalon corrects motor asymmetry in the rat model of Parkinson's disease. Experimental Brain Res 1989;77:329–336.

108. Strecker R, Sharp T, Brundin P, et al. Autoregulation of dopamine release and metabolism by intrastriatal nigral grafts as revealed by intracerebral dialysis. Neuroscience 1987;22:169–178.

109. Gold B, Zeleny-Pooley M, Chaturvedi P, Wang M. Oral administration of a nonimmunosuppressant FKBP12 ligand speeds nerve regeneration. Neuroreport 1998;9:553–558.

110. Steiner JP, Hamilton GS, Ross DT, et al., Neurotrophic immunophilin ligands stimulate structural and functional recovery in neurodegenerative animal models. Proc Nat Acad Sci USA 1997;94:2019–2024.

111. Sauer H, Francis J, Jiang H, et al. Systemic treatment with GPI 1046 improves spatial memory and reverses cholinergic atrophy in the medial septal nucleus of aged mice. Brain Res 1999;842:109–118.

112. Johnson EM, Koike T, Franklin J. The "calcium set-point hypothesis" of neuronal dependence on neurotrophic factor. Exp Neurol 1992;115:163–166.

113. Jayaraman T, Brillantes A, Timerman AP, et al. FK506 binding protein associated with the calcium release channel (ryanodine receptor). J Biol Chem 1992;267:9474–9477.

114. Brillantes AB, Ondrias K, Scott A, et al. Stabilization of calcium release channel (ryanodine receptor) function by FK506-binding protein. Cell 1994;77:513–523.

115. Cameron AM, Steiner JP, Roskams AJ, et al. Calcineurin associated with the inositol 1,4,5-trisphosphate receptor-SKBP12 complex modulates Ca^{2+} flux. Cell 1995;83:463–472.

116. Mattson MP. Calcium and free radicals: Mediators of neurotrophic factor and excitatory transmitter-regulated developmental plasticity and cell death. Perspect Dev Neurobiol 1996;3:79–91.

117. Subramanian K, Meyer T. Calcium-induced restructuring of nuclear envelope and endoplasmic reticulum calcium stores. Cell 1997;89:963–971.

118. Harding MW, Galat A, Uehling DE, Schreiber SL. A receptor for the immunosuppressant FK506 is a cis-trans peptidyl-prolyl isomerase. Nature 1989;341:758–760.

119. Helekar SA, Char D, Neff S, Patrick J. Prolyl isomerase requirement for the expression of functional homo-oligomeric ligand-gated ion channels. Neuron 1994;12:179–189.

120. Peattie DA, Harding MW, Fleming MA, et al. Expression and characterization of human FKBP52, an immunophilin that associates with the 90-kDa heat shock protein and is a component of steroid receptor complexes. Proc Nat Acad Sci USA 1992;89:10,974–10,978.

121. Backman C, Rose GM, Hoffer BJ, et al. Systemic administration of nerve
     growth factor conjugate reverses age-related cognitive dysfunction and pre-
     vents cholinergic neuron atrophy. J Neurosci 1996;16:5437–5442.

4
Effects of Neuroimmunophilin Ligands on Parkinson's Disease and Cognition

Joseph P. Steiner, Douglas T. Ross, Hansjorg Sauer, Theresa Morrow, and Gregory S. Hamilton

INTRODUCTION

Immunophilins are high-affinity receptor proteins for the immunosuppressive drugs FK506 and cyclosporin A. Cyclosporin A (CsA) is a cyclic undecapeptide, whose discovery in the late 1970s and subsequent clinical use has paved the way for highly successful organ transplantation *(1–3)*. It has set the gold standard for immunosuppression therapy to prevent graft rejection and enable transplanted organs to function without rejection. FK506 is a structurally distinct, macrolide antibiotic with a potent immunosuppressant activity. It is also used clinically to suppress immune system activity and facilitate organ transplantation *(1,2,4)*. These clinically relevant actions are mediated via high-affinity interactions of these immunosuppressive drugs with their receptor proteins, the immunophilins. CsA interacts with high affinity to cyclophilin A, while FK506 associates specifically with the FK506 binding protein of 12 kDa, (FKBP12) *(5–7)*. Each of these immunophilins has an inherent enzymatic activity, designated protein foldase, peptidyl prolyl-*cis-trans*-isomerase or rotamase activity *(6–9)*. This enzyme acts to rotate X-prolyl bonds in protein substrates by 180° from the *cis* to the *trans* conformer. Binding of each immunosuppressive drug to its cognate immunophilin potently inhibits this enzymatic activity, with picomolar to low nanomolar potency. However, inhibition of the rotamase activity does not correlate with immunosuppressive activity, as the chemically synthesized 506BD molecule potently inhibits FKBP12 rotamase activity, yet has no effect on immune system function *(10)*. In addition, CsA and FK506 act at nanomolar concentrations, whereas tissue concentrations of immunophilins are at much higher levels, suggesting that only a small fraction of total rotamase activity would be inhibited in intact tissues *(10)*.

From: *Immunosuppressant Analogs in Neuroprotection*
Edited by: C. V. Borlongan, O. Isacson, and P. R. Sanberg © Humana Press Inc., Totowa, NJ

Both FK506 and cyclosporin converge on a common target molecule to elicit their immunosuppressive actions. FK506 binds to FKBP12, and this ligand–receptor complex then associates selectively with the calcium–calmodulin-dependent serine–threonine-specific protein phosphatase, calcineurin. Likewise, CsA associates with cyclophilin A, and this complex interacts with this same calcineurin target protein *(11,12)*. Either FK506/ FKBP or CsA–cyclophilin A can attenuate the phosphatase activity of calcineurin, which results in increased levels of phosphorylated calcineurin substrates. One such target, the nuclear factor of activated T cells (NF-AT), requires calcineurin dephosphorylation to enable it to translocate into the nucleus and target cytokine genes, such as interleukin-2 *(13)*. Blockade of NF-AT dephosphorylation does not enable cytokine expression, leads to inhibition of T-cell proliferation and immunosuppression.

This chapter details our research into the study of immunophilins in the nervous system—the neuroimmunophilins. We present our initial experiments that characterize FKBP12 and its distribution in the brain and its codistribution with calcineurin. We describe the actions of FKBP ligands to elicit neurite outgrowth in neural cells. Experiments are presented that delineated the immunosuppressive actions from the neurotrophic activities of these compounds. Detailed actions of the prototypic FKBP ligand GPI1046 are presented in cell culture and in animal models of neuro-degeneration.

BACKGROUND

Initially, there were three questions to be answered regarding the immunophilins in general, and FKBP12 in particular.

1. Did FKBP12 exist in the brain, and how did brain levels compare to peripheral tissues?
2. If FKBP did possess a brain expression, where was the protein expressed, and what was the brain distribution of FKBP?
3. What was the function of the FKBP12 in the nervous system?

We readily answered the first question by setting up a binding assay utilizing [^{3}H]FK506 and brain tissue homogenates. We found that not only was the FKBP12 immunophilin protein present in the nervous system, but that it was concentrated there. The brain levels of FKBP12 were 10 to 30 times the levels of FKBP12 protein in peripheral tissues, including the thymus, spleen, and tissues of the immune system *(14,15)*. Owing to the elevated disposition of these proteins in the brain, we have called them neuroimmunophilins. Within the brain, FKBP12 was highly colocalized with its putative target protein calcineurin *(15)*. These data were generated by comparing messenger RNA levels of calcineurin and FKBP12 by *in situ* hybridization, as well as protein levels by immunohistochemistry and autoradiography. The highest levels of FKBP were found in the hippocampal formation and corpus striatum, with very high levels in layers of the cerebral cortex, thalamus, and olfactory bulb. FKBP12 is present in significant, but lower, amounts in the cerebellum, brainstem, and spinal cord.

To address the issue of the function of the immunophilin FKBP12 in the brain, we examined brain homogenates for the presence of hyperphosphorylated calcineurin substrate proteins in response to FK506 treatment. In brain homogenates, we identified a number of calcineurin substrates whose phosphorylation levels were elevated with FK506 *(15)*. A few of these proteins were identified as the regulatory subunit of AMP-dependent protein kinase (PKA), the dendritic protein MAP2, neuronal nitric oxide synthase, and the growth-associated protein of 43 kDa (GAP43). We were particularly intrigued by the GAP43 result, especially since GAP43 has been linked to the neuronal regeneration process. Following a nerve lesion, an early cellular response is the upregulation of the mRNA for GAP43. In our own experiments, lesioning of the facial nerve produces a significant upregulation of GAP43 mRNA in the facial nucleus within 24 h *(16)*. Maximal levels of GAP43 are reached by 7 d. These levels remain elevated for another 7 d, and begin to decrease thereafter to reach basal levels by 21 d posttransection. The spatial and temporal disposition of FKBP mRNA in the facial nucleus mimics that of GAP43 in this model *(16)*, suggesting involvement of the neuroimmunophilins in the regenerative process. Additional experiments also suggest the involvement of neuroimmunophilin proteins in regeneration. Lesioning of the sciatic nerve by nerve crush and subsequent analysis of axonal transport suggest that FKBP expression is rapidly upregulated after the crush lesion and transported to the nerve terminal. FKBP12 is transported with fastest rate, that of group I axonal transport *(16)*.

The close correlation of the expression of the neuroimmunophilin FKBP12 with GAP43 in the neuronal regeneration process suggested that perhaps FKBP12 would be involved in another cellular process known to involve GAP43, namely, neuronal regrowth, synaptic targeting of neurons, and neurite outgrowth. We chose to address this issue by evaluating the effects of the neuroimmunophilin ligand FK506 on neurite outgrowth in two model systems, pheochromocytoma cells (PC12) and explant cultures of dorsal root ganglia *(17)*. Treatment of sensory neurons in the DRG explant cultures with FK506 elicited neurite outgrowth in the absence of any exogenously added neurotrophic factor. Maximal neurite outgrowth was observed in cultures treated with 100 n*M* FK506. In additional experiments with PC12 cells, we found that treating latent PC12 cells with FK506 did not affect neurite outgrowth. Neurite outgrowth of PC12 cells treated with the maximal dose of nerve growth factor (50 ng/mL NGF) was also unaffected by FK506 treatment. However, treatment of PC12 cells with a suboptimal dose of NGF (0.5–1 ng/mL) and 100 nM FK506, elicited striking neurite outgrowth that was comparable to 50 ng/mL NGF *(17)*. We quantitated the number of cells bearing processes as a fraction of total PC12 cell number. The data suggested the FK506 increased the sensitivity of the PC12 cells to NGF.

In a series of experiments designed as controls, we intended to antagonize the neurotrophic effects of FK506 with its structural homolog, rapamycin. While rapamycin possesses a potent FKBP12 binding domain similar to FK506, its effector domain is quite different from that of FK506. Therefore, rapamycin does bind to FKBP12 potently, but this complex does not interact with calcineurin. Rapamycin, in the presence of the priming dose of NGF (0.5 ng/mL), elicited striking neurite growth in the PC12 cell cultures *(17)*. Not only did rapamycin not antagonize the effects of FK506, but itself induced neurite outgrowth. These experiments had implications for the neurotrophic mechanism of actions of these compounds. Either FK506–FKBP12–calcineurin and rapamycin–FKBP12–RAFT interactions initiated parallel cascades of events that both resulted in significant neurite outgrowth in these cell culture models, or perhaps a common noncalcineurin neurotrophic pathway was utilized by both neuroimmunophilin ligands.

We chose to evaluate the hypothesis that a common noncalcineurin neurotrophic pathway was utilized by the neuroimmunophilin ligands by testing a number of ligands in these neurite outgrowth assays with differing potencies for calcineurin inhibition and immunosuppressive activity *(18)*. FK506 and its nonimmunosuppressive analog L-685818, rapamycin and its nonimmunosuppressive analog WAY124466, and cyclosporin A (CsA) and its nonimmunosuppressive analog 6-MeAla–CsA were each evaluated for neurite outgrowth promoting activity in chick DRG explant and NGF-primed PC12 cell cultures. Each of these compounds potently elicited neurite outgrowth in both culture models. The neurotrophic effects of these compounds did not parallel inhibition of calcineurin, but neurite outgrowth-promoting activities approximated affinities for binding to their cognate neuroimmunophilin, FKBP12 for FK506 and rapamycin, and cyclophilin A for cyclosporin A. These data effectively indicated that the neurotrophic and immunosuppressive actions of these compounds were separate and distinct.

The data suggested that it should be possible to generate small organic compounds as ligands that bind to these neuroimmunophilins and stimulate neurite outgrowth but lack the immunosuppressive actions of FK506. This distinction is critical in generating treatments and therapies for neuro-degenerative disorders, which would likely require chronic drug treatment. Chronic treatment of the immunosuppressant FK506 may be linked to toxicities such as renal hypertension, which occur as a result of calcineurin inhibition and subsequent effects on Na/K-ATPase. Nonimmunosuppressant neurotrophic ligands of FKBP would not have these likely side effects.

IN VITRO ACTIVITIES

The utility of neuroimmunophilin ligands as neuroprotective agents in tissue culture models was recognized a number of years ago. In our early studies, we found that the immunosuppressive drug FK506 protected primary cortical neuronal cultures from glutamate toxicity*(19)*. In 21-d-old primarily neuronal (70–90%) adult cortical neurons, FK506 dose dependently protected the neurons from NMDA toxicity, with an apparent EC_{50} of 25–100 nM. Maximal neuroprotective effects of FK506 were demonstrated at 0.5–1 µM FK506. The proposed neuroprotective mechanism of action of FK506 in these cultures was to maintain neuronal NOS in a highly phosphorylated and therefore inactive state. These effects on NOS were thought to be mediated primarily via inhibition of calcineurin, since the neuroprotective effects of FK506 were antagonized by the structurally similar macrolide antibiotic, rapamycin. It was interesting to note that the immunosuppressive drug cyclosporin A also protected these neurons from NMDA and glutamate-mediated toxicity. Both FK506 and cyclosporin A together with their cognate immunophilin receptor proteins, FKBP12 and cyclophilin A, potently inhibit the phosphatase activity of calcineurin, possibly providing a mechanism for the neuroprotective effects of these drugs.

A prototypic nonimmunosuppressive FKBP12 ligand, GPI-1046, also elicits increased neurite outgrowth from embryonic and adult sensory neuronal explant cultures *(20,21)*. GPI-1046 treatment elicited an increased number of neurites in sensory ganglion cultures isolated from chick embryos. These effects were evident as a result of picomolar GPI-1046 treatment. This drug also stimulated dose-dependent increases in neurite length from small-, medium- and large-caliber diameter sensory neurons, with half-maximal stimulation at 10–100 nM. Increased branching of neuronal processes also resulted from GPI-1046 treatment. GPI-1046 also protected organotypic spinal cord cultures of motor neurons from excitotoxic lesions *(22)*. This effect appears to be mediated through FKBP12 and GPI-1046 treatment of these cultures results in an upregulation of the astroglial glutamate transporter GLT1, perhaps accounting for the neuroprotective effects. Furthermore, this compound promotes survival of mesencephalic dopamine neurons and protects them from cell death induced by MPP+ and 6-OHDA *(23)*.

Subsequent studies by other researchers have demonstrated in vitro neurotropic effects of neuroimmunophilin ligands. In SY5Y neuroblastoma cells, FK506 promoted neurite outgrowth *(24)*. Likewise, FK506 stimulated neuroprotection and neurite outgrowth in primary hippocampal cultures *(25)*. The work of Costantini and Isacson demonstrated a significant effect of FK506 on increased neurite length in mesenchephalic dopamine neurons *(26,27)*. An additional nonimmunosuppressive ligand for FKBP12, V-10,367, also promoted neurite extension in neuroblastoma and dopamine neurons. They proposed that the immunosuppressant FK506 treatment primarily leads to increased neurite length, while the nonimmuosuppressive V-10,367 elicits increased branching of neuronal processes *(26)*.

PARKINSON'S DISEASE MODELS

Ligands for the neuroimmunophilin FKBP12 have been found to possess both neuroprotective and neurite outgrowth-promoting activites in a number of different culture systems. A plausible next test was to evaluate these compounds in animal models of neurodegenreative diseases. One such model was provided by administering to mice the neurotoxin MPTP, which selectively targets the neurons of the nigrostriatal dopaminergic system *(28,29)*. Data have been presented that show that FK506 may have some utility in this type of model *(30)*. However, a progressive neurodegenerative disorder such as Parkinson's disease may require chronic dosing with a therapeutic agent, and the effects on the immune system as well as the side effect profile (e.g., renal hypertension) caused by the immunosuppressive agent FK506 would not be warranted nor tolerated. However, administration of a neurotropic but nonimmunosuppressive agent for dopamine neurons would provide a likely therapy for the chronic degenerative disease.

In a model in which the MPTP toxin was administered concurrently with the test compound, protection of dopaminergic cell bodies in the substantia nigra and pars compacta, as well as maintenance of striatal tyrosine hydroxylase immunoreactivity, can be assessed. This mouse model of Parkinson's disease is a partial lesion model, in which about 50–60% of nigrostriatal dopamine neurons are targeted, degenerate, and are destroyed, resulting in about a 50–60% decrease in striatal dopamine levels and striatal tyrosine hydroxylase immunoreactive nerve fibers and terminals. Treatment of MPTP-intoxicated mice with the prototypic nonimmunosuppressive neuroimmunophilin ligand GPI-1046 resulted in significant sparing of dopamine neurons and dopaminergic innervation density in the striatum *(31)*. Initial experiments in which the drug was administered systemically (i.e., subcutaneously) demonstrated that the GPI-1046 was highly protective in the model *(31)*, sparing about 60–70% of the vulnerable dopamine neurons in the SNc. Subsequent studies with GPI-1046 revealed that the drug is also highly efficacious following oral administration of the compound *(21,32,33)*. Consistent with GPI-1046-dependent maximal sparing of up to 70% of the intoxicated dopamine neurons, about 75–85% of the striatal TH innervation density was maintained (*see* Fig. 1). GPI-1046 showed dose-dependent increase in sparing of nigral dopamine neurons, with an ED50 of 1–5 mg/kg sc and oral. Neuronal cell counts of dopamine neurons in the SNc and TH staining in the corpus striatum shows that GPI-1046 spares these neurons when the drug is given concurrently with the MPTP neurotoxin. Likewise, the neuroimmunophilin drug treatment maintains the catecholamine neurochemistry as well, since striatal dopamine and metabolite levels are increased in MPTP-lesioned mice treated with drug compared to MPTP–Vehicle-treated animals.

While the strikingly neuroprotective effects of GPI-1046 in the mouse MPTP model of PD were remarkable, another question concerning neuroimmunophilin ligands was being asked. If the degeneration in the dopaminergic system was first allowed to occur following MPTP administration, would neuroimmunophilin drug treatment reverse the neurodegenerative effects and stimulate recovery of the nigrostriatal dopaminergic neurons? The neurodegeneration in this postlesion model of PD was caused by administration of the dopamine neurotoxin MPTP daily on d 1–5, as was the case for the concurrent MPTP model presented above. GPI-1046 treatment was initiated on d 8 of the experiment, allowing most of the degeneration of the nigrostriatal dopaminergic system to occur. Treatment with GPI-1046 systemically (subcutaneous and oral) for 5 d under these conditions resulted in significant increases in TH immunostaining in the striatum of lesioned mice (*see* Fig. 2) *(31)*. While this model remains a partial lesion model and striatal TH staining was reduced by 50–60% in MPTP–vehicle versus vehicle–vehicle treated mice, MPTP-lesioned mice treated with GPI-1046 displayed up to 50% increase in striatal TH immunoreactivity. These increases in striatal TH immunoreactivity were dependent on the administered dose of GPI-1046, with a half-maximal effective dose of 5–10 mg/kg. These increased indices for GPI-1046-dependent striatal innervation density were the result of regenerative actions of the neuroimmunophilin ligand GPI-1046, since the nigral cell counts following drug treatment showed no increase in TH immunoreactivity. Increased stri-

A

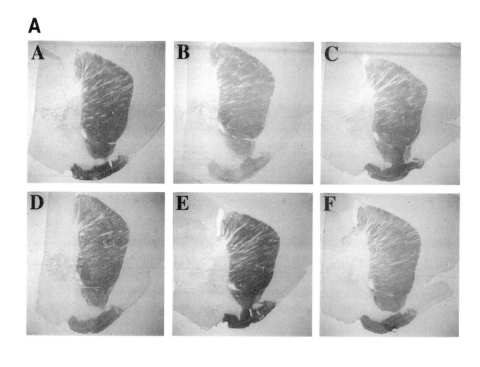

B

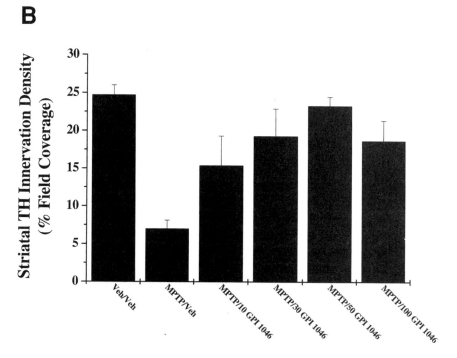

atal innervation density of the dopaminergic fibers, while expressing an equivalent number of dopamine neuronal cell bodies, underlies these neuroanatomical changes.

We hypothesized that the augmented dopamine innervation in the striatum was due to sprouting from spared DA projections into the corpus striatum. Another marker to assess this sprouting event targeted the striatal dopamine transporter protein. The DA transporter resides on the presynaptic nerve terminals of dopamine neurons, and has been shown to decrease following DA lesions and in Parkinson's disease. We found that in both of the mouse MPTP lesion models described above, the striatal DAT immunoreactivity in MPTP–vehicle treated mice was decreased by 50% compared to vehicle/vehicle control animals. Whether GPI-1046 was administered to MPTP-lesioned mice in the concurrent- or post-MPTP-lesion paradigms, striatal DAT immunoreactivity was increased to levels comparable to vehicle–vehicle-treated animals (Fig. 3). This increase in presynaptic dopamine nerve terminal staining by DAT also demonstrates regeneration of the nigrostriatal dopamine system, which correlates well with the increased TH innervation found in these same mice.

In addition to the morphological improvement in the striata of the MPTP-lesioned mice treated with GPI-1046, the neurotransmitter levels were also affected. Striatal dopamine levels were decreased by nearly 50% in the MPTP–vehicle treated mice. GPI-1046-treated MPTP mice displayed 25% higher levels of striatal dopamine than the MPTP–vehicle treated mice. This significant increase in striatal dopamine and its metabolites elicited by GPI-1046 treatment also provides evidence of neurochemical recovery by neuroimmunophilin drug treatment.

Morphologic and neurochemical recovery provided by GPI-1046 to the lesioned animals in these mouse MPTP models of PD is followed by func-

---

Fig. 1. *(opposite page)* Dose dependence of concurrent GPI-1046 mediated protection of striatal dopaminergic markers in MPTP treated mice. (**A**) A-F depict low power tyrosine hydroxylase (TH)-labeled striata following MPTP and concurrent GPI-1046 treatment. The TH immunoreactivity of normal (A, vehicle/vehicle) mice is compared to the TH immunoreactivity in the striata of MPTP-treated mice (B) where labeling is characterized by a sparse network of long TH+ processes and very few TH+ punctae. The dose-dependent recovery of TH+ immunoreactivity is evident in the striata of mice treated with GPI-1046 at 10 mg/kg (C), 30 mg/kg (D), 50 mg/kg (E), and 100 mg/kg (F). (**B**) Quantitation of the dose dependency of GPI-1046-mediated recovery of striatal TH innervation density is shown. At all dose levels TH innervation density was significantly greater than MPTP-treated cases alone, *p* < 0.001.

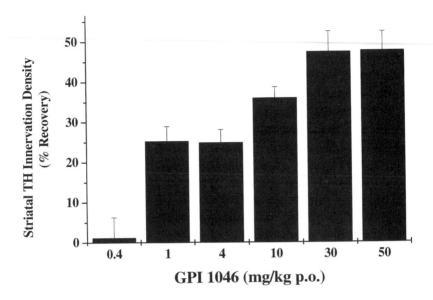

Fig. 2. Dose dependence of GPI-1046-mediated recovery of striatal dopaminergic markers in post-MPTP treated mice. Quantitation of the dose dependancy of therapeutically administered GPI-1046 in recovery of striatal TH innervation density is shown in the graph. At all dose levels TH innervation density was significantly greater than MPTP treated cases alone, $p < 0.001$.

tional recovery as well. Since the mouse MPTP models were partial lesion models, behavioral changes in the injured animals were not obvious. Treatment of MPTP-lesioned mice with haloperidol produced catalepsy and akinesia at doses that are subthreshold in vehicle–vehicle mice. GPI-1046 treatment of MPTP-lesioned mice in both concurrent- and post-MPTP treatment paradigms resulted in attenuation of the cataleptic and akinetic behaviors. These data provide evidence of neuroimmunophilin ligand-dependent functional recovery of these animals as well.

While GPI-1046 protected dopaminergic neurons when administered concurrently with the MPTP neurotoxin and stimulated resprouting and reinnervation of the striatum in the postlesion model, the compound did not induce abnormal sprouting in nonlesioned tissue. We found no evidence of intranigral sprouting from the SNc to SNr in sham animals. Likewise, we saw no evidence of increased innervation of other neurotransmitter containing neurons following GPI-1046 treatment in these Parkinson's disease models.

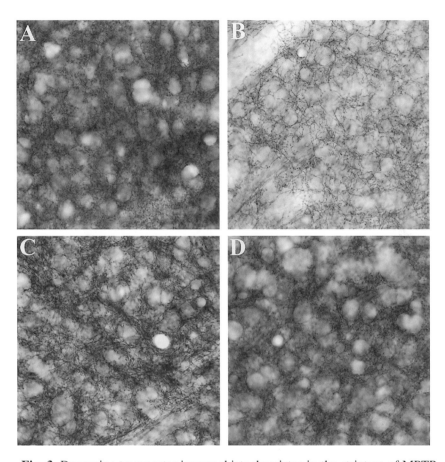

Fig. 3. Dopamine transporter immunohistochemistry in the striatum of MPTP-lesioned mice. Panels A–D depict high power dopamine transporter (DAT) labeled striatal fields (630X) used for quantitative analysis. The dense aggregation of DAT positive punctae and processes in the striatal neuropil of normal (A, vehicle/vehicle) mice is decreased in the striata of MPTP treated mice (B). DAT immunostaining in (C) MPTP/50 mg/kg GPI1046 from concurrent MPTP experiments and (D) MPTP/50 mg/kg GPI1046 from post-MPTP experiments represent the protection and recovery of dopaminergic nerve terminals following GPI-1046 treatment in these models.

The mouse MPTP model of Parkinson's disease provided a model in which a partial lesion of about 50% toxicity was apparent. To evaluate the neuroimmunophilin ligands in a more severe model of dopaminergic toxicity, we evaluated the compounds in the rat 6-hydroxydopamine (6-OHDA) model. In this model, the dopaminergic neurotoxin 6-OHDA is delivered directly to the dopaminergic cell bodies in the SNc by stereotaxic injection. The extent of the lesion in this model was approx 85–90% cell loss in the SNc and a concomitant loss of about 90% of TH innervation density in the striatum. In our initial experiments, we administered GPI-1046 in one of three paradigms: 1 h, 1 wk, or 1 mo after the 6-OHDA injection. The number of dopaminergic cell bodies in the SNc was comparable in each of the treatment groups, showing that no protection of DA neurons was evident in this paradigm. While we found about 90% loss of striatal TH innervation density in vehicle-treated rats, animals treated with 10 mg/kg GPI-1046 had substantially more TH immunoreactivity in each of the three treatment paradigms *(31)*. About 30–40% of vulnerable dopaminergic processes and nerve terminals in the striatum were recovered following drug treatment, even if treatment was delayed for up to a month. In subsequent studies, even with GPI-1046 treatment to these rats delayed up to 3 mo, increased striatal innervation density resulted from drug treatment *(34,35)*.

In an attempt to compare striatal innervation density as a function of DA neuron number across all treatment groups, we found that a three- to fourfold increase in striatal TH innervation density per dopamine neuron number. This provided evidence of striatal sprouting, perhaps from spared projections, with GPI-1046 treatment. These studies also provided evidence that the extent of the lesion was extremely important in determining the outcome of the neuroimmunophilin ligand treatment. Since we hypothesized that these compounds were inducing reinnervation from spared projections, the level of remaining innervation density after 6-OHDA lesions but prior to neuroimmunophilin drug treatment was critical to the success of the treatment. These remaining neuronal cell bodies and striatal projections were the substrate upon which the GPI-1046 acted to stimulate the increased TH innervation density which was observed. If the 6-OHDA lesion destroyed greater than 95% of dopamine neurons and striatal innervation density (an excessive lesion), there was no remaining substrate on which the GPI-1046 could act and the drug treatment was not effective. Operationally, if the VTA was essentially intact and up to about 90% neuronal cell loss in the pars compacta was found, GPI-1046 treatment was effective in stimulating increased TH innervation density (Fig. 4). With more extensive lesions, we, along with other investigators *(36)*, found little effect of GPI-1046 treatment.

The effects of GPI-1046 on sparing dopamine neurons and striatal innervation by dopaminergic projections were evaluated in MPTP-lesioned rhesus monkeys *(37)*. In this study, the GPI-1046 was administered prior to and during MPTP infusion, and also for the following 6 wk. Five groups of five monkeys each treated with either vehicle, 0.3, 1, 3, or 10 mg/kg GPI-1046 were evaluated. Tested parameters included home cage locomotor activity, clinical neurologic rating score and fine motor control in food retrieval as behavioral measures, along with dopamine neuron cell counts in the SNC-and TH-innervation density in the caudate nucleus and putamen. Of the 20 MPTP-lesioned and drug-treated animals, seven displayed evidence of neuroprotection by both neuroanatomical and behavioral measures in each parameter tested. Unfortunately, these monkeys were spread across all four dose-treatment groups, which precluded the finding of a statistically significant effect.

Other laboratories have also demonstrated significant drug effects of neuroimmunophilin ligands in animal models of Parkinson's disease. Costantini and coworkers *(38,39)* found that a neuroimmunophilin ligand V10,367 was quite effective in stimulating neurite outgrowth and protecting dopamine neurons from MPTP toxicity. These results were analogous to the results summarized here with GPI-1046. Harper and coworkers *(38)* evaluated GPI-1046 in a number of in vitro and in vivo models, and found some evidence of neurite outgrowth in cell culture experiments and regeneration in a sciatic nerve crush model with rats and mice. While these workers found little effect in the 6-OHDA lesion model in rats, the lesions they reported were about 95% loss of neurons and striatal innervation density. These lesions were very extensive, and this excessive injury likely precluded the finding of a significant drug treatment effect. Recent studies by two additional groups in the mouse MPTP model of Parkinson's disease found mixed effects of GPI-1046 treatment on striatal dopamine levels, one group finding efficacy *(40,41)* and the other did not *(42)* in essentially the same model. The group that used the GPI-1046 unsuccessfully used a different drug formulation for the compound dosing to mice, which may explain the lack of efficacy in their hands.

Recently, additional ligands of the neuroimmunophilin FKBP have been developed that also possess neuroprotective and neuroregenerative efficacy. One such ligand, called NIL-A, displayed potent neuroprotection and recovery of lesioned dopaminergic neurons and reinnervation of the striatum following MPTP application. This compound displayed improved potency and pharmacokinetic properties compared to the prototypic ligand, GPI-1046. Safety studies with this compound have been completed successfully. Human clinical trials of NIL-A treatment have been initiated in patients with Parkinson's disease.

In an additional aspect of our in vivo work, we assessed the efficacy of our prototypic FKBP ligand GPI-1046 in an animal model of age-related cognitive decline and basal forebrain cholinergic neuron atrophy. Aged

A

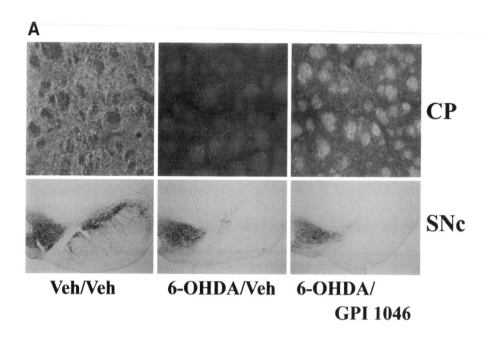

CP

SNc

Veh/Veh   6-OHDA/Veh   6-OHDA/
                                     GPI 1046

B

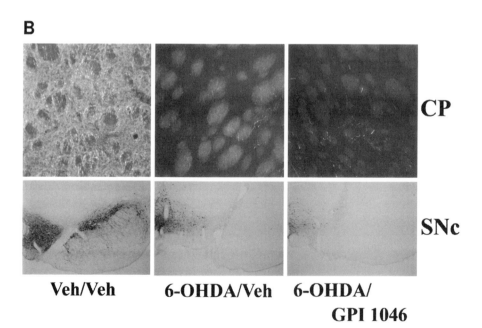

CP

SNc

Veh/Veh   6-OHDA/Veh   6-OHDA/
                                     GPI 1046

rodents exhibit marked individual differences in performance on a variety of behavioral tasks, including two-choice spatial discrimination in single- or multiple-unit T mazes *(43,44)*, spatial discrimination in a circular platform task *(45)*, passive avoidance *(46)*, radial maze tasks *(48)*, and spatial navigation in the Morris water maze *(48)*. In all of these tasks, a proportion of aged rats or mice perform as well as the vast majority of young control animals, while other animals display severe impairments in memory function compared to young animals.

Cholinergic function in the hippocampus has been extensively studied as one neural substrate of spatial learning in rodents, and an age-related decline in hippocampal cholinergic function has been noted in parallel with the development of learning and memory impairments *(49,50)*. Other neurotransmitter systems, such as the dopaminergic and noradrenergic *(51)*, serotonergic *(52)*, and glutamatergic systems *(53)*, have also been shown to contribute to spatial learning, and to decline with age. These findings, as well as reports on age-related deficits of hippocampal long-term potentiation (LTP)–induction *(54)*, a reduction in theta rhythm frequency, a loss of experience-dependent plasticity of hippocampal place-units *(55)*, and reductions in hippocampal protein kinase C *(56)* are in keeping with the concept that no single underlying pathology can be identified as the cause of age-related behavioral impairment in rodents.

Nevertheless, many investigators today believe that there are intriguing parallels between rodents and humans in at least some aspects of learning and memory decline during normal aging. Thus, aged rats and mice have frequently been used in the testing of putative cognition enhancing drugs.

We assessed the effects of chronic systemic treatment with GPI-1046 on the spatial learning and memory, and the medial septal cholinergic neuron atrophy of aged C57BI mice *(see* Fig. 5), *(57)*. To this end, 18-mo-old male mice and young control mice were first screened for their ability to swim, locate, and escape onto a visible platform in a standard Morris water-maze procedure. Subsequently, animals were subjected to a place learning task where the platform was submerged, that is, concealed from view, just beneath the water surface, thus requiring the animals to use distant visual

---

Fig. 4. *(opposite page)* Tyrosine hydroxylase immunostaining in striatum and SNc of 6-OHDA lesioned rats. **(A)** While there is significant cell death of dopaminergic neurons in the SNc, the VTA is relatively intact and striatal innervation density is restored in 6-OHDA lesioned rats treated with GPI-1046 (10 mg/kg s.c.). **(B)** With significant neuronal degeneration in the SNc and VTA, very little TH innervation is found in the striatum following GPI-1046 treatment.

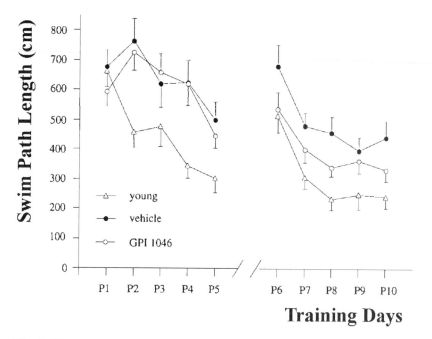

Fig. 5. Water maze swim data for aged mice. Mean swim distance (in centimeters) for young male C57BL6N/Nia control mice ("young", aged 3 mo), aged male C57BL6N/Nia mice systemically treated with 10 mg/kg/d GPI-1046 ("GPI-1046", aged 19 mo), and aged vehicle-treated control mice ("vehicle"). Mice that had previously been trained in a visible platform task were subjected to four swim trials per day in a non-visible platform place learning task. The platform location remained the same during all trials on all days. Daily treatment with vehicle or GPI-1046 was initiated after the first 5 d of place learning (P1-P5). The second set of place learning days (P6-P10) began after 3 wk of GPI-1046 treatment. Error bars indicate standard errors of the mean. Adapted from ref. *57*.

cues in the laboratory to triangulate their position in the water maze. Consistent with previous findings, aged untreated mice in our study were not able to acquire a hidden platform location at the same rate as young control mice even with repeated training. This deficit likely reflected an age-related hippocampal dysfunction, since the same mice had shown good sensory, motivational, and motor function during the preceding visual platform screen. Daily treatment with GPI-1046 was initiated 2 d after completion of 5 d of training in the spatial task.

When the animals were reintroduced to the maze 3 wk later, both young and old animals showed clear signs of attenuation, that is, forgetting, of the previously acquired platform location. However, aged GPI-1046-treated mice located the platform with clearly higher accuracy and displayed significantly less "forgetting" than their vehicle-treated aged counterparts (Fig. 5). Both groups of aged mice as well as the young control mice improved their performance during the second spatial testing period, that is, they relearned the location of the platform over the following 4 d of training. But again, even though aged animals did not learn to locate the submerged platform with the same accuracy as young animals, aged animals treated with GPI-1046 did perform significantly better than their respective aged vehicle controls. In fact, aged mice that had shown the greatest impairment in their spatial learning ability before treatment was initiated were the ones to benefit most from GPI-1046 administration.

We were able to corroborate the effects of GPI-1046 on water-maze place learning by morphometric analysis of medial septal cholinergic neurons in our study animals. Atrophy of these cells during aging has been described in mice and rats *(49,58)*. Our study animals were maintained for an additional 10 mo following water-maze testing to reach late senescence at 29–30 mo of age. During this period, they were treated daily with GPI-1046 or vehicle. We found that, consistent with previous reports, late senescent animals displayed a significant atrophy of cholinergic cell bodies in the medial septal nucleus, which is the origin of the main cholinergic afferent projection to the hippocampus. Remarkably, animals that had been treated with GPI-1046 during the preceding 10 mo showed a significant reversal of cholinergic cell atrophy and were statistically indistinguishable from young control mice.

Our findings bear some similarity to observations made previously with nerve growth factor (NGF) treatment in aged mice and rats. Following intracranial administration of NGF in aged rodents, place learning and memory retention in the water maze is improved and cholinergic cell atrophy is reversed *(58–63)*. Indeed, these and other studies have shown that there may be a link between forebrain cholinergic hypofunction, cell size, cholinergic tone in the hippocampus, and impaired spatial navigation in aged rats. The results obtained with GPI-1046 are intriguing because to date there is little evidence that a systemically available small molecule can have an effect similar to NGF in an aged rodent.

The mechanism by which GPI-1046 exerts this effect is not well understood at this time. FKBP12 is known to play an important physiological role in the regulation of the IP_3 (inositol-1,4,5-triphosphate) and RyR (ryanodine) intracellular calcium release channel complexes. Ryanodine receptors and IP_3 receptors represent two multigene families of channel proteins that mediate the release of Ca^{2+} ions from intracellular stores. Both receptors form very large tetrameric channels and are abundantly expressed in peripheral tissues including heart and skeletal muscle, but also in the cerebellum, hippocampus, neocortex, and basal ganglia *(64–66)*.

FKBP12 interacts specifically with the RyR and IP_3R, and has been shown to exert profound effects on the calcium conductance characteristics of these channels. One molecule of FKBP is bound to each of the four channel subunits; it appears to stabilize the calcium channel complex both in its open and closed states but also decreases the probability of the open state *(67)*. Dissociating FKBP12 from RyR with FK506 or rapamycin, or expressing RyR in the absence of FKBP12, result in an increased open probability of the channel followed by unstable partial opening (subconductance) states and leakage of calcium from the sarcoplasmic reticulum. In isolated muscle preparations, this mobilization of intracellular calcium causes increased muscle tension after application of caffeine. Also, dissociation of FKBP12 from the two calcium channel complexes by the use of FK506 results in reduced calcium accumulation in brain membrane preparations, which was attributed to leakage of calcium through destabilized IP_3R and possibly RyR. Dissociating FKBP12 from the IP_3R by FK506 treatment also markedly enhances IP_3-stimulated calcium efflux from brain synaptosomal preparations, thus indicating a sensitization of the IP_3R to IP_3 *(68)* (for comprehensive reviews, *see* refs *69* and *70*).

In the brain, ryanodine- and IP_3-regulated intracellular calcium release mechanisms are involved in hippocampal long-term potentiation and long-term depression induction *(71–74)*. Cavallaro and colleagues *(75)* in a study on differentially expressed mRNAs following water-maze training of young rats, have found that expression of the mRNA for the type 2 RyR is markedly upregulated in the CA3 and dentate gyrus at 6 and 12 h after spatial acquisition training. This upregulation dropped back to baseline levels at 24 h after training and was not observed in swimming control rats. Also, the observed upregulation was limited to the hippocampal dentate and CA3 regions, and no changes in expression levels were observed in other brain regions.

Reduced postmortem IP_3 binding and reduced IP_3R levels have been demonstrated in cortical and hippocampal tissue samples of patients suffering from Alzheimer's disease *(76,77)*, and the relative loss of IP_3 binding sites correlates with the extent of AD pathology in the subiculum and the hippocampal CA1 region *(78)*. There are thus several lines of evidence that implicate the RyR and IP_3R intracellular calcium channels in physiological processes that underlie learning and memory. It is conceivable that GPI-1046 could alter the conductance characteristics of these channels through a non-calcineurin-dependent mechanism analogous to that of the immunosuppressants FK506 or rapamycin, and that an ensuing mobilization of intracellular neuronal calcium stores could play a role in the observed behavioral effect. Further, since IP_3 formation is coupled to activation of the muscarinic cholinergic receptor, sensitization of the IP_3R to IP_3 could indirectly lead to a potentiation of cholinergic neurotransmission. Finally, the activity of calcineurin, which has been implicated in the postsynaptic regulation of synaptic potentiation and LTP induction, would remain unaffected in this scenario.

Another important role for FKBP12, and a potential physiological target for GPI-1046, could be the regulation of serine/threonine kinase receptors. Lopez-Ilasaca and colleagues *(79)* reported that FKBP12 exerts concentration-dependent inhibitory effects on the autophosphorylation of the epidermal growth factor (EGF) receptor which may be independent of calcineurin, and that this effect appears to depend on the rotamase activity of FKBP12. Treatment with FK506 or rapamycin was found to greatly enhance the autophosphorylation of the EGF receptor.

FKBP12 has previously been found to play a role in signal transduction through another serine–threonine kinase receptor, the type I transforming growth factor-β (TGF-β) receptor. FKBP12 was found to be associated with the cytoplasmic domains of the type I TGF-β receptor. Upon TGF-β binding, the type I TGF-β receptor binds to, and phosphorylates the type I TGF-β receptor. The ensuing activation of the type I receptor kinase is accompanied by the dissociation of FKBP12 from the ligand–bound receptor complex. It was shown that when FKBP12 was dissociated from the type I TGF-β receptor by nonimmunosuppressive FKBP12 ligands, TGF-β signaling was markedly enhanced *(80)*. This suggests that FKBP12 in itself is not required for TGF-β signaling *(80,81)*, but rather serves as an important functional inhibitor of the type 1 TGF β receptor, possibly by recruiting an intracellular phosphatase to the receptor that inhibits phosphorylation *(36,80,82,83)*. Other studies, however, do not support a critical role of FKBP in regulating type I TGF-β receptors *(84,85)*.

If FKBP12 is involved in TGF-β signaling, it is interesting to note that TGF-β-1 has been shown to induce production and secretion of NGF in brain and in cultured astrocytes *(86)*, and astrocytic cell lines *(87)*, but not cultured hippocampal neurons *(88)*. This is interesting in light of our studies, since intracranially infused NGF, as described above, has been shown to enhance septal cholinergic cell size and water-maze performance in aged rodents.

Whether the observed effects of GPI-1046 are direct (by acting on intracellular calcium release channels) or indirect (by enhancing endogenous neurotrophic mechanisms), or both cannot be answered at present. The present results suggest that the septohippocampal cholinergic system deserves further study as a target for GPI-1046. In this context, it is important to bear in mind that Alzheimer's disease, though far from being exclusively a disorder of the cholinergic system, presents with prominent early degeneration of basal forebrain cholinergic neurons, and that patients respond with clinically meaningful cognitive improvements to drugs, such as tacrine and donepezil, which enhance cholinergic tone. The potential usefulness of GPI-1046 in treating memory loss associated with Alzheimer's disease thus deserves further investigation.

REFERENCES

1. Bierer BE, Hollander G, Fruman D, Burakoff SJ. Cyclosporin A and FK506: molecular mechanisms of immunosuppression and probes for transplantation biology. Curr Opin Immunol 1993;5:763–773.
2. Henry ML. Cyclosporine and tacrolimus (FK506): a comparison of efficacy and safety profiles. Clin Transplant 1999;13:209–220.
3. Kahan BD. Cyclosporine: the base for immunosuppressive therapy—present and future. Transplant Proc 1993;25:508–510.
4. Spencer CM, Goa KL, Gillis JC. Tacrolimus: an update of its pharmacology and clinical efficacy in the management of organ transplantation. Drugs 1997;54:925–975.
5. Handschumacher RE, Harding MW, Rice J, et al. Cyclophilin: a specific cytosolic binding protein for cyclosporin A. Science 1984;226:544–547.
6. Harding MW, Galat A, Uehling DE, Schreiber SL. A receptor for the immunosuppressant FK506 is a cis-trans peptidyl- prolyl isomerase. Nature 1989;341:758–760.
7. Siekierka JJ, Hung SH, Poe M, et al. A cytosolic binding protein for the immunosuppressant FK506 has peptidyl-prolyl isomerase activity but is distinct from cyclophilin. Nature 1989;341:755–757.
8. Fischer G, Wittmann-Liebold B, Lang K, et al. Cyclophilin and peptidyl-prolyl cis-trans isomerase are probably identical proteins [see comments]. Nature 1989;337:476–478.
9. Takahashi N, Hayano T, Suzuki M. Peptidyl-prolyl cis-trans isomerase is the cyclosporin A-binding protein cyclophilin. Nature 1989;337:473–475.
10. Schreiber SL. Chemistry and biology of the immunophilins and their immunosuppressive ligands. Science 1991;251:283–287.
11. Friedman J, Weissman I. Two cytoplasmic candidates for immunophilin action are revealed by affinity for a new cyclophilin: one in the presence and one in the absence of CsA. Cell 1991;66:799–806.
12. Liu J, Farmer JD Jr, Lane WS, et al. Calcineurin is a common target of cyclophilin-cyclosporin A and FKBP- FK506 complexes. Cell 1991;66:807–815.
13. Tocci MJ, Matkovich DA, Collier KA, et al. The immunosuppressant FK506 selectively inhibits expression of early T cell activation genes. J Immunol 1989;143:718–726.

14. Dawson TM, Steiner JP, Lyons WE, et al. The immunophilins, FK506 binding protein and cyclophilin, are discretely localized in the brain: relationship to calcineurin. Neuroscience 1994;62:569–580.

15. Steiner JP, Dawson TM, Fotuhi M, et al. High brain densities of the immunophilin FKBP colocalized with calcineurin. Nature 1992;358:584–587.

16. Lyons WE, Steiner JP, Snyder SH., Dawson TM. Neuronal regeneration enhances the expression of the immunophilin FKBP- 12. J Neurosci 1995; 15:2985–2994.

17. Lyons WE, George EB, Dawson TM, et al. Immunosuppressant FK506 promotes neurite outgrowth in cultures of PC12 cells and sensory ganglia. Proc Natl Acad Sci USA 1994;91:3191–3195.

18. Steiner JP, Connolly MA, Valentine HL, et al. Neurotrophic actions of nonimmunosuppressive analogues of immunosuppressive drugs FK506, rapamycin and cyclosporin A. Nat Med 1997;3:421–428.

19. Dawson TM, Steiner JP, Dawson VL, et al. Immunosuppressant FK506 enhances phosphorylation of nitric oxide synthase and protects against glutamate neurotoxicity. Proc Natl Acad Sci USA 1993;90:9808–9812.

20. Khan Z, Kasper M, Connolly MA, et al. GPI-1046 stimulates regenerating axon growth in adult dorsal root ganglion explants. Paper presented at the Society for Neuroscience Abstracts Los Angeles, Society for Neuroscience, 1998.

21. Steiner JP, Ross DT, Valentine HL, et al. The orally active neuroimmunophilin ligand GPI-1046 promotes structural and functional recovery in the mouse MPTP model of Parkinson's disease. Paper presented at the Society for Neuroscience Abstracts New Orleans, Society for Neuroscience, 1997.

22. Steiner, J. P., Ho, T., Lai, M. M, et al. The Neuroimmunophilin ligand GPI-1046 protects motor neurons from chronic excitotoxicity. Paper presented at the Society for Neuroscience Abstracts, Los Angeles, CA, Society for Neuroscience, 1998.

23. Guo X, Dawson VL, Dawson TM. Protective effects of immunophilin ligands on dopaminergic neurons. Paper presented at the Society for Neuroscience Abstracts, Miami, FL, Society for Neuroscience, 1999.

24. Gold BG, Densmore V, Shou W, et al. Immunophilin FK506-binding protein 52 (not FK506-binding protein 12) mediates the neurotrophic action of FK506. J Pharmacol Exp Ther 1999;289:1202–1210.

25. Carreau A, Gueugnon J, Benavides J, Vige X. Comparative effects of FK-506, rapamycin and cyclosporin A, on the in vitro differentiation of dorsal root ganglia explants and septal cholinergic neurons. Neuropharmacology 1997; 36:1755–1762.

26. Costantini LC, Chaturvedi P, Armistead DM, et al. A novel immunophilin ligand: distinct branching effects on dopaminergic neurons in culture and neurotrophic actions after oral administration in an animal model of Parkinson's disease. Neurobiol Dis 1998;5:97–106.

27. Costantini LC, Isacson O. Immunophilin ligands and GDNF enhance neurite branching or elongation from developing dopamine neurons in culture. Exp Neurol 2000;164:60–70.

28. Heikkila RE, Hess A, Duvoisin RC. Dopaminergic neurotoxicity of 1-methyl-4-phenyl-1,2,5,6- tetrahydropyridine in mice. Science 1984;224:1451–1453.

29. Langston JW, Langston EB, Irwin I. MPTP-induced parkinsonism in human and non-human primates: clinical and experimental aspects. Acta Neurol Scand Suppl 1984;100:49–54.

30. Kitamura Y, Itano Y, Kubo T, Nomura Y. Suppressive effect of FK-506, a novel immunosuppressant, against MPTP- induced dopamine depletion in the striatum of young C57BL/6 mice. J Neuroimmunol 1994;50:221–224.

31. Steiner JP, Hamilton GS, Ross DT, et al. Neurotrophic immunophilin ligands stimulate structural and functional recovery in neurodegenerative animal models. Proc Natl Acad Sci USA 1997;94:2019–2024.

32. Hamilton GS, Steiner JP. Neuroimmunophilin ligands as novel therapeutics for the treatment of degenerative disorders of the nervous system. Curr Pharm Design 1997;3:405–428.

33. Hamilton GS, Steiner JP. Immunophilins: beyond immunosuppression. J Med Chem 1998;41:5119–5143.

34. Ross DT, Guo H, Howorth P, et al. The small molecule FKBP ligand GPI-1046 induces partial striatal re- innervation after intranigral 6-hydroxydopamine lesion in rats. Neurosci Lett 2001;297:113–116.

35. Ross DT, Guo H, Howorth P, et al. The novel immunophilin ligand GPI-1046 stimulates morphological, biochemical, and behavioral recovery in the rat intranigral 6-OHDA parkinson's disease model. Paper presented at the Society for Neurosciences Abstracts, New Orleans, LA, 1997.

36. Harper S, Bilsland J, Young L, et al. Analysis of the neurotrophic effects of GPI-1046 on neuron survival and regeneration in culture and in vivo. Neuroscience 1999;88:257–267.

37. Emborg ME, Shin P, Roitberg, B., et al. Systemic administration of the immunophilin ligand GPI-1046 in MPTP- treated monkeys. Exp Neurol 2001;168:171–182.

38. Constantini LC, Chaturvedi P, McCaffrey P, et al. Neuroprotective and regenerative effects of immunophilin ligands in an animal model of parkinson's disease. Paper presented at the Society for Neuroscience Abstracts, New Orleans, LA, 1997.

39. Costantini LC, Cole D, Isacson O. Immunophilin ligands can prevent progressive dopaminergic degeneration in animal models of Parkinson's disease. Eur J Neurosci 2001;13:1085–1092.

40. Kondo T. Neuroprotection by dopamine (DA) agonists and potential application of immunophilin ligands. Paper presented at the 5th International Conference on Progress in Alzheimer's and Parkinson's Disease, Kyoto, Japan, 2001.

41. Kondo T, Hironishi M, Kihira T, Mizutani Y. Nonimmunosuppressive immunophilin ligand GPI-1046 protects nigral neurons of C57BL6 mouse from MPTP toxicity. Paper presented at the 5th International Conference on Progress in Alzheimer's and Parkinson's Disease, Kyoto, Japan, 2001.

42. Bocquet A, Lorent G, Fuks B, et al. Failure of GPI compounds to display neurotrophic activity in vitro and in vivo. Eur J Pharmacol 2001;415:173–180.

43. Ingram, DK. (1988). Complex maze learning in rodents as a model of age-related memory impairment. Neurobiol Aging 9, 475–485.
44. Lowy AM, Ingram DK, Olton DS, et al. Discrimination learning requiring different memory components in rats: age and neurochemical comparisons. Behav Neurosci 1985;99:638–651.
45. Barnes CA. Memory deficits associated with senescence: a neurophysiological and behavioral study in the rat. J Comp Physiol Psychol 1979;93:74–104.
46. Bartus RT, Dean RL, Goas JA, Lippa AS. Age-related changes in passive avoidance retention: modulation with dietary choline. Science 1980;209:301–303.
47. Ingram DK, London ED, Goodrick CL. Age and neurochemical correlates of radial maze performance in rats. Neurobiol Aging 1981;2:41–47.
48. Gage FH, Dunnett SB, Bjorklund A. Spatial learning and motor deficits in aged rats. Neurobiol Aging 1984;5:43–48.
49. Fischer W, Chen KS, Gage FH, Bjorklund A. Progressive decline in spatial learning and integrity of forebrain cholinergic neurons in rats during aging. Neurobiol Aging 1992;13:9–23.
50. Gage FH, Chen KS, Buzsaki G, Armstrong D. Experimental approaches to age-related cognitive impairments. Neurobiol Aging 1988;9:645–655.
51. Luine V, Bowling D, Hearns M. Spatial memory deficits in aged rats: contributions of monoaminergic systems. Brain Res 1990;537:271–278.
52. Richter-Levin G, Segal M. Serotonin, aging and cognitive functions of the hippocampus. Rev Neurosci 1996;7:103–113.
53. Zhang WQ, Mundy WR, Thai L, et al. Decreased glutamate release correlates with elevated dynorphin content in the hippocampus of aged rats with spatial learning deficits. Hippocampus 1991;1:391–397.
54. Deupree DL, Turner DA, Watters CL. Spatial performance correlates with in vitro potentiation in young and aged Fischer 344 rats. Brain Res 1991;554:1–9.
55. Shen J, Barnes CA, McNaughton BL, et al. The effect of aging on experience-dependent plasticity of hippocampal place cells. J Neurosci 1997;17:6769–6782.
56. Fordyce DE, Wehner JM. Effects of aging on spatial learning and hippocampal protein kinase C in mice. Neurobiol Aging 1993;14:309–317.
57. Sauer H, Francis JM, Jiang H, et al. Systemic treatment with GPI-1046 improves spatial memory and reverses cholinergic neuron atrophy in the medial septal nucleus of aged mice. Brain Res 1999;842:109–118.
58. Fischer W, Bjorklund A, Chen K, Gage FH. NGF improves spatial memory in aged rodents as a function of age. J Neurosci 1991;11:1889–1906.
59. Chen KS, Masliah E, Mallory M, Gage FH. Synaptic loss in cognitively impaired aged rats is ameliorated by chronic human nerve growth factor infusion. Neuroscience 1995;68:19–27.
60. Fischer W, Wictorin K, Bjorklund A, et al. Amelioration of cholinergic neuron atrophy and spatial memory impairment in aged rats by nerve growth factor. Nature 1987;329:65–68.
61. Gallagher M, Pelleymounter MA. An age-related spatial learning deficit: choline uptake distinguishes "impaired" and "unimpaired" rats. Neurobiol Aging 1988;9:363–369.

62. Markowska AL, Koliatsos VE, Breckler SJ, et al. Human nerve growth factor improves spatial memory in aged but not in young rats. J Neurosci 1994;14:4815–4824.

63. Pelleymounter MA, Cullen MJ, Baker MB, et al. The effects of intra-hippocampal BDNF and NGF on spatial learning in aged Long Evans rats. Mol Chem Neuropathol 1996;29:211–226.

64. Martin C, Chapman KE, Seckl JR, Ashley RH. Partial cloning and differential expression of ryanodine receptor/calcium-release channel genes in human tissues including the hippocampus and cerebellum. Neuroscience 1998;85:205–216.

65. Nakanishi S, Maeda N, Mikoshiba K. Immunohistochemical localization of an inositol 1,4,5-trisphosphate receptor, P400, in neural tissue: studies in developing and adult mouse brain. J Neurosci 1991;11:2075–2086.

66. Nakashima Y, Nishimura S, Maeda A, et al. Molecular cloning and characterization of a human brain ryanodine receptor. FEBS Lett 1997;417:157–162.

67. Brillantes AB, Ondrias K, Scott A, et al. Stabilization of calcium release channel (ryanodine receptor) function by FK506-binding protein. Cell 1994; 77:513–523.

68. Cameron AM, Steiner JP, Sabatini DM, et al. Immunophilin FK506 binding protein associated with inositol 1,4,5-trisphosphate receptor modulates calcium flux. Proc Natl Acad Sci USA 1995;92:1784–1788.

69. Marks AR. Cellular functions of immunophilins. Physiol Rev 1996;76:631–649.

70. Snyder, SH, Sabatini DM. Immunophilins and the nervous system. Nat Med 1995;1:32–37.

71. Reyes M, Stanton PK. Induction of hippocampal long-term depression requires release of Ca^{2+} from separate presynaptic and postsynaptic intracellular stores. J Neurosci 1996;16:5951–5960.

72. Schiegg A, Gerstner W, Ritz R, van Hemmen JL. Intracellular Ca^{2+} stores can account for the time course of LTP induction: a model of Ca^{2+} dynamics in dendritic spines. J Neurophysiol 1995;74:1046–1055.

73. Wang Y, Rowan MJ, Anwyl R. Induction of LTD in the dentate gyrus in vitro is NMDA receptor independent, but dependent on Ca^{2+} influx via low-voltage-activated Ca^{2+} channels and release of Ca^{2+} from intracellular stores. J Neurophysiol 1997;77:812–825.

74. Wang Y, Wu J, Rowan MJ, Anwyl R. Ryanodine produces a low frequency stimulation-induced NMDA receptor- independent long-term potentiation in the rat dentate gyrus in vitro. J Physiol 1996;495:755–767.

75. Cavallaro S, Meiri N, Yi CL, et al. Late memory-related genes in the hippocampus revealed by RNA fingerprinting. Proc Natl Acad Sci USA 1997; 94:9669–9673.

76. Haug LS, Ostvold AC, Cowburn RF, et al. Decreased inositol (1,4,5)-trisphosphate receptor levels in Alzheimer's disease cerebral cortex: selectivity of changes and possible correlation to pathological severity. Neurodegeneration 1996;5:169–176.

77. Young LT, Kish SJ, Li PP, Warsh JJ. Decreased brain [3H]inositol 1,4,5-trisphosphate binding in Alzheimer's disease. Neurosci Lett 1988;94:198–202.

78. Kurumatani T, Fastbom J, Bonkale WL, et al. Loss of inositol 1,4,5-trisphosphate receptor sites and decreased PKC levels correlate with staging of Alzheimer's disease neurofibrillary pathology. Brain Res 1998;796:209–221.
79. Lopez-Ilasaca M, Schiene C, Kullertz G, et al. Effects of FK506-binding protein 12 and FK506 on autophosphorylation of epidermal growth factor receptor. J Biol Chem 1998;273:9430–9434.
80. Wang T, Li BY, Danielson PD, et al. The immunophilin FKBP12 functions as a common inhibitor of the TGF beta family type I receptors. Cell 1996;86:435–444.
81. Okadome T, Oeda E, Saitoh M, et al. Characterization of the interaction of FKBP12 with the transforming growth factor-beta type I receptor in vivo. J Biol Chem 1996;271:21,687–21,690.
82. Chen YG, Liu F, Massague J. Mechanism of TGFbeta receptor inhibition by FKBP12. Embo J 1997;16:3866–3876.
83. Wang T, Donahoe PK, Zervos AS. Specific interaction of type I receptors of the TGF-beta family with the immunophilin FKBP-12. Science 1994;265:674–676.
84. Bassing CH, Shou W, Muir S, et al. FKBP12 is not required for the modulation of transforming growth factor beta receptor I signaling activity in embryonic fibroblasts and thymocytes. Cell Growth Differ 1998;9:223–228.
85. Shou W, Aghdasi B, Armstrong, DL, et al. Cardiac defects and altered ryanodine receptor function in mice lacking FKBP12. Nature 1998;391:489–492.
86. Lindholm D, Hengerer B, Zafra F, Thoenen H. Transforming growth factor-beta 1 stimulates expression of nerve growth factor in the rat CNS. Neuroreport 1990;1:9–12.
87. Hahn M, Lorez H, Fischer G. The immortalized astroglial cell line RC7 is a new model system for the study of nerve growth factor (NGF) regulation: stimulation by interleukin-1 beta and transforming growth factor-beta 1 is additive and affected differently by dibutyryl cyclic AMP. Glia 1994;10:286–295.
88. Zafra F, Lindholm D, Castren E, et al. (1992). Regulation of brain-derived neurotrophic factor and nerve growth factor mRNA in primary cultures of hippocampal neurons and astrocytes. J Neurosci 1992;12:4793–4799.

Improved Survival of Grafted Dopamine Neurons by Calcineurin Inhibitors

Roger F. Castilho, Oskar Hansson, and Patrik Brundin

INTRODUCTION

Parkinson's disease (PD) is characterized by a progressive degeneration of dopamine neurons in the substantia nigra, resulting in severe dopamine depletion in the striatum (for recent reviews *see* refs. *1* and *2*). The loss of dopaminergic neurotransmission is considered the primary and major underlying cause of the disruption of motor function in PD patients *(1,2)*. Around 20 years ago, intrastriatal implants of embryonic nigral tissue were proposed as an alternative therapeutic approach for PD *(3,4)*. During the last decade there have been several reports describing successful clinical application of the technique in a small number of PD patients *(5–7* and refs. therein). In the most successful cases, patients who initially have been severely incapacitated due to the disease have eventually been able to return to their professions after receiving nigral transplants. However, only a minority of PD patients have exhibited this degree of improvement after surgery *(5–7* and refs. therein).

There appear to be several essential conditions that need to be fulfilled for the grafts to exert marked functional effects in patients.

1. Patient selection appears to be crucial. Patients that suffer from one of the Parkinson Plus syndromes are unlikely to experience major benefit, even when graft survival is good *(8)*.
2. It is possible that immunological factors can play a role for graft outcome *(9)*. It is still not clear to what degree immunosuppression is necessary when human embryonic neural allografts are implanted into the brains of PD patients, and different centers have adopted varying approaches on this issue.
3. The choice of transplantation site is likely to be of great importance *(6)*. Based on the pattern of dopaminergic denervation of the PD striatum and normal connectivity of the putamen, there are reasons to believe that the putamen

From: *Immunosuppressant Analogs in Neuroprotection*
Edited by: C. V. Borlongan, O. Isacson, and P. R. Sanberg © Humana Press Inc., Totowa, NJ

should be the primary target in attempts to reverse motor symptoms, but the role of grafts in the caudate remain to be established.

4. The extent to which the grafted neurons are able to generate axons and innervate the new host brain is likely to be crucial *(10)*. Results obtained in rats show a correlation between the degree of functional recovery and the extent of reinnervation of the host brain by the grafted neurons.

5. One decisive factor governing whether a mesencephalic transplant is successful at ameliorating symptoms in a PD patient is probably the number of dopamine neurons that survive in the graft (for a recent review, *see* ref. *11*).

There is increasing evidence from rats that a large number of surviving neurons support more rapid and extensive behavioral recovery, and in the few patients that have been operated on there appears to be a correlation between increases in fluorodopa uptake in postoperative positron emission scans and the extent of symptomatic relief *(8,12)*.

In theory, the use of calcineurin inhibitors during embryonic nigral tissue transplantation may improve the graft outcome by immunossupressing the host *(13)* and by enhancing both neurite elongation *(14,15)* and survival of grafted dopamine neurons *(16)*. In this chapter we discuss the beneficial role of the calcineurin inhibitors FK506 (tacrolimus, Prograf®) and cyclosporin A (Sandimmun®) in nigral tissue transplantation by improving the survival of grafted embryonic dopamine neurons.

POOR SURVIVAL OF EMBRYONIC DOPAMINE NEURONS GRAFTED IN ANIMAL MODELS OF PARKINSON'S DISEASE: MECHANISMS OF CELL DEATH

It is estimated that only 1–20% of grafted dopamine neurons survive in rodents and in PD patients *(11)*. During the embryonic nigral tissue transplantation procedure, the cell death process may be initiated by distinct insults and occurs during different temporal phases. For practical reasons, four distinct hypothetical phases when neural death may occur have been identified.

First phase: When the donor embryo is removed from its maternal blood supply, this part of the procedure will result in oxygen and glucose deprivation in the embryonic brain tissue.

Second phase: Characterized mainly by mechanical trauma of the embryonic brain tissue dissection and dissociation, and death is induced by storage under nonphysiological conditions.

Third phase: Cell death may occur during the implantation procedure itself and the immediate period after injection of the grafted tissue into the novel adult host environment.

Fourth phase: When the graft matures in the recipient host, it is conceivable that grafted neurons die.

One or several triggers may initiate cell death, by necrosis or apoptosis, during each of these phases, such as mechanical disruption of plasma membrane, cytoplasmic calcium accumulation, oxidative stress, activation of the mitochondrial pathway of apoptosis, and activation of plasma membrane cell death receptors (for a recent review *see* ref. *11*).

It has been estimated that around 30% of the embryonic mesencephalic dopamine neurons die during the dissection of ventral mesencephalon and preparation of the cell suspension *(17,18)*. Probably this cell death is mainly due to mechanical disruption of the plasma membrane and a transient deprivation of glucose and oxygen. Cytoplasmic calcium accumulation is also a potential important phenomenon involved in death of nigral embryonic neurons. By administration of flunarizine, a calcium channel blocker, during dissection and cell suspension preparation, Kaminski Schierle and collaborators *(19)* obtained increased survival of grafted dopamine neurons to 260% of control values. However, it seems that activation of N-methyl-D-aspartate (NMDA) receptors, which promotes calcium and sodium influx to the cytoplasm, does not play an important role in the death of embryonic grafted dopamine neurons *(20)*. Indeed, a recent report suggests that NMDA receptors are not yet expressed on the nigral dopamine neurons in the 14-d-old rat embryo *(21)*. The participation of oxidative stress in grafted nigral neurons' death was demonstrated by improved survival (to 170–260% of control values) of grafted nigral neurons when one of the antioxidant lazaroids U-74389G, U-83836G, or tirilazad mesylate, was added to the graft tissue *(21–24)*. Finally, a recent study by Schierle and collaborators *(25)* has revealed an important role of caspase activation in grafted nigral neurons' death. Caspases are intracellular proteases involved in the apoptotic process *(26)*. The precise intracellular pathways involved in caspase activation and death of grafted dopamine neurons are currently being elucidated *(16,18,27)*.

FK506 AND CYCLOSPORIN A ENHANCE THE SURVIVAL OF GRAFTED RAT EMBRYONIC DOPAMINE NEURONS: POSSIBLE MECHANISMS OF ACTION

Several reports suggest that most of the embryonic dopamine neurons die during the cell suspension preparation and during the first 1–3 d after implantation procedure (for a recent review *see* ref. *11*). In fact, many publications report interventions that successfully improved survival of grafted dopamine neurons when administering pharmacological treatment only during the tissue dissection and cell suspension preparation *(11)*. This indicates that death of dopamine neurons in nigral transplants is marked during the period when neuroprotective pharmacological interventions are most easily applied. Two interesting compounds, that could potentially be neuroprotective for grafted embryonic dopamine neurons are the immunophilin ligands and calcineurin inhibitors FK506 and cyclosporin A. These drugs have been described to act through binding to intracellular immunophilins FKBPs (FK506-binding proteins) for FK506 and cyclophilins for cyclosporin A (for a recent review *see* ref. *28*).

In order to find the appropriate concentration of FK506 and cyclosporin A to test on grafts of nigral neurons, we examined the efffects of a wide range of concentrations of these compounds on cultured mesencephalic embryonic neurons exposed to serum deprivation. Under this condition, only around 20% of both dopamine [identified as tyrosine hydroxylase (TH)-immunoreactive] and total cells remain viable after 5 d in vitro. We observed a protective effect of FK506 (1–3 μM) and cyclosporin A (0.2–0.5 μM) when these compounds were present from the withdrawal of serum from the cultured cells *(16)*. We chose monolayer cultures of dissociated mesencephalic tissue subjected to serum deprivation as an in vitro model of cell transplantation. This model readily permits titration of optimal drug concentrations and also provides information specifically on the survival of TH-immunoreactive neurons. Recent reports from our group suggest that assessments of DNA fragmentation and lactate dehydrogenase release in mesencephalic cell suspensions may also constitute useful methods to evaluate neuroprotective compounds that are to be applied in intracerebral grafts *(18,25)*.

Based on the results obtained with cultured mesencephalic neurons subjected to serum deprivation, we chose the concentrations of FK506 (3 μM) and cyclosporin A (0.5 μM) for the grafting experiments. The drugs were present during dissection and dissociation of the embryonic ventral mesencephalon and in the final cell suspension for intrastriatal grafting in adult rats. In rats grafted with control cell suspensions we observed a survival of 20% of the TH-immunoreactive neurons [≈35,000 TH-immunoreactive neurons, with one-half embryonic ventral mesencephalon implantated in each recipient rat, i.e., 17,500 TH neurons *(22)*] (Fig. 1). When either FK506 or cyclosporin A was added during the preparation and in the final cell suspension used for grafting, we observed a significant increase in survival of TH-immunoreactive neurons of around 85% *(16)* (Fig. 1). In a second in vivo experiment, the graft-recipient rats (but not the graft tissue itself) were treated with FK506 or cyclosporin A. Immunosuppressive concentrations of FK506 (1 mg/kg, im) and cyclosporin A (10 mg/kg, ip) were administered from 1 d before transplantation surgery until 7 d after the operation, with one injection made 30 min before graft implantation. Treatment of graft-recipient animals with FK506 or cyclosporin A did not improve the survival

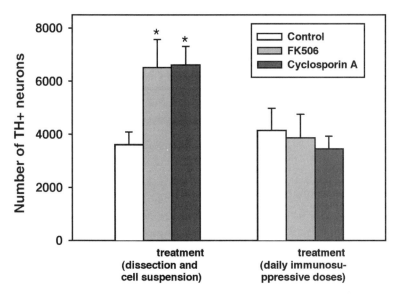

Fig. 1. In vitro, but not in vivo, treatment with either FK506 or cyclosporin A increases the survival of grafted TH-immunoreactive neurons. In vitro treatment: FK506 (3.0 μ*M*) or cyclosporin A (0.5 μ*M*) was present when dissecting the embryonic ventral mesencephalon and in the final cell suspension used for grafting (control, *n* = 10; FK506, *n* = 9; cyclosporin A, *n* = 10). In vivo treatment: graft-recipient rats received daily injections of FK506 (1 mg/kg, im) or cyclosporin A (10 mg/kg, ip) starting 1 d before grafting and continuing for 7 d after transplantation (control, *n* = 6; FK506, *n* = 7; cyclosporin A, *n* = 7). *Statistically significant, *p* < 0.05. (Modified from ref. *16*).

of grafted embryonic TH-immunoreactive neurons (Fig. 1). In this paradigm, when only the grafted recipient animal received FK506 or cyclosporin A, it is possible that the implanted embryonic neurons are exposed to the immunophilins only at a late stage in the cell death process. At this stage, it may not be possible to inhibit the cell death process that may be initiated already during preparation of the cell suspension *(11)*. It is important to emphasize that FK506 normally crosses the blood–brain barrier and that the insertion of a implantation cannula into the brain parenchyma during nigral graft injection disrupts the blood–brain barrier for at least 1 wk *(29)*, facilitating cyclosporin A's access to the brain *(30)*.

Based on our results, we can speculate on several mechanisms underlying the observed increase in survival of grafted embryonic dopamine neurons promoted by FK506 and cyclosporin A. They include inhibition of nitric oxide synthase activity, blockage of the mitochondrial permeability transi-

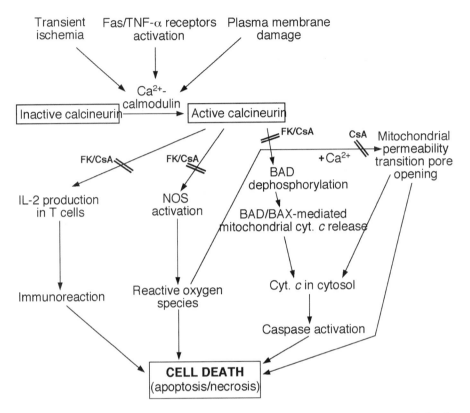

Fig. 2. Scheme summarizing FK506- and cyclosporin A-sensitive cell death mechanisms in transplanted mesencephalic neurons. Descriptions of the various mechanisms can be found in the text and cited references. CsA, cyclosporin A; Cyt. *c*, cytochrome *c*; FK, FK506; IL-2, interleukin-2; NOS, nitric oxide synthase; TNF-α, tumor necrosis factor-alpha.

tion pore, inhibition of cell death process initiated by BAD (a proapoptotic member of the Bcl-2 family), immunosuppression, and neurotrophic action (Fig. 2).

Both FK506 and cyclosporin A are potent inhibitors of calcineurin, a calcium–calmodulin-dependent phosphatase that is involved in distinct mechanisms of cell death (for reviews *see* refs. *28* and *31*). When activated, calcineurin dephosphorylates neuronal nitric oxide synthase and thereby activating the production of nitric oxide (NO•) in the cytosol. Nitric oxide is a physiological intracellular messanger. However, in some situations nitric oxide may cause cellular toxicity by reacting with proteins and inactivating critical metabolic enzymes. In addition, nitric oxide can react with superoxide ($O_2^{\bullet-}$) to form an even more potent oxidant, peroxynitrite ($ONOO^{\bullet-}$) *(32,33)*. Peroxynitrite can induce protein oxidation and dysfunction, lipid peroxidation, oxidation of DNA with strand breaks, and activation of poly(ADP-ribose) polymerase, all of which are processes involved in cell death *(32,33)*. However, a recent study by Van Muiswinkel and collaborators *(34)* has shown that treatment of the mesencephalic cell suspension and chronic treatment of the graft-recipient rat with the nitric oxide synthase inhibitor N^{ω}-nitro-L-arginine methyl ester (L-NAME) do not improve survival of grafted dopamine neurons. These results suggest that activation of nitric oxide synthase with increased production of NO[*] are not important steps in the death of grafted dopamine neurons.

Cyclosporin A is a potent inhibitor of the mitochondrial permeability transition (MPT) pore (for a recent review, *see* ref. *35*). MPT is defined as a Ca^{2+}-dependent, nonspecific permeabilization of the inner mitochondrial membrane. This process begins with a mitochondrial membrane permeabilization to protons and small ions and progresses with permeabilization to small sugars and osmotic support, finally resulting in permeabilization of the membrane to low-molecular-mass proteins (<1500 Da), which is accompanied by irreversible mitochondrial dysfunction *(36)*. MPT can be enhanced by various agents (inducers), including prooxidants, thiol crosslinking reagents, inorganic phosphate and uncouplers (for a recent review, *see* ref. *35*). MPT pore opening may induce cell death by necrosis due to mitochondrial dysfunction and cellular energy depletion. However, recently it has been proposed that MPT pore opening is also related to induction of apoptotic cell death by release of apoptogenic proteins from the mitochondrial intermembrane space, including cytochrome c, apoptosis-inducing factor, and some procaspases (for reviews *see* refs. *35* and *37*). It is known that the inhibitory property of cyclosporin A on mammalian MPT is related to its binding to cyclophilin D in the inner mitochondrial membrane in a process associated with inhibition of the peptidylprolyl-*cis-trans*-isomerase activity *(38)*. This implies that cyclophilin is a structural component of the mammalian MPT pore *(38)* or catalyses mammalian MPT opening via peptide bond isomerization. In contrast to cyclosporin A, FK506 is not able to inhibit MPT pore opening *(39)*. Cyclosporin A-inhibited cell death mediated by MPT pore opening does not appear important in grafted neurons in view of the fact that cyclosporin A did not provide additional protection beyond that observed with FK506 treatment. In addition, implants of nigral tissue from transgenic mice overexpressing Bcl-2, an antiapoptotic protein that inhibits MPT pore opening, exhibit similar survival of dopamine neurons to those derived from control embryos *(19)*.

Recently, Wang and collaborators *(40)* have shown that calcineurin activation can start the process of hippocampal neuron death by dephosphorylating cytosolic BAD. This process promotes the translocation of BAD to the mitochondrial membranes where it interacts with Bcl-xL to initiate the release of proapoptotic proteins from the mitochondrial intermembranous space (e.g.: cytochrome *c*, apoptosis-inducing factor) *(37)*. Interestingly, it has been shown that activation of Fas (APO-1/CD95) receptors of lymphocytes results in mobilization of Ca^{2+} from intracellular stores and BAD dephosphorylation by calcineurin A *(41)*. It is possible that similar mechanisms take place in death of embryonic grafted dopamine neurons, since Kaminski Schierle and collaborators *(27)* recently observed that death of embryonic dopamine neurons in nigral grafts is, in part, mediated via the Fas (APO-1/CD95) receptor activation. Calcineurin-mediated dephosphorylation of other target proteins or enzymes, whose roles in cell death pathways have not yet been elucidated, could also be involved in death of grafted embryonic dopamine neurons.

Immunossupression is unlikely to be the mechanism by which cyclosporin A and FK506 improve the survival of grafted embryonic dopamine neurons in our paradigm. The experiments were performed using Sprague-Dawley rat donors and recipients that come from a colony that is outbred from an originally inbred strain. Previous studies with intracerebral neural grafts indicate that immune reactions do not play a role in this syngeneic (grafts between genetically identical individuals) setting *(42)*. Following syngeneic neural transplantation to the striatum, there is astrogliosis and activation of microglia around the graft for at least 6 wk after transplantation *(42,43)*. However, in vitro *(44)* and in vivo *(45)* studies suggest that the microglia reaction occurring after transplantation may actually be beneficial for graft survival. Moreover, in our experiments *(16)*, when the grafted adult rats received immunosuppressive doses of FK506 or cyclosporin A from 1 d before transplantation surgery until 7 d after the operation, we did not observe any increase in survival of grafted embryonic dopamine neurons.

Finally, it is likely that trophic support in the adult brain plays an important role in survival of grafted embryonic dopamine neurons (for a recent review, *see* ref. *11)*. In fact, injections of rat glial cell line-derived neurotrophic factor (GDNF) adjacent to grafted embryonic dopamine neurons increase survival, growth, and function of the intrastriatal graft *(46)*. Several other protocols for delivery of GDNF to grafts have also been employed successfully *(47–50)*. Both FK506 and cyclosporin A can exert neurotrophic effects in cultured embryonic dopamine neurons by binding to immunophilins, in a mechanism independent of calcineurin inhibition

(14,15,27) (*see* also Chapters 3 and 4). In our experiments, demonstrating neuroprotective effects of FK506 and cyclosporin A, embryonic neurons were exposed to the compounds only for 2–6 h, during cell suspension preparation and graft implantation. It seems unlikely that this short period of exposure could result in trophic support and, consequently, increased survival of embryonic dopamine neurons. In conclusion, FK506 and cyclosporin A are useful compounds to consider as agents that can improve survival of nigral transplants, and it remains to be seen if their neuroprotective effects will be additive to those seen with other drug treatments that improve the survival of grafted dopamine neurons.

ACKNOWLEDGMENTS

Roger F. Castilho is currently supported by grants from the Brazilian agencies CNPq, FAEP-UNICAMP, and FAPESP. This work was supported by grants from the Swedish Medical Research Council, The Söderberg Foundation, and Swedish National Network in Neuroscience.

REFERENCES

1. Dunnett SB, Björklund A. Prospects for new restorative and neuroprotective treatments in Parkinson's disease. Nature 1999;399(Suppl):A32–A39.
2. Olanow CW, Tatton WG. Etiology and pathogenesis of Parkinson's disease. Annu Rev Neurosci 1999;22:123–144.
3. Björklund A, Stenevi U. Reconstruction of the nigralstriatal dopamine pathway by intracerebral nigral transplants. Brain Res 1979;177:555–560.
4. Perlow MJ, Freed WJ, Hoffer BJ, et al. Brain grafts reduce motor abnormalities produced by destruction of nigrostriatal dopamine system. Science 1979;204:643–647.
5. Tabbal S, Fahn S, Frucht S. Fetal tissue transplantation in Parkinson's disease. Curr Opin Neurol 1998;11:341–349.
6. Lindvall O. Neural transplantation: a hope for patients with Parkinson's disease. Neuroreport 1997;8:iii–x.
7. Lindvall O. Cerebral implantation in movement disorders: state of the art. Mov Disord 1999;14:201–205.
8. Hagell P, Schrag A, Piccini P, et al. Sequential bilateral transplantation in Parkinson's disease: effects of the second graft. Brain 1999;122:1121–1132.
9. Kordower JH, Styren S, Clarke M, et al. Fetal grafting for Parkinson's disease: expression of immune markers in two patients with functional fetal nigral implants. Cell Transplant 1997;6:213–219.
10. Björklund A, Dunnett SB, Stenevi U, et al. Reinnervation of the denervated striatum by substantia nigra transplants: functional consequences as revealed by pharmacological and sensorimotor testing. Brain Res 1980;199:307–333.

11. Brundin P, Karlsson J, Emgard M, et al. Improving the survival of grafted dopaminergic neurons: a review over current approaches. Cell Transplant 2000;9:179–195.

12. Remy P, Samson Y, Hantraye P, et al. Clinical correlates of [18F]fluorodopa uptake in five grafted parkinsonian patients. Ann Neurol 1995;38:580–588.

13. Wennberg L, Czech KA, Larsson LC, et al. Effects of immunosuppressive treatment on host responses and survival of porcine neural xenografts in rats. Transplantation 2001;71:1797–1806.

14. Costantini LC, Chaturvedi P, Armistead DM, et al. A novel immunophilin ligand: distinct branching effects on dopaminergic neurons in culture and neurotrophic actions after oral administration in an animal model of Parkinson's disease. Neurobiol Dis 1998;5:97–106.

15. Costantini LC, Isacson O. Immunophilin ligands and GDNF enhance neurite branching or elongation from developing dopamine neurons in culture. Exp Neurol 2000;164:60–70.

16. Castilho RF, Hansson O, Brundin P. FK506 and cyclosporin A enhance the survival of cultured and grafted rat embryonic dopamine neurons. Exp Neurol 2000;164:94–101.

17. Fawcett JW, Barker RA, Dunnett SB. Dopaminergic neuronal survival and the effects of bFGF in explant, three dimensional and monolayer cultures of embryonic rat ventral mesencephalon. Exp Brain Res 1995;106:275–282.

18. Schierle GS, Leist M, Martinou JC, et al. Differential effects of Bcl-2 overexpression on fibre outgrowth and survival of embryonic dopaminergic neurons in intracerebral transplants. Eur J Neurosci 1999;11:3073–3081.

19. Kaminski Schierle GS, Hansson O, Brundin P. Flunarizine improves the survival of grafted dopaminergic neurons. Neuroscience 1999;94:17–20.

20. Schierle GS, Karlsson J, Brundin P. MK-801 does not enhance dopaminergic cell survival in embryonic nigral grafts. Neuroreport 1998;9:1313–1316.

21. Yung KK. Localization of ionotropic and metabotropic glutamate receptors in distinct neuronal elements of the rat substantia nigra. Neurochem Int 1998;33:313–326.

22. Nakao N, Frodl EM, Duan WM, et al. Lazaroids improve the survival of grafted rat embryonic dopamine neurons. Proc Natl Acad Sci USA 1994;91:12,408–12,412.

23. Karlsson J, Love RM, Clarke DJ, Brundin P. Effects of anaesthetics and lazaroid U-83836E on survival of transplanted rat dopaminergic neurones. Brain Res 1999;821:546–550.

24. Hansson O, Castilho RF, Kaminski Schierle GS, et al. Additive effects of caspase inhibitor and lazaroid on the survival of transplanted rat and human embryonic dopamine neurons. Exp Neurol 2000;164:102–111.

25. Schierle GS, Hansson O, Leist M, et al. Caspase inhibition reduces apoptosis and increases survival of nigral transplants. Nat Med 1999;5:97–100.

26. Pettmann B, Henderson CE. Neuronal cell death. Neuron 1998;20:633–647.

27. Kaminski Schierle GS, Keep MF, Brundin P. Death of dopaminergic neurons in nigral transplants is in part mediated via the CD95 receptor. Soc Neurosci Abstr 2000; 209:50.

28. Snyder SH, Lai MM, Burnett PE. Immunophilins in the nervous system. Neuron 1998;21:283–294.
29. Brundin P, Widner H, Nilsson OG, et al. Intracerebral xenografts of dopamine neurons: the role of immunosuppression and the blood-brain barrier. Exp Brain Res 1989;75:195–207.
30. Uchino H, Elmer E, Uchino K, et al. Amelioration by cyclosporin A of brain damage in transient forebrain ischemia in the rat. Brain Res 1998;812:216–226.
31. Morioka M, Hamada J, Ushio Y, Miyamoto E. Potential role of calcineurin for brain ischemia and traumatic injury. Prog Neurobiol 1999;58:1–30.
32. Bredt DS. Endogenous nitric oxide synthesis: biological functions and pathophysiology. Free Radic Res 1999;31:577–596.
33. Pryor WA, Squadrito GL. The chemistry of peroxynitrite: a product from the reaction of nitric oxide with superoxide. Am J Physiol 1995;268:L699–L722.
34. Van Muiswinkel FL, Drukarch B, Steinbusch HW, De Vente J. Sustained pharmacological inhibition of nitric oxide synthase does not affect the survival of intrastriatal rat fetal mesencephalic transplants. Brain Res 1998; 792:48–58.
35. Crompton M. The mitochondrial permeability transition pore and its role in cell death. Biochem J 1999;341:233–249.
36. Castilho RF, Kowaltowski AJ, Vercesi AE. The irreversibility of inner mitochondrial membrane permeabilization by Ca^{2+} plus prooxidants is determined by the extent of membrane protein thiol cross-linking. J Bioenerg Biomembr 1996;28:523–529.
37. Green DR, Reed JC. Mitochondria and apoptosis. Science 1998;281:1309–1312.
38. Nicolli A, Basso E, Petronilli V, et al. Interactions of cyclophilin with the mitochondrial inner membrane and regulation of the permeability transition pore, and cyclosporin A-sensitive channel. J Biol Chem 1996;271:2185–2192.
39. Griffiths EJ, Halestrap AP. Further evidence that cyclosporin A protects mitochondria from calcium overload by inhibiting a matrix peptidyl-prolyl cis-trans isomerase. Implications for the immunosuppressive and toxic effects of cyclosporin. Biochem J 1991;274:611–614.
40. Wang HG, Pathan N, Ethell IM, et al. Ca^{2+}-induced apoptosis through calcineurin dephosphorylation of BAD. Science 1999;284:339–343.
41. Jayaraman T, Marks AR. Calcineurin is downstream of the inositol 1,4,5-trisphosphate receptor in the apoptotic and cell growth pathways. J Biol Chem 2000;275:6417–6420.
42. Duan WM, Widner H, Brundin P. Temporal pattern of host responses against intrastriatal grafts of syngeneic, allogeneic or xenogeneic embryonic neuronal tissue in rats. Exp Brain Res 1995;104:227–242.
43. Blunt SB, Jenner P, Marsden CD. Motor function, graft survival and gliosis in rats with 6-OHDA lesions and foetal ventral mesencephalic grafts chronically treated with L-dopa and carbidopa. Exp Brain Res 1992;88:326–340.
44. Zietlow R, Dunnett SB, Fawcett JW. The effect of microglia on embryonic dopaminergic neuronal survival in vitro: diffusible signals from neurons and glia change microglia from neurotoxic to neuroprotective. Eur J Neurosci 1999;11:1657–1667.

45. Duan WM, Widner H, Cameron RM, Brundin P. Quinolinic acid-induced inflammation in the striatum does not impair the survival of neural allografts in the rat. Eur J Neurosci 1998;10:2595–2606.

46. Rosenblad C, Martinez-Serrano A, Björklund A. Glial cell line-derived neurotrophic factor increases survival, growth and function of intrastriatal fetal nigral dopaminergic grafts. Neuroscience 1996;75:979–985.

47. Sautter J, Tseng JL, Braguglia D, et al. Implants of polymer-encapsulated genetically modified cells releasing glial cell line-derived neurotrophic factor improve survival, growth, and function of fetal dopaminergic grafts. Exp Neurol 1998;149:230–236.

48. Sullivan AM, Pohl J, Blunt SB. Growth/differentiation factor 5 and glial cell line-derived neurotrophic factor enhance survival and function of dopaminergic grafts in a rat model of Parkinson's disease. Eur J Neurosci 1998;10:3681–3688.

49. Yurek DM. Glial cell line-derived neurotrophic factor improves survival of dopaminergic neurons in transplants of fetal ventral mesencephalic tissue. Exp Neurol 1998;153:195–202.

50. Wilby MJ, Sinclair SR, Muir EM., et al. A glial cell line-derived neurotrophic factor-secreting clone of the Schwann cell line SCTM41 enhances survival and fiber outgrowth from embryonic nigral neurons grafted to the striatum and to the lesioned substantia nigra. J Neurosci 1999;19:2301–2312.

6

Possible Mechanisms Underlying the Protective Action of Immunosuppressants Against Parkinson's Disease

The Mitochondrial Permeability Transition Pore Hypothesis

L.V. P. Korlipara and A. H. V. Schapira

INTRODUCTION

Current therapies for Parkinson's disease (PD) alleviate symptoms but do not ameliorate the progressive selective loss of dopaminergic neurons in the substantia nigra pars compacta (SNpC) characteristic of the disease. Traditionally they may be associated with a long-term reduction in efficacy and the development of disabling side effects. Interest has therefore diverted to the development of neuroprotective strategies that halt or retard disease progression.

The exact mechanisms and etiology of cell death in PD remain unknown. The parkinsonian syndrome, similar but not identical to idiopathic PD, induced by the meperidine analog 1-methyl-4-phenyltetrahydropyridine (MPTP) initially focused attention on potential environmental toxic agents. Although MPTP has provided a good model for elucidating bioenergetic and pathogenic mechanisms in PD, intense scrutiny has failed to identify nigral toxins that may account for the majority of cases of idiopathic PD.

More recently, mutations in genes encoding α-synuclein, ubiquitin carboxyl-terminal hydrolase L1, and parkin have been described in a number of patients with familial PD *(1–3)*. First-degree relatives of patients with PD have a significantly increased risk of developing the disease *(4,5)*. Patients with identified genetic mutations, however, account for a small percentage of PD patients.

The concept that PD may be caused by diverse genetic or environmental factors, either by themselves or in combination, with common clinicopathological consequences has focused attention onto downstream pathways of

From: *Immunosuppressant Analogs in Neuroprotection*
Edited by: C. V. Borlongan, O. Isacson, and P. R. Sanberg © Humana Press Inc., Totowa, NJ

nigral neuronal death. Apoptotic cell death has increasingly been implicated in PD and other neurodegenerative diseases. Mitochondria play a key role in both necrotic and apoptotic cell death and are considered to be mediated by the opening of a large nonselective proteinaceous pore complex, the mitochondrial membrane permeability transition pore (PTP). Bioenergetic abnormalities described in PD, increased oxidative stress and excitotoxicity, are also known to affect PTP opening. The effects of the immunosuppressant cyclosporin A (CsA), a selective PTP inhibitor, on ameliorating apoptotic and pathological changes has been described in some animal and cellular PD models; therefore, an attractive hypothesis is that PTP opening is a key step in the pathway leading to cell death in PD.

This chapter discusses the PTP and its role in apoptosis and attempts to relate this to pathogenic mechanisms known to be involved in the neuronal death characteristic of PD. The relevance of this in the context of neuroprotective strategies is examined.

MITOCHONDRIAL PERMEABILITY TRANSITION

Mitochondria have traditionally been regarded as cellular power plants, generating ATP for the metabolic needs of the cell. However, this simple view has been modified whereby mitochondria would appear to play active roles in calcium homeostasis and in cell death pathways. An electrical ($\Psi\Delta_M$) and pH gradient exists across the inner mitochondrial membrane, which together generate a proton-motive force. Modulation of this gradient by the PTP plays an essential part of mitochondrial involvement in cell death and calcium cycling. Opening of the PTP under certain conditions results in the collapse of the $\Psi\Delta_M$, uncoupling of oxidative phosphorylation, equilibration of gradients of ions and small solutes across the mitochondrial membrane, and mitochondrial swelling. Such events represent early changes that may occur in necrotic and some forms of apoptotic cell death.

Historical Aspects

The first description of mitochondrial permeability transition followed work by Hunter and Haworth in the 1970s *(6–9)*. They observed that isolated mitochondria could undergo an abrupt calcium-dependent increase in permeability under certain conditions. Using calcium- and phosphate-treated mitochondria suspended in polyethylene glycols of varying molecular masses, they showed that the permeability increase had an abrupt cutoff to solutes greater than 1500 Da. Mitochondrial permeability transition was shown to be promoted by Ca^{2+}, phosphate, and prooxidants and to be inhibited by Mg^{2+}, ADP/ATP, matrix acidification, and high $\Psi\Delta_M$ *(6–8)*.

It was postulated that the abrupt increase in permeability to solutes less than 1500 Da could be effected by either a generalized dysfunction of the lipid membrane or by channels in the mitochondrial membrane. The latter view gained credence for a number of reasons. The discrete size limitation in permeability was more in keeping with the presence of a pore. Then, the discovery that the immunosuppressant CsA inhibited permeability transition with saturable kinetics implied that a specific protein may be inhibited by this agent *(10,11)*.

A CsA-sensitive pore was subsequently identified in mitochondrial membranes, using patch clamp-techniques *(12)*, and this correlated with a previously identified high-conductance channel, the mitochondrial megachannel (MCC) in rat liver mitoplasts *(13,14)*. The MCC was shown to exhibit Ca^{2+} dependence, CsA sensitivity, and large conductance (≥ 1 nS), making it likely to be the channel involved in permeability transition. The pore radius was estimated to be 1.0–1.3 nm. Agents that promote mitochondrial permeability transition keep the pore in an open state, including Ca^{2+}, phosphate, and prooxidants; conversely, low-matrix pH, ADP, and high $\Psi\Delta_M$ promote pore closure.

The physiological function of the PTP is as yet not known. One theory is that it serves as an efflux channel for mitochondrial Ca^{2+}, maintaining homeostasis and thus regulating the actvitiy of Ca-dependent enzymes. As its function is modulated by reactive oxygen species, matrix pH, Ca^{2+}, and membrane potential, it may serve an important role in reacting to changes in cellular and mitochondrial function, and in homeostatic mechanisms. The PTP can open in a low-conductance state under matrix pH modulation, allowing the diffusion of ions, but without the catastrophic consequences for the cell of PTP opening in the traditional high-conductance mode, and this may represent its physiological role *(15)*.

Pore Constituents

The exact molecular composition and conformation of the PTP remains a matter of some debate. Much of current knowledge regarding its constituents was originally inferred from ligands that are known to affect PTP activity. Consequently, a number of key components have been identified, including the adenine nucleotide translocator (ANT) in the inner membrane, voltage-dependent anion channel (VDAC, porin), cyclophilin D (CYP-D) in the mitochondrial matrix, and a number of associated protein kinases. Current models suggest that the PTP resides as a protein complex in the contact sites between the inner and outer mitochondrial membranes *(16)*. In support of this notion, mitochondrial membrane contact sites reconstituted into liposomes exhibited behavior typical of the PTP *(17)*.

Adenine Nucleotide Translocator

The ANT exists in the inner mitochondrial membrane, and, as its name suggests, it is responsible for the antiport transfer of the adenine nucleotides, ADP and ATP, across the mitochondrial inner membrane. Its role in the PTP was first suggested when ligands of the ANT, bongkrekic acid and actractyloside, were shown to inhibit and activate, respectively, permeability transition and pore activity *(7,17)*. Following reconstitution into liposomes and lipid bilayers under the influence of Ca^{2+}, ANT was reversibly transformed into a nonselective pore *(18,19)*. Similarities were observed between ANT pore activity and the PTP, including pH and membrane potential modulation. ANT exists in two conformational states, the *m* state in which the nucleotide binding site is exposed to the matrix side of the inner membrane, and the *c* state whereby the active site is exposed to the cytoplasmic side. The observation that *c* mode ligands such as atractylate activated the PTP suggested that this mode was necessary for PTP opening *(17)*.

Voltage Dependent Anion Channel

CsA-sensitive channels identified in patch-clamped mitochondrial membranes exhibit some properties similar to those of mitochondrial porins *(20)*. When pore components were extracted from heart mitochondrial membranes solubilized with CHAPS detergent using a CYP-D affinity matrix, ANT was identified along with equal amounts of VDAC *(21)*. VDAC is located in the outer membrane and highest concentrations are to be found in the inner/ outer membrane contact sites. This evidence, in conjunction with the observation that VDAC binds to several proteins that are known to influence pore behavior, suggests the involvement of VDAC in the pore complex.

Cyclophilin D: Interactions with Cyclosporin A

Cyclophilin D (CYP-D) is the mitochondrial isoform of a group of proteins that possess peptidylprolyl-*cis-trans*-isomerase activity. It is a water-soluble protein that exists in a free state in the mitochondrial matrix. As with the ANT, the role of CYP-D became apparent by virtue of the activity of its ligand on PTP activity. CsA was found to block PTP activity at submicromolar concentrations *(11)*, and the amount required for inhibition was noted to be the same as that required for inhibition of the enzymic activity of CYP-D *(22)*. The similar sensitivities of the PTP and CYP-D to CsA analogs further implicated CYP-D as the CsA ligand in this setting *(23,24)*.

CsA is a cyclic entity with 11 amino acids with largely unmodified alkyl side chains. Its activity against cell-mediated immunity has given it widespread clinical use in transplantation medicine. This action is effected by the formation of a CsA–cyclophilin A–calcineurin complex. By contrast,

CsA binds to a hydrophobic pocket in the CYP-D molecule, and it is likely that occupancy of this active site is sufficient for its actions without the recruitment of other proteins *(23)*. The function of CYP-D is not known, although its enzymic activity would suggest a role in the folding of mitochondrially imported proteins. Immunoassays for CYP-D of mitochondrial membranes suggest that it is recruited into the membrane PTP complex, binding to ANT in the inner mitochondrial membrane, under conditions that induce pore opening *(25)*.

It is not certain how CsA blocks pore opening. The most accepted theory is that CsA binds to CYP-D, thus preventing it from binding to ANT in the PTP complex. In support of this theory, CsA blocked ANT binding to CYP-D affinity matrices *(26)*. However, other work has shown that CsA does not prevent CYP-D from binding to ANT–VDAC complexes *(21)*. This would imply an alternative model whereby CsA forms a stable complex with the PTP. Conceptually this could block pore activity by either stearically hindering solute movement or by inducing an inhibitory conformational change in the pore complex. These issues will need to be the focus of future work.

Other PTP Components

The VDAC–ANT complex is able to recruit a number of other proteins, including protein kinases *(27)*, the peripheral benzodiazepine receptor *(28)*, and members of the Bcl-2 protein family, which can regulate apoptosis. Hexokinase oligomers, in association with VDAC, ANT, and CYP-D, extracted from rat brain membranes, exhibit PTP behavior, and this is inhibited by hexokinase substrates, suggesting that the functional pore complex contained the kinase *(27)*. Similar preparations with creatine kinase showed pore behavior only when the octamers were dissociated. Hexokinase and creatine kinase associate with VDAC at the outer membrane and intermembrane space, respectively, lending further evidence for the presence of VDAC in the active pore complex *(29)*. These kinase–VDAC–ANT interactions are thought to provide a means of coupling ATP production by oxidative phosphorylation with its utilization by kinases.

Conformation of the Pore

Given the information discussed above, a schematic depiction of the PTP complex is shown in Fig. 1. The likely complex involves entities from the mitochondrial matrix (CYP-D), inner mitochondrial membrane (ANT), intermembrane space (creatine kinase), outer mitochondrial membrane (VDAC), and cytoplasm (hexokinase).

Which moiety actually confers channel properties on the complex is not known. The estimated radius of the open pore is 1–1.3 nm *(30)*, and its chan-

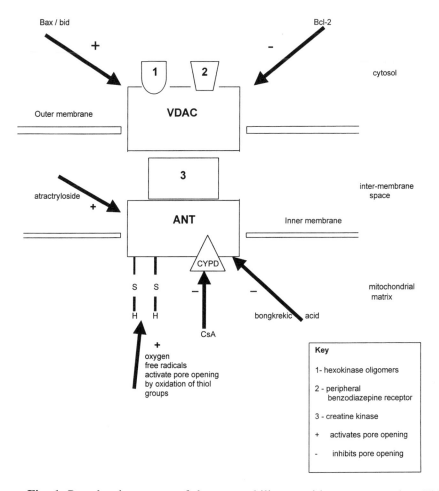

Fig. 1. Postulated structure of the permeability transition pore complex. This schematic depiction takes into account molecules spanning both mitochondrial membranes and the intermembrane space. The number of each molecule recruited into the pore complex, their precise relationship to each other, and the pore conferring moiety is not fully understood. The sites of action of a number of agents that regulate pore behavior are shown (*thick arrows*).

nel conductance is approx 1.2 nS *(13)*. Halestrap argued that the ANT represented the PTP, given its modulation by the ANT ligands, actractyloside and bongkrekic acid. This notion was supported by the behavior of reconstituted ANT into liposomes, which exhibited pore behavior under high [Ca^{2+}] with a conductance equivalent to 900 pS *(18)*. Fully open VDAC in planar lipid bilayers displayed a conductance of 600 pS *(31)*, leading to suggestions that the PTP may be a consequence of cooperation between two VDAC proteins

(32). Estimations of the size of open VDAC show it to be similar in size to PTP. Therefore, ANT, VDAC, or a combination of both may be the functional channel in the PTP.

CELL DEATH AND THE PERMEABILITY TRANSITION PORE

Neuronal death in neurodegenerative diseases was traditionally considered, until recently, to occur by necrosis. Tissue necrosis is the result of passive cell destruction invoked by noxious stimuli, including toxic agents, infective agents, and ischemia. Such agents induce a rapid cellular respiratory failure with acute ATP depletion, massive ionic shifts, cellular swelling, enzyme degradation of cellular constituents, and cell lysis.

"Apoptosis" was a term first used by Kerr and colleagues *(33)* to describe a specific morphological appearance, initially observed in shrunken dying cells in ischemic liver. Ultrastructural features were the condensation of nuclear chromatin into electron-dense masses, preservation of plasma and nuclear membranes, appearance of apoptotic bodies, and the lack of inflammatory changes. Apoptosis has become synonymous with the concept of programmed cell death, whereby cell death is enacted by intrinsic cellular programs and is thought to play an important role in tissue development and maturation. Apoptotic cell death, in contrast to necrosis, may take hours to days and may involve gene transcription and new protein expression.

PTP opening is thought to play a role in both necrotic and apoptotic cell death. The in vitro conditions that lead to PTP opening in isolated mitochondria, including mitochondrial calcium overload, depletion of ATP, increased oxidative stress, and mitochondrial membrane potential changes, are key features of cell injury and death in a variety of situations. Indirect evidence of PTP involvement is provided by protection by CsA such as is descibed in models of ischemia–reperfusion and excitotoxicity. However the possibility that CsA exerts its effects by means other than those on CYP-D cannot be discounted. The effects of these pseudopathological conditions on PTP function will be discussed in turn in the context of bioenergetic deficits known to play a role in PD.

Mitochondrial Ca^{2+} Overload

Ca^{2+} is the principal inducing stimulus in virtually all described models of PTP opening. Mitochondria act physiologically to buffer changes in cytosolic Ca^{2+} (reviewed in ref. *34*). Slow, maintained increases in cytosolic Ca^{2+} is a feature of a number of pathological states, including ischemia, excitotoxicity, and oxidative stress, and results in mitochondrial Ca^{2+} overload. Intramitochondrial Ca^{2+} activates the PTP by binding to low-affinity sites that are modulated by the presence of adenine nucleotides *(35)*.

Cellular ATP and PTP Opening

A key feature of necrotic cell death is the severe depletion of cellular ATP caused by inducing noxious stimuli. PTP opening induced by Ca^{2+} and phosphate or by Ca^{2+} and prooxidants is inhibited by the adenine nucleotides, ADP and ATP, in isolated mitochondria *(17,36,37)*. Experiments in intact heart mitochondria reveal that membranes become vulnerable to PTP opening when two-thirds of cellular ATP has dissipated *(38)*. Cellular ATP may play a role in determining cell fate following PTP opening.

Oxidative Stress and PTP

Oxidative stress has been implicated in the pathogenesis of a number of neurodegenerative diseases. The appreciation that the metabolism of dopamine can generate highly reactive free radicals led to the hypothesis that dopaminergic neurons may be selectively susceptible to such agents *(39,40)*. Dopamine is metabolized by monoamine oxidase, leading to the formation of hydrogen peroxide (H_2O_2). Reduced glutathione inactivates H_2O_2, thus preventing its reaction from reacting with iron to form the reactive hydroxyl free radical. In addition, autooxidation of dopamine generates an array of other free radicals.

An appreciation for the role of oxidative stress in PD was derived from three lines of evidence: the findings of increased levels of products of prooxidant-induced damage; complex I deficiency in mitochondria, and evidence of altered antioxidant defenses in PD. Products of oxidative damage, including protein carbonyls *(41)*, malondialdehydes *(42)*, and oxidation-induced DNA base changes *(43,44)* have all been shown to be increased in SNpC in PD brains, although levels of these were increased in other brain regions studied. Although the possibility exists that these changes were due to the effects of levodopa, they were not found in levodopa-treated monkeys. Increased SNpC iron levels can promote reactive oxidative species (ROS) generation via the Fenton reaction. However, it is not certain whether the increased iron content observed in PD substantia nigra *(45–47)* is present in a free and reactive form. Perry and colleagues *(48)* first described low levels of reduced glutathione (GSH) in PD SNpC. Subsequently, other groups confirmed these findings, reporting a decrease of GSH of approx 30–40%. This was not found in other brain regions and was present in preclinical Lewy body brains *(49–54)*. Reduced glutathione represents the major antioxidant defense against hydrogen peroxide-induced cell injury in the brain, and so this was considered to be a highly significant finding.

Oxidative stress is an important cause of PTP opening in mitochondrial membranes, in living cells, and in animal models of ischemia–reperfusion.

t-Butylhydroperoxide (*t*-BuOOH) can be used to induce conditions of oxidative stress in vitro and causes lethal injury to cells in culture. In isolated mitochondria peroxides can cause PTP opening in the presence of mitochondrial Ca^{2+} overload *(55)*. Additionally, PTP opening induced by Ca^{2+} and phosphate was partially blocked by catalase, suggesting that the action of inducing phospate may be exerted through the generation of hydrogen peroxide *(56)*.

Study of the PTP in living cells has utilized techniques involving cellular labeling with calcein esters, which become entrapped in the cytoplasm. The dye distribution may be observed with confocal microscopy, showing exclusion from mitochondria in healthy cells. On PTP opening, calcein was observed to redistribute into the mitochondrial space. Lemaster's group used this approach in conjunction with labeling with the fluorophore tetramethylrhodamine methylester (TMRME), whose accumulation varies as a function of inner membrane potential *(57,58)*. Induction of conditions of oxidative stress in hepatocytes with *t*-BuOOH showed CsA-sensitive calcein redistribution and collapse of the mitochondrial membrane, suggestive of PTP opening. These events preceded ATP depletion and cell death. *t*-BuOOH exerts its effects through the oxidation of GSH and mitochondrial pyridine nucleotides and the subsequent generation of ROS *(59)*. The in vitro conditions required for PTP opening would suggest similar requirements in vivo.

The question remains as to how ROS induce pore opening. It is emerging that this may be mediated via the oxidation of *vicinal* thiols in the PTP. In systems involving photogenerated ROS, PTP opening may be suppressed by thiol-reducing agents such as reduced glutathione *(60)*. Arsenite, which targets *vic*-thiols can coactivate PTP opening with Ca^{2+} *(61)*. Reduced mitochondrial glutathione may act to prevent such oxidation, maintaining the pore in the closed state. Halestrap's group postulated that the ANT contains the target *vic*-thiols, and this was reinforced by the ability of thiol oxidants to reduce the inhibitory effects of adenine nucleotides on pore opening *(36)*.

Thus, it is apparent that redox status is a key factor regulating PTP opening. Therefore, the PD subtantia nigra appears to exist in an environment that would favor pore opening. Although this may be insufficient in itself to cause PTP opening and commit neurons to cell death pathways, it may render them vulnerable in combination with other bioenergetic or pathogenic factors.

Mitochondrial Membrane Potential and the PTP

Pivotal to mitochondrial function, including the production of ATP, apoptosis, and PTP modulation, is the proton-motive force that exists across the inner mitochondrial membrane. Enzyme complexes I–IV mediate the transfer of electrons along a series of carrier molecules in a series of redox reactions in the electron transport chain (ETC), resulting in the reduction of oxygen to water and the conversion of ADP to ATP. Energy derived from electron transfer is used by complexes I, III, and IV to actively pump protons out of the mitochondrial matrix across the inner mitochondrial membrane. This results in the creation of a pH gradient and a potential difference across the inner mitochondrial membrane. The proton-motive force created drives the conversion of ADP to ATP by complex V, ATP synthase. The greater component of this force is the transmembrane potential and therefore approximates to the ATP/ADP ratio. Dysfunction in the ETC therefore has two consequences: 1) The incomplete electron transfer and reduction of oxygen gives rise to highly reactive oxygen free radicals, and 2) reduced proton extrusion results in reduction of the transmembrane potential and reduced ATP synthesis.

The mitochondrial respiratory chain was first implicated in the pathogenesis of PD after work into the effects of MPTP. MPTP caused a clinicopathological phenomenon similar but not identical to idiopathic PD *(62,63)*. MPP[+], the toxic metabolite of MPTP, was found to be an inhibitor of complex I of the ETC *(64)* and α-ketoglutarate dehydrogenase *(65)*, reducing ATP production and causing the generation of free radicals *(66)*. Subsequent analysis of complex I activity in postmortem PD substantia nigra pars compacta demonstrated a 30–40% deficiency in complex I activity *(67,68)*. This provided a direct parallel between the MPTP model and sporadic PD. The defect was not demonstrated in other brain regions or in multisystem atophy. Studies of complex I activities in peripheral tissues in PD patients have yielded conflicting results. Complex I, the largest complex of the ETC, comprises 41 subunits, 7 of which are encoded by mitochondrial DNA (mtDNA), the remainder by nuclear DNA. Cybrid fusions of A549 tumor cell lines with mitochondrial DNA from PD patients perpetuated the complex I deficiency, suggesting that its origin was encoded by mitochondrial rather than nuclear DNA *(69)*. However, no mitochondrial DNA mutations have thus far been identified in PD.

PTP opening is actively modulated by the inner mitochondrial membrane potential. Manipulation of the membrane potential using uncoupling agents demonstrated that PT opening increased with depolarization *(70,71)*. Dissipation of membrane potential appears to increase the propensity for PTP opening under suitable opening conditions, rather than directly inducing pore opening itself.

ANT in liposomes also showed a similar voltage sensitivity, suggesting a potential site for the voltage sensitivity of the PTP *(18)*. Therefore, it is apparent that a complex I deficiency, through the effects on mitochondrial transmembrane potential, could render nigral neurons vulnerable to PTP opening in the presence of suitable conditions, such as increased Ca^{2+} and oxidative stress. To this effect, Chavez and coworkers *(72)* showed that dysfunction of the ETC, induced by antimycin A, in the presence of Ca^{2+} induced CsA-sensitive mitochondrial permeability transition. Complex I deficiency can result in the increased production of ROS and ROS can cause further dysfunction of the electron-transport chain. Thus once such conditions are established their effects may be amplified.

Mitochondrial Control of Apoptosis

Until recently, mitochondria were not considered to play an important role in apoptosis. The original morphological descriptions were dominated by nuclear changes, while mitochondria did not appear to undergo significant change.

The importance of mitochondria in apoptosis was suggested from results in cell-free systems, where it was observed that nuclear chromatin condensation and DNA fragmentation could be induced by mitochondria or their products *(73)*. Mitochondria from healthy cells exerted such effects if they were treated with cytosolic extracts from dying cells or inducers of permeability transition *(74,75)*. PTP opening was further implicated, using cationic fluorophores, which provide an index of mitochondrial membrane polarization, when it was observed that dissipation of $\Psi\Delta_M$ was one of the earliest changes to occur in apoptotic cell death *(76)*. This occurred before the development of any of the morphological nuclear and DNA changes. Apoptosis-regulating members of the Bcl-2 protein family appeared to exert their effects at the mitochondrial level. Therefore, it became apparent that mitochondria play a central role in many of the pathways to apoptotic cell death.

The disruption of $\Psi\Delta_M$ is considered to be due to opening of the PT pore. As well as the conditions already described, a considerable array of cell death-inducing agents can cause $\Psi\Delta_M$ prior to apoptosis (reviewed in ref. 77). Therefore, PTP opening may represent a central integrative point that many different apoptotic pathways feed into, thus committing the cell to an apoptotic fate. In this respect, ANT and cyclophilin D ligands, which block PTP opening, inhibit $\Psi\Delta_M$ dissipation and subsequent signs of apotosis in several models of apoptosis, which adds weight to this hypothesis.

Mitochondrial Proapoptogenic Factors

Further evidence of mitochondrial involvement in apoptosis was derived from the fact that the water-soluble electron carrier cytochrome *c* translocates to the cytosol in models of apoptosis. Cytochrome c normally exists in the mitochondrial intermembrane space but can be detected in subcellular cytosolic fractions on induction of apoptosis *(78,79)*. Therefore, its translocation implies a perturbation in the barrier function of the outer mitochondrial membrane. Electron microscopy of apoptotic changes in Jurkat cells reveal breaks in the outer mitochondrial membrane *(80)*. In addition, various other proapoptogenic factors are known to reside in this compartment, including the apoptosis initiating factor (AIF), a 57-kDa flavoprotein *(81)*. PTP pore opening in mitochondria leads to matrix swelling and unfolding of the inner membrane. This can lead to outer membrane rupture, which would cause the release of these and other apoptogenic proteins from the intermembrane space. Whether this mechanism is responsible for the changes that occur in apoptosis is not known for certain. However, PTP opening by a range of inducing agents were shown to induce mitochondrial swelling, cytochrome c release, and apoptotic changes in cell-free systems *(75,82–85)*.

Both cytochrome c and AIF can induce apoptotic changes in nuclei in cell-free systems and following intracytoplasmic injection *(78,81,85,86)*. They are also both present in the cytosol in the early phases of apoptosis. The temporal link with PTP opening was questioned, however, on the basis of work showing that cytochrome c release may occur prior to any decrease in $\Psi\Delta_M$ *(87)*. In a model involving TNF-α-induced apoptosis in rat hepatocytes doubly labeled with calcein and TMRME, it was clear that PTP opening initially commenced in only a fraction of mitochondria within a single cell, resulting in a mixed mitochondrial population in terms of polarity. However, after 1–2 h virtually all mitochondria had depolarized. CsA blocked the onset of depolarization in this system, confirming that it was due to PTP opening *(88)*. Therefore a situation may arise whereby polarized mitochondria may be observed while cytochrome c is detected in the cytosol. This does not, however, necessarily mean that cytochrome c release and PTP opening are not temporally related at the level of the individual mitochondrion.

Apoptotic Effector Mechanisms: Activation of Caspases

Apoptotic pathways are executed by caspases, a family of cysteine proteases active at aspartic acid residues. Increasing numbers of caspases have been identified, but these will not be reviewed in this chapter. They exist in the cytosol as inactive procaspases, and are activated by cleavage either by other caspases or following aggregation into complexes with subsequent self-cleavage. Cytochrome c binds to Apaf-1 and procaspases, particularly procaspase 4, 8, and 9, are recruited into the resultant complex, and are subsequently activated *(89,90)*. Such caspases activate downstream effector caspases 3, 6, and 7 in a sequential cascade, which can then exert their effects on endonucleases and other effectors of apoptosis *(91,92)*. Similarly AIF activates caspase-9 and can cause a positive feedback loop by the activation of cytochrome *c (85)*.

Regulation of Apoptosis and PTP Opening: The Bcl-2 Family

The PTP may play a further important part in the regulation of apoptosis via functional interactions with proteins that can regulate the induction and progression of apoptosis. The Bcl-2 family of oncoproteins contains both inhibitors of apoptosis, including Bcl-2 and Bcl-X_L, and promoters of apoptosis, including BAX and BID.

Functionally and spatially there is good reason to suspect an interaction between Bcl-2 and the PTP. Bcl-2 exists in the outer mitochondrial membrane through insertion of its c-terminal domain *(93)*. Like the PTP, Bcl-2 localization is enriched in contact sites between the inner and outer mitochondrial membranes *(94)*. Functionally, Bcl-2 prevents signs of PTP opening in cells, and mitochondria and reconstituted PTP complexes in liposomes *(95)*. Furthermore, in cell-free systems Bcl-2 prevented the release of proapoptogenic factors from the intermembrane space, and nuclear apoptotic nuclear changes in response to PTP-inducing agents *(75,80,81,95–99)*. This evidence directly linked the antiapoptotic effects of Bcl-2 with its effects on PTP opening.

BID and BAX reside in the cytosol in resting cells. Both translocate to the mitochondria in response to apototic stimuli *(100–103)*. They act to induce the release of cytochrome *c* and proapoptogenic factors from the intermembrane space. Exposure to apoptotic stimuli causes a strong interaction between BID and BAX, which induces a conformational change in the latter, enabling it to insert into the mitochondrial membrane *(104,105)*. There is evidence that BAX binds to the PTP pore complex, in that BAX coimmunoprecipitates with VDAC and binds to purified VDAC in proteoliposomes *(106,107)*. Mitoplasts, stripped of the outer membrane other than at contact sites, bound Bcl-2 and BAX *(108)*. Confocal microscopy using fluorescently labeled Bcl-2 and BAX, suggested a tight interaction between the two *(109)*. Therefore the relative amounts of Bcl-2, BAX, and BID in the outer mitochondrial membrane may regulate the apoptogenic potential of mitochondria and possibly PTP opening. The fact that immunodepletion of BAX from PTP complexes rendered them unresponsive to the pore activator, atractryloside, suggests a functional effect of BAX on PTP function *(108)*. However, the exact mechanism by which BAX may induce the release of proapoptogenic factors and whether this is via PTP activation and outer membrane rupture is not known; BAX can exhibit pore properties in lipid bilayers *(110)*, although there is no other evidence to suggest a role for a protein channel in cytochrome *c* release.

Mode of Cell Death: Necrosis Versus Apoptosis

It is clear that the same stimuli can induce both necrosis and apoptosis. Thus in models of ischemia in the heart and brain, the central ischemic area undergoes necrotic cell death, whereas cells in the penumbra may undergo slower apoptotic death as well as necrosis *(111,112)*. Many insults, including Ca^{2+} overload, excitotoxins, and drugs, induce necrosis at high levels and apoptosis at lower levels of exposure. Therefore apoptosis generally appears to be a consequence of exposure to weaker pathological apoptosis.

Cellular ATP is a crucial determinant of the mode of cell death following PTP opening. Necrosis is associated with an early depletion of cellular ATP, whereas this is maintained, and is actually required, in the early stages in apoptosis. A strong inducing stimulus may therefore engage massive PTP opening, with an abrupt bioenergetic collapse and catastrophic consequences for the cell leading to necrosis. Therefore, in this setting the relative dependence of a cell on glycolytic versus respiratory ATP production would be expected to affect a cell's tendency to undergo necrotic change. "Milder" insults could induce a more protracted or lower level of PTP opening within the mitochondrial population, resulting in ATP being initially maintained by the remaining polarized mitochondria, thus allowing the activation of proteases. Therefore the availability of caspases and their state of activation would be expected to affect the propensity of a cell to undergo apoptosis in response to a given stimulus.

MECHANISMS OF CELL DEATH IN PD: ROLE OF PTP

Apoptosis in PD

The appreciation that neurons undergo programmed cell death in the development and maturation of the prenatal and postnatal central nervous system raised the question as to whether the same mechanisms could operate under pathological conditions. Neuronal apoptosis can be induced by a wide range of inducing stimuli, many of which are relevant to PD, including glutamate *(113)*, MPTP and its metabolites *(114,115)*, 6-hydroxydopamine (6-OHDA) *(116)*, complex I inhibitors *(117)*, prooxidants *(118)*, high levels of dopamine *(119)*, and levodopa *(120)*. Furthermore, dopaminergic neurons of the SNpC are able to undergo apoptosis. Changes in the expression of proteins that regulate apoptosis have been noted in SNpC. Bcl-2 is increased in surviving neurons of the SNpC in PD, which suggests a possible compensatory survival strategy *(121)*, whereas proapoptotic BAX expression is increased in neurons after MPTP treatment *(122)*, before they have entered changes suggestive of apoptosis. Activated caspase 3 is found to be increased in PD SNpC *(123)*, suggesting an involvement for this protease in downstream pathways leading to neuronal apoptosis.

Apoptosis has been described in a variety of neurodegenerative diseases, including PD, Alzheimer's disease, amyotrophic lateral sclerosis and Huntington's disease *(124)*. Cell culture and animal models, in conjunction with postmortem brain analysis have attempted to define the role of apoptosis in PD. Many groups have demonstrated that MPP^+ can induce apoptosis in vitro in cultured neurons *(115)* and neuronal cell lines *(117,125)*. Furthermore, in a mouse model involving chronic MPTP administration for 5 d, apoptosis was observed in dopaminergic neurons *(114)*. Similarly, rats lesioned with the prooxidant 6-OHDA exhibited apoptotic changes in nigral dopaminergic neurons *(126)*.

Analysis of postmortem brain has yielded conflicting results. This has been due in part to the fact that methods used to detect apoptotic changes in tissue sections have been problematic. *In situ* end labeling (ISEL) techniques have been used widely for this purpose, whereby the 3' ends of cleaved DNA are labeled with a chromagen or fluorophore. One report used this method to detect positive staining in four of seven patients with typical idiopathic PD *(127)*. However, it has become apparent that ISEL can yield false-positive results in necrotic cell death. Therefore it is considered essential to combine this technique with one that demonstrates characteristic morphological appearances, in order to unequivocally detect apoptosis. One group demonstrated apoptotic changes in PD and diffuse Lewy body disease brains *(128)*. Another study failed to show apoptotic changes in PD brain despite positive ISEL detection *(129)*. However, one group ,using a double labeling fluorescence technique with ISEL and the cyanine DNA binding dye, YOYO1, detected apoptosis in 1–2% of dopaminergic neurons of the SNpC *(130)*. The fact that results in this area have been conflicting may be a reflection of the fact that apoptotic cells are rapidly phagocytosed; in a chronic disease the appearance of a few apoptotic cells may in fact belie a much more significant pathological involvement of this form of cell death.

Mitochondrial PTP in the Central Nervous System

Much of the work that defined the PTP, its constituents, and behavior was elucidated following work in liver and heart. An obvious and fundamental issue in a hypothesis invoking PTP opening in a neurodegenerative disease is the ability of neurons to undergo permeability transition.

The effects of calcium-rich medium in the presence of a calcium ionophore were studied in the mitochondria of astrocytes and cultured hippocampal neurons. In astrocytes, *in situ* visualization with the mitochondrial dye 5,5',6,6'-tetrachloro-1,1'3,3'-tetraethylbenzimidazolocarbocyanine (JC-1) revealed changes of mitochondrial swelling *(131)*. These changes were reversible with Ca^{2+} chelation and were inhibited by various agents, including CsA and other pore inhibitors. Morphological changes were also observed in cultured hippocampal neurons and were preceded by membrane depolarization *(132)*. Such changes were explained by Ca^{2+}-induced PTP opening, although in astrocytes the potency of CsA inhibition of Ca^{2+}-induced mitochondrial changes was relatively low *(131)*. Ca^{2+} mitochondrial swelling in rat brain was inhibited by adenine nucleotides, low matrix pH, and CsA, and promoted by thiol reagents, indicating that PTP activity was present and qualitatively similar to that observed in heart and liver *(133)*.

A role for PTP opening can be inferred in vivo by CsA protection in animal disease models. CsA exerts protective effects in models of cerebral ischemia in hypoglycemic and hyperglycemic rats *(134,135)*, intrastriatal NMDA injections *(136)*, ischemia–reperfusion *(137)*, and traumatic brain injury *(138)*. Single excitotoxic insults to cultured neurons are partially protected by CsA *(139)*. Excitotoxicity is of particular relevance to PD, and CsA exerts protective effects in some animal PD models.

Excitoxicity Models and PD

Excitotoxicity remains one of the principal models of mitochondrially mediated neuronal death. It is implicated in a variety of neurological conditions including neurodegenerative diseases and cerebral ischemia. The term refers to the persistent overstimulation of *N*-methyl-D-aspartate (NMDA) glutamate receptors leading to massive cellular calcium influx and ensuing neuronal death.

The description of bioenergetic defects in PD, principally complex I deficiency, provided a model for the role of excitotoxicity. As already discussed, dysfunction of the ETC leads to impairment of the mitochondrial inner transmembrane potential and disruption of ATP synthesis. The normal resting cell membrane potential, which is usually approx $-90\,mV$, relies on ATP for its maintenance. The NMDA receptor exhibits a voltage-dependent Mg^{2+} block at resting cell membrane potential. Therefore reduction in cellular ATP and depolarisation of the cell membrane potential beyond a voltage threshold will relieve this block, leading to persistent NMDA receptor stimulation. The effects of membrane potential modulation were demonstrated using inhibitors of glycolysis, oxidative phosphorylation, or sodium–potassium ATPase, which rendered neurons vulnerable to glutamate at previously nontoxic concentrations *(140–142)*.

NMDA overstimulation leads to Ca^{2+} influx, and this event correlates closely with consequent neuronal death. Glutamate-induced Ca^{2+} overload is then buffered by mitochondria. The implication of mitochondrial involvement was strengthened following the observation that excitoxicity is initiated in areas with high mitochondrial density *(143)*, resulting in mitochondrial calcium influx in these areas and collapse of the mitochondrial transmembrane potential *(144–147)*. Additionally, calcium overload is associated with increased production of highly reactive free radicals, either directly or through the activation of nitric oxide synthase (NOS) *(148)*. Nitric oxide reacts with superoxide to form peroxynitrite, which leads to oxidative damage of cellular constituents *(149)*. Peroxynitrite has been reported to induce pore opening in liver mitochondria *(150,151)*, although nitric oxide has been reported to exert both stimulatory and inhibitory effects on PTP opening, cytochrome c release, and apoptosis, which is cell type- and concentration-specific *(152)*. It is, however, not certain how such peroxynitrite-mediated PTP opening occurs, although oxidation of thiol groups in the pore complex may play a role, as previously discussed. Therefore, the conditions produced by NMDA receptor overstimulation provide the ideal cellular environment for PTP opening, and this would appear to be corroborated by the changes observed in inner membrane potential in the several models. In these models, CsA enabled membrane potential recovery and prevented subsequent cell death. Furthermore, more recently Budd and associates *(153)* showed that NMDA receptor-mediated apoptosis in cultured cerebrocortical neurons was preceded by depolarization of $\Psi\Delta_M$ and cytochrome c release, which was prevented by bongkrekic acid and inhibition of caspase-3 activation.

Evidence for a role of excitoxic cell death in PD has largely been provided by MPTP models in animals. Substantia nigral neurons possess NMDA receptors *(154)*. Despite the lack of protection against MPP+ afforded to dopaminergic neurons in vitro by NMDA antagonists *(155)*, such agents protected against MPP+ or MPTP striatal dopamine depletion in rats, mice, and primates *(156–160)*. Furthermore, administration of MPTP significantly upregulated the expression of inducible NOS *(161)*, while inhibition of NOS protected against MPTP neurotoxicity in mice and baboons *(162,163)*. MPP+-induced neuronal degeneration and striatal 3-nitrotyrosine concentrations (a marker of peroxynitrite-mediated damage) are reduced in mutant mice lacking neuronal NOS *(164,165)*. Therefore, given the bioenergetic anomalies and oxidative stress described in PD, conceptually there is good reason to suspect excitoxicity as a pathogenic mechanism in PD.

Cyclosporin A and PD Models

The properties of CsA in binding to CYP-D causing inhibition of PTP opening make it an attractive candidate for neuroprotective strategies in our hypothesis. CsA sensitivity in vivo and in vitro models is often used to infer the involvement of PTP opening. Some of the wide array of situations whereby CsA prevents PTP opening or pathological changes to both endogenous and exogenous agents have already been referred to.

Evidence of PTP involvement has been demonstrated in cell models relevant to PD. Studies of the effects of the neuorotoxin MPP+ on liver and brain mitochondria, in the presence of Ca^{2+} and phosphate, observed permeability transition, mitochondrial swelling, and cytochrome *c* release *(166)*. These phenomena were inhibited by CsA and free radical scavengers, and synergized with nitric oxide, atractyloside, and thiol oxidizing agents. Dopamine metabolites, quinone, and reactive oxygen species can also induce CsA-sensitive swelling of brain and liver mitochondria *(167)*. Seaton and coworkers *(168)* demonstrated the antiapoptotic protective action of CsA on PC12 cells treated with MPP+ and other complex I inhibitors. *N*-Methyl-4-valine cyclosporin is an analog of CsA that inhibits PTP opening but lacks its immunosuppressant properties. The observation, however, that *N*-methyl-4-valine cyclosporin afforded similar protection against the complex I inhibitors rotenone and tetrahydroisoquinolone but not MPP+ may suggest that additional factors may be involved other than opening of the PTP. However, Zamzami and associates *(169)* demonstrated that, although both CsA and *N*-methyl-4-valine cyclosporin prevented dexamethasone-induced loss of $\Psi\Delta_M$ in lymphocytes, the former was approx 30% more effective in preventing PTP opening.

The use of CsA in animal PD models has yielded encouraging results. In mice with 6-OHDA induced nigrostriatal neuronal injury, Matsuura's group *(170,171)* showed that CsA, given either at repeated high dose or as a single administration protected against striatal depletion of dopamine and its metabolites. Similarly, in 6-OHDA-treated rats, CsA similarly protected against striatal dopamine depletion, attenuated the decrease of tyrosine hydroxylase staining cells in the SNpC *(172)*, and improved motor performance *(173)*, suggesting a functional correlate of the neuroprotective effects.

Other Effects of CsA and Immunophilin Ligands

This chapter has focused on the neuroprotective effects of CsA via its modulation of mitochondrial permeability transition, by binding to cyclophilin D. Its actions extend beyond this, however, and may be responsible for its effects in neurological disease. The first identified CsA-binding protein, named cyclophilin (later named cyclophilin A), was shown to be an enzyme, PPIase, that catalyzes the interconversion of *cis* and *trans* rotamers of amide bonds adjacent to proline residues *(174)*. Similarly, another PPIase, structurally unrelated to cyclophilin, that bound the immunosuppressant

FK506, was described and named FKBP (later FKBP12) *(175)*. A large number of PPIases, termed immunophilins, have subsequently been described and belong to three highly conserved families of proteins, the cyclophilins, the FKBPs and noncyclophilin, non-FKBP immunophilins. The biological and immunosuppresant effects of CsA and FK506 are not mediated via their inhibition of PPIase activity but through the interaction of the drug–immunophilin complex with target proteins, such as the calmodulin-dependent phosphatase, calcineurin, in the case of CsA–cyclophilin A and FK506–FKBP12 and modulation of Ca^{2+} signaling pathways *(176)*.

Interest in immunophilins in the central nervous system developed when it was shown that FKBP12 expression was 40 times greater in the brain than in the immune system *(177)*. Subsequent studies revealed a high level of neuronal expression of cyclophilin A and FKBP12 in the brain, particularly in cerebellar granule cells, hippocampus, and nigrostriatal dopaminergic pathways *(178)*. Snyder identified proteins from brain homogenates whose phosphorylation levels were affected by treatment with CsA and FK506. Among the identified proteins were nitric oxide synthase (NOS) *(179)* and GAP43 *(177)*. NOS plays an important role in excitotxicity models of PD. Phosphorylated NOS is inactive and therefore the phosphatase, calcineurin, may regulate its activity *(180)*. Thus calcineurin inhibition by FK506–FKBP12 or CsA–cyclophilin A may keep NOS in its inactive phosphorylated state. To this effect, CsA and FK506 were potent inhibitors of NMDA excitoxicity in cortical cultures *(181)*.

GAP43 has been linked to neuronal growth and neurite extension *(182)*. This generated interest in the use of immunophilin ligands as neurotrophic factors. FK506 and CsA potentiated neurite extension in nerve growth factor–treated PC12 pheochromocytoma cell lines *(183)* and primary dopaminergic cultured neurons *(184)*. The high levels of FKBP ligands in the nigrostriatal pathway stimulated interest in FKBP ligands in mouse and rat PD models *(185)*. When they were administered concurrently in mice with MPTP, a marked neuroprotective effect on tyrosine hydroxylase dopaminergic neurons was observed. FKBP ligands given days after destruction of the nigrostriatal pathway by MPTP, showed an increase in TH+ neurons, regeneration of striatal dopamine and its metabolites, and a behavioral recovery. Similar effects were seen in 6-OHDA-lesioned rats, indicating a regenerative role of FKBP ligands in these models.

CONCLUDING REMARKS

A model has been described where the central critical event in neuronal death in PD is PTP opening. A schematic depiction of the hypothesis is

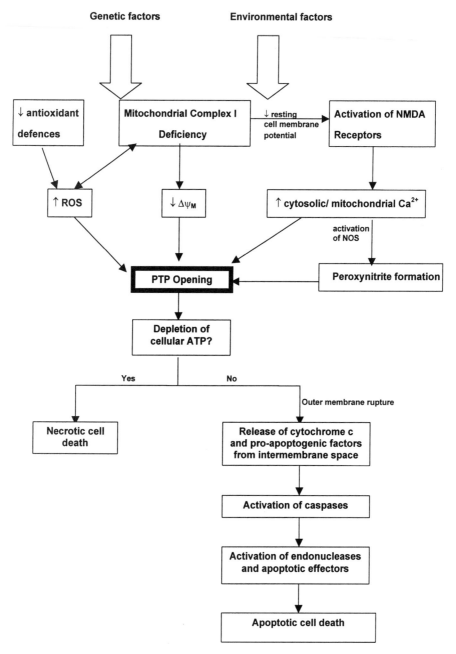

Fig. 2. Pathogenesis of PD and the PTP hypothesis.

shown in Fig. 2. Bioenergetic defects, for example, ETC dysfunction, oxidative stress, excitotoxicity, and calcium overload all feed synergistically into the system. The strength of the insult and the metabolic consequences may then determine the mode of cell death that the cell undergoes. The description of mutations in the gene encoding α-synuclein, a major constituent of Lewy bodies in sporadic PD, ubiquitin carboxyl-terminal hydrolase L1, and parkin, which acts as a ubiquitin protein ligase, implicates dysfunction of the proteosomal system of protein degradation in the pathogenesis of PD, causing toxic protein accumulation within cells. How this relates to the described bioenergetic phenomena is not certain.

Much, however, needs to be explained. Most of the models described involve neuronal degeneration over hours to weeks. How this relates to the chronic progressive neuronal degeneration over years in idiopathic PD is not known. One possibility is that the bioenergetic abnormalities described in PD may keep neurons in a dormant but vulnerable preapoptotic state, entering into full-blown apoptosis when suitable additional conditions develop. In addition, some in vitro models suggest that the effects of CsA are modest and at high doses CsA has even been reported to induce apoptosis. Other neuroprotective and regenerative actions of CsA and related proteins may be important, via their interactions with their cognate immunophilins.

Much hope remains, however, that uncovering the pathways that lead to neuronal death in PD will provide targets for future neuroprotective strategies. If PD has multiple etiologies and PTP opening signals the start of a common pathway leading to cell death, the PTP and the consequent downstream pathways represent conceptually attractive targets for future work.

REFERENCES

1. Polymeropoulos MH, Lavedan C, Leroy E, et al. Mutation in the α-synuclein gene identified in families with Parkinson's disease. Science 1997;276: 2045–2047.
2. Leroy E, Boyer R, Auburger G, et al. The ubiquitin pathway in Parkinson's disease. Nature 1998;395:415–452.
3. Kitada T, Asakawa S, Hattori N, et al. Mutations in the parkin gene cause autosomal recessive juvenile parkinsonism. Nature 1998;392:605–608.
4. Payami H, Larsen K, Bernard S, Nutt J. Increased risk of Parkinson's disease in parents and siblings of patients. Ann Neurol 1994;36:659–661.
5. Marder K, Tang MX, Mejia H, et al. Risk of Parkinson's disease among first degree relatives: a community based study. Neurology 1996;47:155–160.
6. Hunter DR, Haworth RA, Southard JH. Relationship between configuration, function and permeability in calcium treated mitochondria. J Biol Chem 1976;251:5069–5077.

7. Hunter DR, Haworth RA. The Ca^{2+}-induced membrane transition in mito-chondria. I. The protective mechanisms. Arch Biochem Biophys 1979; 195:453–459.

8. Hunter DR, Haworth RA. The Ca^{2+}-induced membrane transition in mito-chondria. II. Nature of the Ca^{2+} trigger site. Arch Biochem Biophys 1979;195:460–467.

9. Hunter DR, Haworth RA. The Ca^{2+}-induced membrane transition in mito-chondria. III. Transitional Ca^{2+} release. Arch Biochem Biophys 1979; 195:468–477.

10. Fournier N, Ducet G, Crevat A. Action of cyclosporine on mitochondrial cal-cium fluxes. J Bioenerg Biomembr 1987;19:297–303.

11. Crompton M, Ellinger H, Costi A. Inhibition by cyclosporin A of a Ca^{2+} dependent pore in heart mitochondria activated by inorganic phosphate and oxidative stress. Biochem J 1988;255:357–360.

12. Szabo I, Zoratti M. The giant channel of the inner mitochondrial membrane is inhibited by cyclosporin A. J Biol Chem 1991;266:3376–3379.

13. Petronilli V, Szabo I, Zoratti M. The inner mitochondrial membrane contains ion-conducting channels similar to those found in bacteria. FEBS Lett 1989;259:137–143.

14. Kinally KW, Campo ML, Tedeschi H. Mitochondrial channel activity studied by patch-clamping mitoplasts. J Bioenerg Biomembr 1989;21:497–506.

15. Brdiczka D, Beutner G, Ruck A, et al. The molecular structure of mitochon-drial contact sites. Their role in regulation of energy metabolism and perme-ability transition. Biofactors 1998;8:235–242.

16. Moran O, Sandri G, Panfili E, et al. Electrophysiological characterization of contact sites in brain mitochondria. J Biol Chem 1990;265:908–913.

17. Le Quoc K, Le Quoc D. Involvement of the ADP/ ATP carrier in calcium induced perturbations of the mitochondrial inner membrane permeability: importance of the orientation of the nucleotide binding site. Arch Biochem Biophys 1988;265:249–257.

18. Brustovetsky N, Klingenberg M. Mitochondrial ADP/ATP carrier can be reversibly converted into a large channel by Ca^{2+}. Biochemistry 1996;35: 8483–8488.

19. Ruck A, Dolder M, Wallimann T, Brdiczka D. Reconstituted adenine nucle-otide translocase forms a channel for small molecules comparable to the mito-chondrial permeability transition pore. FEBS Letts 1998;426:97–101.

20. Kinally KW, Campo ML, Tedeschi H. Mitochondrial channel activity studied by patch-clamping mitoplasts. J Bioenerg Biomembr 1989;21:497–506.

21. Crompton M, Virji S, Ward JM. Cyclophilin-D binds strongly to complexes of the voltage-dependent anion channel and the adenine nucleotide trans-locase to form the permeability transition pore. Eur. J. Biochem. 1998; 258:729–735.

22. Halestrap AP, Davidson AM. Inhibition of Ca2(+)-induced large-amplitude swelling of liver and heart mitochondria by cyclosporin is probably caused by the inhibitor binding to mitochondrial-matrix peptidyl-prolyl cis-trans

isomerase and preventing it interacting with the adenine nucleotide translocase. Biochem J 1990;268:153–160.

23. Nicolli A, Basso E, Petronilli V, et al. Interactions of cyclophilin with the mitochondrial inner membrane and regulation of the permeability transition pore, and cyclosporin A-sensitive channel. J Biol Chem 1996;271:2185–2192.

24. Griffiths EJ, Halestrap AP. Further evidence that cyclosporin A protects mitochondria from calcium overload by inhibiting a matrix peptidyl-prolyl cis-trans isomerase. Implications for the immunosuppressive and toxic effects of cyclosporin. Biochem J 1991;274:611–614.

25. Halestrap AP, Woodfield KY, Connern CP. Oxidative stress, thiol reagents, and membrane potential modulate the mitochondrial permeability transition by affecting nucleotide binding to the adenine nucleotide translocase. J Biol Chem 1997;272:3346–3354.

26. Woodfield K, Ruck A, Brdiczka D, Halestrap AP. Direct demonstration of a specific interaction between cyclophilin-D and the adenine nucleotide translocase confirms their role in the mitochondrial permeability transition. Biochem J 1998;336:287–290.

27. Buetner G, Ruck A, Riede B, Brdiczka D. Complexes between porin, hexokinase, mitochondrial creatine kinase and adenylate translocator display proerties of the permeability trnasition pore. Implication for the regulation of permeability transition by the kinases. Biochim Biophys Acta 1998;1368:7–18.

28. Kinnally KW, Zorov DB, Antonenko YN, et al. Mitochondrial benzodiazepine receptor linked to inner membrane ion channels by nanomolar actions of ligands. Proc Natl Acad Sci USA 1993;90:1374–1378.

29. Moynagh PN. Contact sites and transport in mitochondria. Essays Biochem 1995;30:1–14.

30. Crompton M, Costi A. A heart mitochondrial Ca2(+)-dependent pore of possible relevance to re-perfusion-induced injury. Evidence that ADP facilitates pore interconversion between the closed and open states. Biochem J 1990;266:33–39.

31. Rostovtseva T, Colombini M. VDAC channels mediate and gate the flow of ATP: implications for the regulation of mitochondrial function. Biophys J 1997;72:1954–1962.

32. Szabo I, De Pinto V, Zoratti M. The mitochondrial permeability transition pore may comprise VDAC molecules. II. The electrophysiological properties of VDAC are compatible with those of the mitochondrial megachannel. FEBS Lett 1993;330:206–210.

33. Kerr JFR, Wyllie AH, Currie AR. Apoptosis: a baisc biological phenomenon with wide ranging implications in tissue kinetics. Br J Cancer 1972;26:239–257.

34. Crompton M. The mitochondrial permeability transition pore and its role in cell death. Biochem J 1999;341:233–249.

35. Al-Nasser I, Crompton M. The reversible Ca^{2+}-induced permeabilization of rat liver mitochondria. Biochem J 1986;239:19–29.

36. Halestrap AP, Woodfield KY, Connern CP. Oxidative stress, thiol reagents, and membrane potential modulate the mitochondrial permeability transition

by affecting nucleotide binding to the adenine nucleotide translocase. J Biol Chem 1997;272:3346–3354.

37. Crompton M, Costi A. Kinetic evidence for a heart mitochondrial pore activated by Ca^{2+}, inorganic phosphate and oxidative stress. A potential mechanism for mitochondrial dysfunction during cellular Ca^{2+} overload. Eur J Biochem 1998;178:489–501.

38. Duchen MR, McGuinness O, Brown LA, Crompton M. On the involvement of a cyclosporin A sensitive mitochondrial pore in myocardial reperfusion injury. Cardiovasc Res 1993;27:1790–1794.

39. Halliwell B, Gutteridge J. Oxygen radicals and the nervous system. Trends Neurosci 1985;8:22–29.

40. Olanow CW. Oxidation reactions in Parkinson's disease. Neurology 1990;40:32–37.

41. Alam ZI, Daniel SE, Lees AJ, et al. A generalised increase in protein carbonyls in the brain in Parkinson's but not incidental Lewy body disease. J Neurochem 1997;69:1326–1329.

42. Dexter DT, Carter CJ, Wells FR, et al. Basal lipid peroxidation in substantia nigra is increased in Parkinson's disease. J Neurochem 1989;52:381–389.

43. Sanchez-Ramos J, Overik E, Ames BN. A marker of oxyradical-mediated DNA damage (8-hydroxy-2' deoxyguanosine is increased in nigro-striatum of Parkinson's disease. Neurodegeneration 1994;3:197–204.

44. Alam ZI, Jenner A, Daniel SE, et al. Oxidative DNA damage in the parkinsonian brain: an apparent selective increase in 8-hydroxyguanine levels in substantia nigra. J Neurochem 1997;69:1195–1203.

45. Olanow CW. Magnetic resonance imaging in parkinsonism. Neurol Clin 1992;10:405–420.

46. Dexter DT, Wells FR, Lees AJ, et al. Increased nigral iron content and alterations in other metal ions occurring in brain in Parkinson's disease. J Neurochem 1989;52:1830–1836.

47. Sofic E, Paulus W, Jellinger K, et al. Selective increase of iron in substantia nigra zona compacta of parkinsonian brains. J Neurochem 1991;56:978–982.

48. Perry TL, Godin DV, Hansen S. Parkinson's disease: a disorder due to nigral glutathione deficiency. Neurosci Letts 1982;33:305–310.

49. Perry TL, Yong VW. Idiopathic Parkinson's disease, progressive supranuclear palsy and glutathione metabolism in the substantia nigra of patients. Neurosci Lett 1986;67:269–274.

50. Perry TL, Hansen S, Jones K. Brain amino acids and glutathione in progressive supranuclear palsy. Neurology 1988;38:943–946.

51. Riederer P, Sofic E, Rausch W-D. Transition metals, ferritin, glutathione, and ascorbic acid in parkinsonian brains. J Neurochem 1989;52:515–520.

52. Sian J, Dexter DT, Lees AJ, et al. Alterations in glutathione levels in Parkinson's disease and other neurodegenerative disorders affecting basal ganglia. Ann Neurol 1994;36:348–355.

53. Sofic E, Lange KW, Jellinger K, Riederer P. Reduced and oxidised glutathione in the substantia nigra of patients with parkinson's disease. Neurosci Letts 1992;142:128–130.

54. Dexter DT, Sian J, Rose J, et al. Indices of oxidative stress and mitochondrial function in individuals with incidental Lewy body disease. Ann Neurol 1994;35:38–44.

55. Crompton M, Costi A, Hayat L. Evidence for the presence of a reversible Ca^{2+}-dependent pore activated by oxidative stress in heart mitochondria. Biochem J 1987;245:915–918.

56. Kowaltowski AJ, Castilho RF, Vercesi AE. Opening of the mitochondrial permeability transition pore by uncoupling or inorganic phosphate in the presence of Ca^{2+} is dependent on mitochondrial-generated reactive oxygen species. FEBS Lett 1996;378:150–152.

57. Nieminen AL, Saylor AK, Tesfai SA, et al. Contribution of the mitochondrial permeability transition to lethal injury after exposure of hepatocytes to t-butylhydroperoxide. Biochem J 1995;307:99–106.

58. Imberti R, Nieminen AL, Herman B, Lemasters JJ. Mitochondrial and glycolytic dysfunction in lethal injury to hepatocytes by t-butylhydroperoxide: protection by fructose, cyclosporin A and trifluoperazine. J Pharmacol Exp Ther 1993;265:392–340.

59. Nieminen AL, Byrne AM, Herman B, Lemasters JJ. Mitochondrial permeability transition in hepatocytes induced by t-BuOOH: NAD(P)H and reactive oxygen species. Am J Physiol 1997;272:1286–1294.

60. Huser J, Rechenmacher CE, Blatter LA. Imaging the permeability pore transition in single mitochondria. Biophys J 1998;74:2129–2137.

61. Chernyak BV, Bernardi P. The mitochondrial permeability transition pore is modulated by oxidative agents through both pyridine nucleotides and glutathione at two separate sites. Eur J Biochem 1996;238:623–630.

62. Langston JW, Ballard P, Tetrud JW, Irwin I. Chronic parkinsonism in humans due to a product of meperidine-analogue synthesis. Science 1983;219:979–980.

63. Langston JW, Forno LS, Robert CS, Irwin I. MPTP causes selective damage to the zona compacta of the substantia nigra in the squirrel monkey. Brain Res 1984;292:390–394.

64. Nicklas WJ, Vyas I, Heikkila RE. Inhibition of NADH-linked oxidation in brain mitochondria by 1-methyl-4-phenylpyridine, a metabolite of the neurotoxin 1-methyl-4-phenyl-1,2,5,6 tetrahydropyridine. Life Sci 1985;36:2503–2508.

65. Mizuno Y, Saitoh T, Sone N. (1987) Inhibition of mitochondrial alpha-ketoglutarate dehydrogenase by 1-methyl-4-phenyl-pyridinium ion. Biochem Biophys Res Commun 1987;143:971–976.

66. Rosetti ZL, Sotgui A, Sharp DE, et al. 1-methyl-4-phenyl-1,2,3,6-tetrahydropyridine (MPTP) and free radicals in vitro. Biochem Pharmacol 1988; 37:4573–4574.

67. Schapira AHV, Cooper JM, Dexter D, et al. Mitochondrial complex I deficiency in Parkinson's disease. J Neurochem 1990;54:823–827.

68. Mizuno Y, Ohta S, Tanaka M, et al. Deficiencies in complex I subunits of the respiratory chain in Parkinson's disease. Biochem Biophys Res Commun 1989;163:1450–1455.

69. Schapira AHV, Gu M, Taanman JW, et al. Mitochondria in the aetiology and pathogenesis of Parkinson's disease. Ann Neurol 1998;44:S89–S98.

70. Petronilli V, Cola C, Bernardi P. Modulation of the mitochondrial cyclosporin A-sensitive permeability transition pore. II. The minimal requirements for pore induction underscore a key role for transmembrane electrical potential, matrix pH, and matrix Ca^{2+}. J Biol Chem 1993;268:1011–1016.
71. Petronilli V, Cola C, Massari S, et al. Physiological effectors modify voltage sensing by the cyclosporin A-sensitive permeability transition pore of mitochondria. J Biol Chem 1993;268:21,939–21,945.
72. Chavez E, Melendez E, Zazueta C, et al. Membrane permeability transition as induced by dysfunction of the electron transport chain. Biochem Mol Biol Int 1997;41:961–968.
73. Newmeyer DD, Farschon DM, Reed JC. Cell-free apoptosis in Xenopus egg extracts: inhibition by Bcl-2 and requirement for an organelle fraction enriched in mitochondria. Cell 1994;79:353–364.
74. Martin SJ, Newmeyer DD, Mathias S, et al. Green DR Cell-free reconstitution of Fas-, UV radiation-and ceramide-induced apoptosis EMBO J 1995;14:5191–5200.
75. Zamzami N, Susin SA, Marchetti P, et al. Mitochondrial control of nuclear apoptosis. J Exp Med 1996;183:1533–1544.
76. Wadia JS, Chalmers-Redman RME, Ju WJH, et al. Mitochondrial membrane potential and nuclear changes in apoptosis caused by serum and nerve growth factor withdrawal: time course and modification by (-)-deprenyl. J Neurosci 1998;18:932–947.
77. Susin SA, Zamzami N, Kroemer G. Mitochondria as regulators of apoptosis: doubt no more. Biochim Biophys Acta 1998;1366:151–165.
78. Liu X, Kim CN, Yang J, et al. Induction of apoptotic program in cell-free extracts: requirement for dATP and cytochrome *c*. Cell 1996;86:147–157.
79. Yang J, Liu X, Bhalla K, et al. Prevention of apoptosis by Bcl-2: release of cytochrome *c* from mitochondria blocked. Science 1997;275:1129–1132.
80. Vander Heiden, MG, Chandel NS, Williamson EK, et al. Bcl-xL regulates the membrane potential and volume homeostasis of mitochondria. Cell 1997;91:627–637.
81. Susin SA, Zamzami N, Castedo M, et al. Bcl-2 inhibits the mitochondrial release of an apoptogenic protease. J Exp Med 1996;184:1331–1341.
82. Marchetti P, Castedo M, Susin SA, et al. Mitochondrial permeability transition is a central coordinating event of apoptosis. J Exp Med 1996;184: 1155–1160.
83. Kantrow SP, Piantadosi CA. Release of cytochrome c from liver mitochondria during permeability transition. Biochem Biophys Res Commun 1997;232:669–671.
84. Ellerby HM, Martin SJ, Ellerby LM, et al. Establishment of a cell-free system of neuronal apoptosis: comparison of premitochondrial, mitochondrial, and postmitochondrial phases. J Neurosci 1997;17:6165–6178.
85. Susin, SA, Lorenzo HK, Zamzami N, et al. Molecular characterization of mitochondrial apoptosis-inducing factor. Nature 1999;397:441–446.
86. Li F, Srinivasan A, Wang Y, et al. Cell-specific induction of apoptosis by microinjection of cytochrome *c*. Bcl-xL has activity independent of cytochrome *c* release. J Biol Chem 1997;272:30,299–30,305.

87. Kluck RM, Bossy-Wetzel E, Green DR, Newmeyer DD. The release of cytochrome c from mitochondria: a primary site for Bcl-2 regulation of apoptosis. Science 1997;275:1132–1136.

88. Bradham CA, Qian T, Streetz K, et al. The mitochondrial permeability transition is required for tumor necrosis factor alpha-mediated apoptosis and cytochrome *c* release. Mol Cell Biol 1998;18:6353–6364.

89. Srinivasula SM, Ahmad M, Fernandes-Alnemri T, Alnemri ES. Autoactivation of procaspase-9 by Apaf-1-mediated oligomerization. Mol Cell 1998;1:949–957.

90. Pan G, O'Rourke K, Dixit VM. Caspase-9, Bcl-XL, and Apaf-1 form a ternary complex. J Biol Chem 1998;273:5841–5845.

91. Zou H, Henzel WJ, Liu X, et al. Apaf-1, a human protein homologous to C. elegans CED-4, participates in cytochrome *c*-dependent activation of caspase-3. Cell 1997;90:405–413.

92. Liu X, Zou H, Slaughter C, Wang X. DFF, a heterodimeric protein that functions downstream of caspase-3 to trigger DNA fragmentation during apoptosis. Cell 1997;89:175–184.

93. Nguyen M, Millar DG, Yong VW, et al. Targeting of Bcl-2 to the mitochondrial outer membrane by a COOH-terminal signal anchor sequence. J Biol Chem 1993;268:25,265–25,268.

94. Riparbelli MG, Callaini G, Tripodi SA, et al. Localization of the Bcl-2 protein to the outer mitochondrial membrane by electron microscopy. Exp Cell Res 1995;221:363–369.

95. Marzo I, Brenner C, Zamzami N, et al. The permeability transition pore complex: a target for apoptosis regulation by caspases and Bcl-2 related proteins. J Exp Med 1998;8:1261–1271.

96. Shimizu S, Eguchi Y, Kamiike W, et al. Bcl-2 blocks loss of mitochondrial membrane potential while ICE inhibitors act at a different step during inhibition of death induced by respiratory chain inhibitors. Oncogene 1996;13:21–29.

97. Decaudin D, Geley S, Hirsch T, et al. Bcl-2 and Bcl-XL antagonize the mitochondrial dysfunction preceding nuclear apoptosis induced by chemotherapeutic agents. Cancer Res 1997;57:62–67.

98. Zamzami N, Marchetti P, Castedo M, et al. Sequential reduction of mitochondrial transmembrane potential and generation of reactive oxygen species in early programmed cell death. J Exp Med 1995;182:367–377.

99. Marchetti P, Hirsch T, Zamzami N, et al. Mitochondrial permeability transition triggers lymphocyte apoptosis. J Immunol 1996;157:4830–4836.

100. Wolter KG, Hsu YT, Snith YL, et al. Movement of BAX from mitochondria to cytosol during apoptosis. J Cell Biol 1997;139:1281–1292.

101. Gross A, Jockel J, Wie MC, Korsmeyer SJ. Enforced dimerisation of BAX results in its translocation, mitochondrial dysfunction and apoptosis. EMBO J 1998;17:3878–3885.

102. Luo X, Budihardjo I, Zou N, et al. BID, a Bcl-2 interacting protein mediates cytochrome c release from mitochondria in response to activation of cell surface death receptors. Cell 1998;94:481–490.

103. Li H, Zhu H, Xu CJ, Yuan J. Cleavage of BID by caspase-8 mediates mitochondrial damage in the fas pathway of apoptosis. Cell 1998;94;491–501.

104. Desagher S, Osend-Sand A, Nichols A, et al. BID induced conformational change of BAX is responsible for mitochondrial cytochrome *c* release during apoptosis. J Cell Biol 1999;144:891–901.

105. Goping IS, Gross A, Lavoie N, et al. Regulated targetting of BAX to mito-chondria. J Cell Biol 1998;143:207–215.

106. Narita M, Shimuzu S, Ito T, et al. BAX interacts with the permeability transition pore to induce the permeability transition and cytochrome *c* release in isolated mitochondria. Proc Natl Acad Sci USA 1998;95:14,681–14,689.

107. Shimizu S, Narita N, Tsujimoto Y. Bcl2 family proteins regulate the release of apoptogenic cytochrome *c* by the mitochondrial channel VDAC. Nature 1999;399:483–487.

108. Marzo I, Brenner C, Zamzami N, et al. BAX and adenine nucleotide translocator cooperate in the mitochondrial control of apoptosis. Science 1998;281:2027–2031.

109. Mahajan NP, Linder K, Berry G, et al. Bcl-2 and BAX interactions in mito-chondria probed with green fluorescent protein and fluorescence resonance energy transfer. Nature Biotechnol 1998;16:547–552.

110. Antonsson B, Conti F, Ciavatta A, et al. Inhibition of BAX channel-forming activity by Bcl-2. Science 1997;277:370–372.

111. Charriaut-Marlangue C, Margaill I, Represa A, et al. Apoptosis and necrosis after reversible focal ischemia: an *in situ* DNA fragmentation analysis. J Cereb Blood Flow Metab 1996;16:186–194.

112. Veinot JP, Gattinger DA, Fliss H. Early apoptosis in human myocardial infarcts. Hum Pathol 1997;28:485–492.

113. Mitchell IJ, Lawson S, Moser B, et al. Glutamate-induced apoptosis results in a loss of striatal neurons in the parkinsonian rat. Neuroscience 1994;63:1–5.

114. Tatton NA, Kish SJ. *In situ* detection of apoptotic nuclei in the substantia nigra compacta of 1-methyl-4-phenyl-1,2,3,6-tetrahydropyridine-treated mice using terminal deoxynucleotidyl transferase labelling and acridine orange staining. Neuroscience 1997;77:1037–1048.

115. Dipasquale B, Marini AM, Youle RJ. Apoptosis and DNA degradation induced by 1-methyl-4-phenylpyridinium in neurons. Biochem Biophys Res Commun 1991;181:1442–1448.

116. Walkinshaw G, Waters CM. Neurotoxin-induced cell death in neuronal PC12 cells is mediated by induction of apoptosis. Neuroscience 1994;63:975–987.

117. Hartley A, Stone JM, Heron C, et al. Complex I inhibitors induce dose-dependent apoptosis in PC12 cells: relevance to Parkinson's disease. J Neurochem 1994;63:1987–1990.

118. Slater AF, Nobel CS, Orrenius S. The role of intracellular oxidants in apoptosis. Biochim Biophys Acta 1995;1271:59–62.

119. Ziv I, Melamed E, Nardi N, et al. Dopamine induces apoptosis-like cell death in cultured chick sympathetic neurons: a possible novel pathogenetic mecha-nism in Parkinson's disease. Neurosci. Lett. 1994;170:136–140.

120. Walkinshaw G, Waters CM. Induction of apoptosis in catecholaminergic PC12 cells by L-DOPA (1995) Implications for the treatment of Parkinson's disease. J Clin Invest 1995;95:2458–2464.

121. Mogi M, Harada M, Kondo T, et al. Bcl-2 protein is increased in the brain from parkinsonian patients. Neurosci Letts 1996;215:137–139.

122. Hassouna I, Wickert H, Zimmermann M, Gillardon F. Increase in BAX expression in substantia nigra following 1-methyl-4-phenyl-1,2,3,6-tetrahydropyridine (MPTP) treatment of mice. Neurosci Letts 1996;204:85–88.

123. Hartmann A, Hunot S, Michel PP, et al. Caspase-3: A vulnerability factor and final effector in apoptotic death of dopaminergic neurons in Parkinson's disease. Proc Natl Acad Sci USA 2000;97:2875–2880.

124. Stefanis L, Burke RE, Greene LA. Apoptosis in neurodegenerative disorders. Curr Opin Neurol 1997;10:299–305.

125. Itano Y, Nomura Y. 1-methyl-4-phenyl-pyridinium ion (MPP+) causes DNA fragmentation and increases the Bcl-2 expression in human neuroblastoma, SH-S5Y cells, through different mechanisms. Brain Res 1995;704:240–245.

126. He Y, Lee T, Leong SK. 6-Hydroxydopamine induced apoptosis of dopaminergic cells in the rat substantia nigra. Brain Res 2000;858:63–66.

127. Mochizuki H, Goto K, Mori H, Mizuno Y. Histochemical detection of apoptosis in Parkinson's disease. J Neurol Sci 1996;137:120–123.

128. Kosel S, Egensperger R, von Eitzen U, et al. On the question of apoptosis in the parkinsonian substantia nigra. Acta Neuropathol 1997;93:105–108.

129. Tompkins MM, Basgall EJ, Zamrini E, Hill WD. Apoptotic-like changes in Lewy-body-associated disorders and normal aging in substantia nigral neurons. Am J Pathol 1997;150:119–131.

130. Tatton NA, Maclean-Fraser A, Tatton WG, et al. A fluorescent double-labeling method to detect and confirm apoptotic nuclei in Parkinson's disease. Ann Neurol 1998;44:S142–S148.

131. Kristal BS, Dubinsky JM. Mitochondrial permeability transition in the central nervous system: induction by calcium cycling-dependent and -independent pathways. J Neurochem 1997;69:524–538.

132. Dubinsky JM, Levi Y. Calcium-induced activation of the mitochondrial permeability transition in hippocampal neurons. J Neurosci Res 1998;53: 728–741.

133. Friberg H, Connern C, Halestrap AP, Wieloch T. Differences in the activation of the mitochondrial permeability transition among brain regions in the rat correlate with selective vulnerability. J Neurochem 1999;72:2488–2497.

134. Friberg H, Ferrand-Drake M, Bengtsson F, et al. Cyclosporin A, but not FK 506, protects mitochondria and neurons against hypoglycaemic damage and implicates the mitochondrial permeability transition in cell death, J Neurosci 1998;18:5151–5159.

135. Li PA, Uchino H, Elmer E, Siesjo BK. Amelioration by cyclosporin A of brain damage following 5 or 10 min of ischemia in rats subjected to preischemic hyperglycemia. Brain Res 1997;753:133–140.

136. Zaidan E, Nilsson M, Sims NR. Cyclosporin A-sensitive changes in mitochondrial glutathione are an early response to intrastiatal NMDA or forebrain ischemia in rats. J Neurochem 1999;73:2214–2217.

137. Matsumoto S, Friberg H, Ferrand-Drake M, Wieloch T. Blockade of the Mitochondrial permeability transition pore diminishes infarct size in the rat

after transient middle cerebral artery occlusion. J Cereb Blood Flow Metab 1999;19:736–741.

138. Sullivan PG, Thompson MB, Scheff SW. Cyclosporin A attenuates acute mitochondrial dysfunction in traumatic brain injury. Exp Neurol 1999; 160:226–234.

139. Novelli A, Reilly JA, Lysko PG, Henneberry RC. Glutamate becomes neuortoxic via the n-methyl-D-aspartate receptor when intracellular energy levels are reduced. Brain Res 1988;451:205–212.

140. Zeevalk GD, Nicklas WJ. Chemically induced hypoglycaemia and anoxia: relationship to glutamate receptor-mediated toxicity in retina. J Pharmacol Exp Ther 1990;253:1285–1292.

141. Zeevalk GD, Nicklas WJ. Mechanisms underlying initiation of excitoxicity associated with metabolic inhibition. J. Pharmacol Exp Ther 1991;257: 870–878.

142. Choi DW. Ionic dependence of glutamate neurotoxicity. J Neurosc 1987; 7:369–379.

143. Bindokas VP, Miller RJ. Excitotoxic degeneration is initiated at non-random sites in cultured rat cerebellar neurons. J Neurosci 1995;15:6999–7011.

144. White RJ, Reynolds IJ. Mitochondrial depolarization in glutamate-stimulated neurons: an early signal specific to excitotoxin exposure. J Neurosci 1996;16:5688–5697.

145. Schinder AF, Olson EC, Spitzer NC, Montal M. Mitochondrial dysfunction is a primary event in glutamate neurotoxicity. J Neurosci 1996;16:6125–6133.

146. Ankarcrona M, Dypbukt JM, Orrenius S, Nicotera P. Calcineurin and mito-chondrial function in glutamate-induced neuronal cell death. FEBS Letts 1996;394:321–324.

147. Nieminen AL, Petrie TG, Lemasters JJ, Selman WR. Cyclosporin A delays mitochondrial depolarization induced by N-methyl-D-aspartate in cortical neu-rons: evidence of the mitochondrial permeability transition. Neuroscience 1996;75:993–997.

148. Dykens JA. Isolated cerebral and cerebellar mitochondria produce free radi-cals when exposed to elevated $Ca(+)$ and $Na(+)$: implications for neuro-degeneration. J Neurochem 1994;63:584–591.

149. Beckman JS, Crow JP. Pathological implications of nitric oxide superoxide and peroxynitrite formation. Biochem Soc Trans 1993;21:330–334.

150. Packer MA, Murphy MP. Peroxynitrite causes calcium efflux from mitochon-dria which is prevented by cyclosporin A. FEBS Letts 1994;345:237–240.

151. Packer MA, Scarlett JL, Martin SW, Murphy MP. Induction of the mitochon-drial permeability transition by peroxynitrite. Biochem Soc Trans 1997; 25:909–914.

152. Brookes PS, Salinas EP, Darley-Usmar K, et al. Concentration-dependent effects of nitric oxide on mitochondrial permeability transition and cyto-chrome c release. J Biol Chem 2000;275:20,474–20,479.

153. Budd SL, Tenneti L, Lishnak T, Lipton SA. Mitochondrial and extramito-chondrial apoptotic signaling pathways in cerebrocortical neurons. Proc Natl Acad Sci USA 2000;97:6161–6166.

154. Difazio MC, Hollingsworth Z, Young JB, Penney J. Glutamate receptors in the substantia nigra of Parkinson's disease. Neurology 1992;42:402–406.
155. Finiels-Markier F, Marini AM, Williams P, Paul SM. The N-methyl-D-aspartate antagonist MK-801 fails to protect dopaminergic neurons from 1-methyl-4-phenylpyridinium toxicity in vitro. J Neurochem 1993;60:1968–1971.
156. Srivastava R, Brouillet E, Beal MF, et al. Blockade of 1-methyl-4phenylpyridinium (MPP+) nigral toxicity in the rat by prior decortication or MK-801 treatment: a stereological estimate of neuronal loss. Neurobiol Aging 1993;14:295–301.
157. Chan P, Langston JW, Di Monte DA. MK-801 temporarily prevents MPTP-induced acute dopamine depletion and MPP+ elimination in the mouse striatum. J Pharmacol Exp Ther 1993;267:1515–1520.
158. Brouillet E, Beal MF. NMDA antagonists partially protect against MPTP neurotoxicity in mice. Neuroreport 1993;4:387–390.
159. Zuddas A, Oberto G, Vaglini F, et al. MK-801 prevents 1-methyl-4-phenyl-1,2,3,6-tetrahydropyridine-induced parkinsonism in primates. J Neurochem 1992;59:733–739.
160. Lange KW, Loschman PA, Sofic E, et al. The competitive NMDA antagonist CPP protects substantia nigra neurons from MPTP-induced degeneration in primates. Naunyn Schmiedebergs Arch Pharmaco. 1993;348: 586–592.
161. Liberatore GT, Jackson-Lewis V, Vukosavic S, et al. Inducible nitric oxide synthase stimulates dopaminergic neurodegeneration in the MPTP model of Parkinson disease. Nature Med 1999;5:1403–1409.
162. Schulz JB, Matthews RT, Muqit MM, et al. Inhibition of neuronal nitric oxide synthase by 7-nitroindazole protects against MPTP-induced neurotoxicity in mice. J Neurochem 1995;64:936–939.
163. Hantraye P, Brouillet E, Ferrante R, et al. Inhibition of neuronal nitric oxide synthase prevents MPTP-induced parkinsonism in baboons. Nature Med 1996;2:1017–1021.
164. Matthews RT, Beal MF, Fallon J, et al. MPP+ induced substantia nigra degeneration is attenuated in nNOS knockout mice. Neurobiol Dis 1997;4:114–121.
165. Schulz JB, Huang PL, Matthews RT, et al. Striatal malonate lesions are attenuated in neuronal nitric oxide synthase knockout mice. J Neurochem 1966;67:430–433.
166. Cassarino DS, Parks JK, Parker Jr, WD, Bennett Jr, JP. The parkinsonian neurotoxin MPP+ opens the mitochondrial membrane permeability transition pore and releases cytochrome c in isolated mitochondria via an oxidative mechanism. Biochim Biophys Acta 1999;1453:49–62.
167. Berman SB, Hastings TG. Dopamine oxidation alters mitochondrial respiration and induces permeability transition in brain mitochondria: implications for Parkinson's disease. J Neurochem 1999;73:1127–1130.
168. Seaton TA, Cooper JM, Schapira AHV. Cyclosporin inhibition of apoptosis induced by mitochondrial complex I toxins. Brain Res 1998;809:12–17.
169. Zamzami N, Marchetti P, Castedo M, et al. Inhibitors of permeability transition interfere with the disruption of the mitochondrial transmembrane potential during apoptosis. FEBS Letts 1996;384:53–57.

170. Matsuura K, Kabuto H, Makino H, Ogawa N. Initial cyclosporin A but not glucocorticoid treatment promotes recovery of striatal dopamine concentration in 6-hydroxydopamine lesioned mice. Neurosci Letts 1997;230: 191–196.

171. Ogawa N. Cyclosporin A attenuates degeneration of dopaminergic neurons induced by 6-hydroxydopamine in the mouse brain. Brain Res 1996;733: 101–104.

172. Matsuura K, Makino H, Ogawa N. Cyclosporin A attenuates the decrease in tyrosine hydroxylase immunoreactivity in nigrostriatal dopaminergic neurons and in striatl dopamine content in rats with intrastriatal injection of 6-hydroxydopamine. Exp Neurol 1997;146:526–535.

173. Borlongan CV, Freeman TB, Hauser RA, et al. Cyclosporine-A increases locomotor activity in rats with 6-hydroxydopamine-induced hemiparkinsonism: relevance to neural transplantation. Surg Neurol 1996;46:384–388.

174. Takahashi N, Hayano T, Suzuki M. Peptidyl-prolyl cis-trans isomerase is the cyclosporin A-binding protein cyclophilin. Nature 1989;337:473–475.

175. Harding MW, Galat A, Uehling DE, Schreiber SL. A receptor for the immunosuppressant FK506 is a cis-trans peptidyl-prolyl isomerase. Nature 1989;341:758–760.

176. Schreiber SL. Chemistry and biology of the immunophilins and their immunosuppressant ligands. Science 1991;251:283–287.

177. Steiner JP, Dawson TM, Fotuhi M, et al. High brain densities of the immunophilin FKBP colocalized with calcineurin. Nature 1992;358: 584–587.

178. Dawson TM, Steiner JP, Lyons WE, et al. The immunophilins, FK506 binding protein and cyclophilin, are discretely localized in the brain: relationship to calcineurin. Neuroscience 1994;62:569–580.

179. Dawson TM, Steiner JP, Dawson VL, et al. Immunosuppressant FK506 enhances phosphorylation of nitric oxide synthase and protects against glutamate neurotoxicity. Proc Natl Acad Sci USA 1993;90:9808–9812.

180. Bredt DS, Ferris CD, Snyder SH. Nitric oxide synthase regulatory sites. Phosphorylation by cyclic AMP-dependent protein kinase, protein kinase C, and calcium/calmodulin protein kinase; identification of flavin and calmodulin binding sites. J Biol Chem 1992;267:10,976–10,981.

181. Dawson VL, Kizushi VM, Huang PL, et al. Resistance to neurotoxicity in cortical cultures from neuronal nitric oxide synthase-deficient mice. J Neurosci 1996;16:2479–2487.

182. Meiri KF, Bickerstaff LE, Schwob JE. Monoclonal antibodies show that kinase C phosphorylation of GAP-43 during axonogenesis is both spatially and temporally restricted in vivo. J Cell Biol 1991;112:991–1005.

183. Steiner JP, Connolly MA, Valentine HL, et al. Neurotrophic actions of nonimmunosuppressive analogues of immunosuppressive drugs FK506, rapamycin and cyclosporin A. Nature Med 1997;3:421–428.

184. Costantini LC, Isacson O. Immunophilin ligands and GDNF enhance neurite branching or elongation from developing dopamine neurons in culture. Exp. Neurol 2000;164:60–70.

185. Steiner JP, Hamilton GS, Ross DT, et al. Neurotrophic immunophilin ligands stimulate structural and functional recovery in neurodegenerative animal models. Proc Natl Acad Sci USA 1997;94:2019–2024.

III

Immunosuppressants and Other Age-Related Disorders

7

Immunosuppressants and Alzheimer's Disease

Mark P. Mattson

CELLULAR AND MOLECULAR MECHANISMS UNDERLYING NEURONAL DEGENERATION IN ALZHELMER'S DISEASE

The two major histopathological abnormalities in the brains of patients with Alzheimer's disease (AD) are extensive extracellular deposits of amyloid β-peptide (Aβ) and degenerating neurons that contain abnormal hyperphosphorylated filaments composed mainly of the microtubule-associated protein tau *(1)*. Aβ is a 40–42 amino acid peptide that is generated by proteolytic processing of a much larger, membrane-associated amyloid precursor protein (APP). A cleavage of APP in the middle of the Aβ sequence by an enzyme activity called α-secretase results in release of a secreted form of APP called sAPPα, Alternatively, APP can be cleaved at the N and C termini of the Aβ sequence by β-secretase and γ-secretase, respectively. A shift in processing of APP in favor of increased production of neurotoxic forms of Aβ , and decreased production of neuroprotective sAPPα, appears to play a seminal role in the initiation of the neurodegenerative process in AD *(2)*. Indeed, mutations in the APP gene (located on chromosome 21), which are causally linked to a small percentage of cases of early-onset inherited AD, result in increased production of Aβ, particularly the highly neurotoxic long form of Aβ (Aβ1–42). Moreover, mutations in two other proteins called presenilin-1 (PS1; chromosome 14) and presenilin-2 (PS2; chromosome 1) that cause dominantly inherited early-onset forms of AD result in aberrant APP processing *(3,4)*. PS1 and PS2 mutations enhance γ-secretase cleavage of APP and may thereby increase production of Aβ1-42 *(5)*. PS1 mutations may also perturb calcium homeostasis in the endoplasmic reticulum (ER), which results in increased neuronal vulnerability to (age-related) increases in oxidative and energetic stress, and thereby promote a form of programmed cell death called apoptosis *(4)* (Fig. 1).

From: *Immunosuppressant Analogs in Neuroprotection*
Edited by: C. V. Borlongan, O. Isacson, and P. R. Sanberg © Humana Press Inc., Totowa, NJ

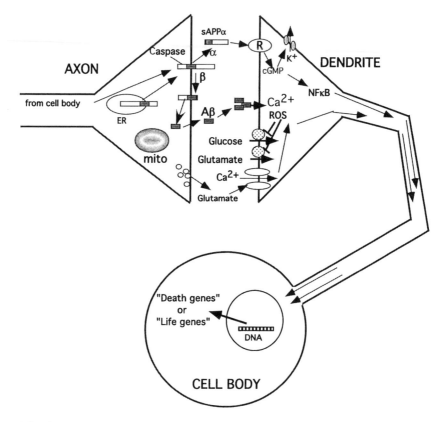

Fig. 1. Roles for alterations in amyloid precursor protein processing and synaptic signaling in the neurodegenerative process in AD. *See* text and ref. *2* for descriptions.

Studies of postmortem brain tissues from AD patients, and of experimental cell culture and animal models of AD, suggest that oxidative stress and perturbed regulation of intracellular calcium levels play central roles in the neurodegenerative process. Increased protein, lipid and DNA oxidation occur in association with neurofibrillary tangles and neuritic plaques, and are also increased in the cerebrospinal fluid of AD patients (*see* for review, ref. *6*). Aβ can induce membrane lipid peroxidation in neurons, which impairs the function of ion-motive ATPases, and glucose and glutamate transporters, resulting in membrane depolarization and elevation of intracellular calcium levels; these alterations render neurons vulnerable to excitotoxicity and apoptosis *(2)*. By impairing glucose transport, Aβ may contribute to the decreased glucose availability to brain cells and mitochondrial dysfunction documented in studies of AD patients *(6,7)*. In cases of sporadic AD, increased oxidative stress and compromised energy metabolism may trigger altered APP processing and perturbed cellular calcium homeostsis, whereas in the case of PS1 mutations perturbed calcium homeostasis may induce oxidative stress and altered APP processing (Fig. 1). A role for perturbed calcium homeostasis in AD is suggested by data showing that levels of Ca^{2+}-dependent protease activity are increased in neurons exhibiting neurofibrillary changes *(8)*. In addition, levels of ryanodine binding are increased in vulnerable neuronal populations in the hippocampus of AD patients in the early stages of the disease, but are then decreased in end-stage patients *(9)*, suggesting that neurons with relatively large pools of ER calcium release sites may be prone to degeneration in AD *(10)*. Our studies of cultured cells and knockin mice expressing PS1 mutations have provided direct evidence for enhanced calcium release from ryanodine-sensitive ER calcium pools being an abnormality that is central the neurodegenerative process *(11)*. Data showing that Aβ disrupts neuronal calcium homeostasis, and that APP and presenililin-1 mutations also perturb neuronal calcium homeostasis in a manner that increases neuronal vulnerability to excitotoxicity and apoptosis, strongly support a pivotal role for aberrant regulation of intracellular calcium levels in the pathogenesis of AD *(12,13)*.

A prominent biochemical alteration in degenerating neurons in AD is the accumulation of filaments composed of hyperphosphorylated forms of the microtubule-associated protein tau *(14)*. Such neurofibrillary tangles are not unique to AD, and their presence in other disorders such as frontal lobe dementias and Guam syndrome, and in normal aging suggests that the mechanism of neuronal degeneration in AD is shared with other disorders. A variety of alterations have been proposed to result in tau hyperphosphorylation and aggregation, including increased kinase activity and/or decreased phosphatase activity *(15)*, oxidative stress *(16)* and perturbed calcium homeostasis *(17)*. Although it is not yet clear as to whether tau hyperphosphorylation and/or aggregation is necessary for the death of neurons in AD, it is of considerable interest that mutations in tau can cause a disorder called frontal lobe dementia in which neurofibrillary tangle formation is associated with cell death *(18)*.

Synapses are believed to be sites where the neurodegenerative process begins in AD *(19)*. Studies of synaptosomes and cultured neurons have provided evidence that insults relevant to AD can induce apoptotic biochemical cascades (caspase activation, loss of plasma membrane phospholipid asymmetry, and mitochondrial dysfunction) in synaptic compartments and neurites (Fig. 2). Synaptic degeneration in AD likely involves membrane lipid peroxidation, and impairment of ion-motive ATPases and glucose

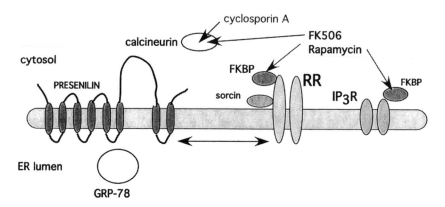

Fig. 2. Actions of immunophilins and immunosuppressant drugs at the level of the endoplasmic reticulum membrane. FKBP, FK506 binding protein; GRP-78, glucose-regulated protein-78; RR, ryanodine receptor. See text for description.

transporters *(2)*. A protein called prostate apoptosis response-4 (Par-4) may play a particularly important role in synapse degeneration because Par-4 levels are rapidly increased in cortical synaptosomes and in dendrites of cultured hippocampal neurons in response to exposure to Fe^{2+} and Aβ *(20)*. The protein synthesis inhibitor cycloheximide or Par-4 antisense oligonucleotides attenuate insult-induced mitochondrial dysfunction and caspase activation, and prevent synaptic damage and neuronal death in experimental models of AD *(20,21)*. Cortical synaptosomes from PS1 mutant mice exhibit enhanced elevations of cytoplasmic calcium levels and mitochondrial depolarization in response to depolarization and exposure to Aβ compared to synaptosomes from nontransgenic mice and mice overexpressing wild-type PS1 *(22)*. Drugs that buffer cytoplasmic calcium or prevent calcium release from the ER can protect against the adverse effects of the PS1 mutations *(23,24)*.

CALCINEURIN AND AD

The protein phosphatase calcineurin, also called protein phosphatase 2B, is a target of the immunosuppressant drugs cyclosporin A and FK506 *(25)*. Calcineurin is a calcium- and calmodulin-sensitive enzyme that can dephosphorylate several protein substrates of relevance to the pathogenesis of AD, prominent among which is tau *(26)*. A role for alterations in calcineurin activity in the process of neurofibrillary tangle formation is suggested by several findings. Suppression of calcineurin levels using antisense technology in adult rats results in a persistent increase in tau phosphorylation at residues Thr191 and Thr231 *(27)*. Hyperphosphorylated tau accumulates in the brains of mice that lack calcineurin Aα *(28)*. The magnitude of the increase in phosphorylated tau levels was greatest in hippocampal dentate cells, which normally contain the highest content of calcineurin of any neuronal population in the brain. Exposure of cultured PC12 cells to maitotoxin resulted in calcium-mediated dephosphorylation of tau and calpain-mediated degradation of tau *(29)*. When cells were treated with the calcineurin inhibitor FK520, both the dephosphorylation and degradation of tau were inhibited, suggesting that tau dephosphorylation by calcineurin normally prevents aggregation of tau. These experimental data suggest that abnormalities in calcineurin activity might contribute to the pathogenesis of neurofibrillary degeneration in AD. Measurements of calcineurin activity in brain tissue homogenates from AD patients and age-matched control patients using the substrate *p*-nitrophenyl phosphate provide support for the latter hypothesis. Thus, levels of calcineurin activity were decreased by 30–60% in temporal cortex of AD patients, and the magnitude of the decrease in calcineurin activity was inversely correlated with numbers of neurofibrillary tangles and neuritic plaques *(30)*. Immunohistochemical analyses of AD brain tissue sections using calcineurin antibodies reveal that calcineurin is present in dendrites and cell bodies of undamaged neurons and in many, but not all, neurofibrillary tangle-bearing neurons *(31,32)*. There did not appear to be a major decrease in calcineurin levels in neurons in AD, suggesting that, although calcineurin activity may decrease in AD, decreased expression of calcineurin may not occur.

A second line of investigation that supports a role for calcineurin in AD involves studies of mechanisms of neuronal apoptosis. Overexpression of calcineurin in cultured neural cells increases their vulnerability to apoptosis induced by withdrawal of trophic support and exposure to a calcium ionophore; preincubation with either cyclosporin A or FK506 reduces susceptibility of the neurons to apoptosis *(33)*. Calcineurin may activate the apoptotic process at a premitochondrial stage because Bcl-2 and caspase inhibitors block calcineurin-mediated apoptosis. Survival of embryonic chick forebrain neurons cultured under suboptimal conditions is also enhanced by several different calcineurin inhibitors including FK506 and cypermethrin *(34)*. An indirect neurotoxic effect of calcineurin is suggested by studies showing that calcineurin can promote Aβ production and that calcineurin inhibitors such as cyclosporin A can inhibit Aβ production *(35)*. Moreover, both cyclosporin A and FK506 can prevent glutamate-induced death of cultured neurons *(36)*; overactivation of glutamate receptors may contribute to the neurodegenerative process in AD *(12,17,37)*. Thus, although the data on calcineurin and cell death suggest that calcineurin can promote death, the data on calcineurin and tau suggest that calcineurin may prevent neurofibrillary degeneration. The role of calcineurin in the pathogenesis of AD therefore remains very unclear. Nevertheless, the data described below suggest that immunosuppressants may protect neurons against death, by mechanisms independent of calcineurin, in experimental models relevant to AD.

IMMUNOSUPPRESSANTS, MITOCHONDRIAL MEMBRANE PERMEABILITY TRANSITION, AND AD

Formation of "permeability transition pores" (PTP) that span both the inner and outer mitochondrial membranes appears to be a key event in neuronal apoptosis in many different neurodegenerative disorders, including AD (38). Studies of brain tissue from AD patients have revealed several alterations consistent with an apoptotic mechanism of neuronal death: DNA damage and activation of genes known to respond to DNA damage (39,40), caspase activation (41), and increased production of proteins known to participate in neuronal apoptosis, including Bax (42), Par-4 (21) and cell cycle-associated proteins (43). Aβ can induce neuronal apoptosis, which involves mitochondrial oxyradical production and membrane permeability transition (44). Cyclosporin A, which prevents formation of PTP (45), protects neurons against Aβ-induced apoptosis (44). By contrast, FK506 (which inhibits calcineurin, but does not prevent PTP formation) affords no protection against Aβ-induced apoptosis. The latter findings are similar to those obtained in studies of neuronal death induced by hypoglycemia and cerebral ischemia in which cyclosporin A, but not FK506, is neuroprotective (46). A cyclosporin A analog that selectively blocks PTP without inhibiting calcineurin was recently reported to be effective in reducing ischemic neuronal injury in a rat model of stroke (47), suggesting that compounds that inhibit PTP may prove effective in limiting brain damage and improving behavioral outcome in several different neurodegenerative conditions.

Studies of "cybrid" cells in which endogenous mitochondria were replaced with mitochondria from platelets of AD and control patients have provided evidence for a major role for alterations in mitochondrial metabolism and calcium buffering in AD (48). The latter study demonstrated a decrease in mitochondrial complex IV activity and an increase in levels of oxyradicals in AD cybrids. These findings suggest a role for mitochondrial dysfunction in the pathogenesis of AD, and further suggest that such mitochondrial dysfunction occurs not only in brain cells, but also in peripheral cells. A decrease in mitochondrial membrane potential occurs in AD cybrids, and the decrease is recovered by treatment with cyclosporin A, suggesting that mitochondria in AD exhibit a tonic low-grade permeability transition (49). Mitochondrial calcium uptake may play a pivotal role in both apoptotic and necrotic death of neurons in various experimental models, and cyclosporin A can prevent both types of cell death *(50)*, suggesting a tight link between mitochondrial calcium uptake and PTP formation.

Studies in which AD-linked PS1 mutations are expressed in cultured neurons and transgenic mice provide further evidence that apoptosis is the predominant form of neuronal death in AD. Thus, neurons expressing mutant PS1 are exquisitely sensitive to apoptosis induced by Aβ, oxidative insults, and trophic factor withdrawal *(13,23,51)*. PS1 mutations promote neuronal apoptosis by causing enhanced release of calcium from ER stores, and, accordingly, drugs that suppress calcium release (such as dantrolene and xestospongin) can counteract the proapoptotic action of mutant PS1. Cells expressing mutant PS1 exhibit increased vulnerability to apoptosis induced by the succinate dehydrogenase (complex IV) inhibitors 3-nitropropionic acid and malonate, and such cell death is prevented by cyclosporin A (*see* Fig. 3) *(24)*.

Indirect support for a role for mitochondrial PTP formation in the cognitive dysfunction in AD comes from studies of hippocampal slices from APP and PS1 mutant mice, and from rats subjected to traumatic brain injury, a risk factor for AD (*see* Fig. 4.) Long-term potentiation (LTP) of synaptic transmission is impaired in APP mutant mice *(52)*. On the other hand, LTP is increased in hippocampal slices from PS1 mutant mice *(53,54)*, consistent with enhanced calcium release from ER *(11,22)* and/or enhanced influx through plasma membrane channels *(12,55)*. LTP was markedly impaired, whereas long-term depression (LTD) was enhanced, 48 h after traumatic brain injury in rats when compared to unoperated and sham-operated control rats *(56)*. Postinjury administration of cyclosporin A resulted in a highly significant amelioration of the impairment of LTP, completely prevented the enhancement of LTD, and reduced the extent of brain injury *(56,57)*. These kinds of data suggest that alterations in hippocampal synaptic plasticity may be responsible for learning and memory deficits resulting from traumatic brain injury and AD, and that agents such as cyclosporin A that stabilize mitochondrial function may be effective treatments for TBI and possibly AD.

ENDOPLASMIC RETICULUM CALCIUM RELEASE CHANNELS, IMMUNOSUPPRESSANTS, AND AD

In addition to actions on calcineurin and proteins associated with the mitochondrial PTP, certain immunosuppressants bind to proteins involved in the control of calcium release from the ER. The 12,000-Da FK506 binding protein FKBP12 is a proline isomerase that associates with the ryanodine

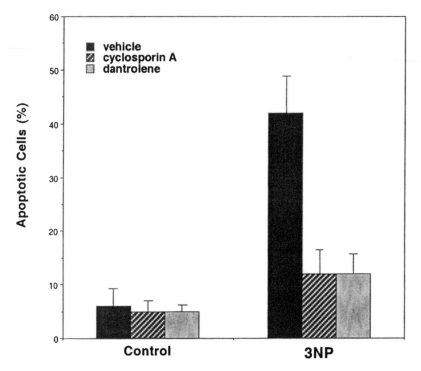

Fig. 3. Cultures of PC12 cells expressing human presenilin-1 with the AD-linked L286V mutation were pretreated for 1 h with 1 μ*M* cyclosporin A, 1 μ*M* dantrolene or 0.5% dimethylsulfoxide (vehicle). Cultures were then exposed to 2 m*M* 3-nitropropionic acid (3NP) or saline (control) for 48 h, and numbers of cells with apoptotic nuclei were quantified. Values are the mean and SEM of determinations made in 6 to 8 cultures. Adapted from data in ref. *24*.

receptor, a 565,00-Da protein with four subunits that forms calcium release channels in the ER *(58)*. The interaction of FKBP12 with ryanodine receptors results in stabilization of the receptor channels in an open state resulting in increased channels with full conductance levels and increased mean open time. This facilitation of ryanodine receptor channel opening by FKBP12 is inhibited by FK506 and rapamycin *(58)*. The cell survival-promoting effects of FK506 and rapamycin in experimental models of excitotoxicity *(59)* are consistent with a role for inhibition of ER calcium release in the neuroprotective actions of these drugs. However, additional actions of FK506 and related immunosuppressants are likely. For example, studies have shown that FKBP12 binds strongly to inositol trisphosphate (IP$_3$) receptors, an interaction that may reduce calcium flux through the receptor channel *(60)*. In addition, studies of digitonin-permeabilized SY5Y neuro-

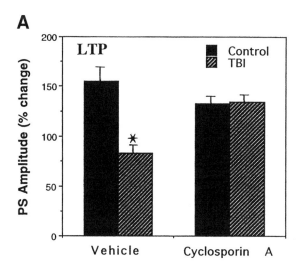

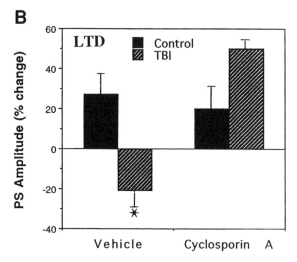

Fig. 4. Traumatic brain injury impairs synaptic correlates of learning and memory in the hippocampus: amelioration by cyclosporin A. Rats were given cyclosporin A intraperitoneally 15 min after traumatic brain injury. Forty eight hours later hippocampal slices were prepared and population spikes were recorded in area CA1 in response to stimulation of input axons. Values for population spike amplitudes recorded 20 min following stimulation at a high frequency that normally induces long-term potentiation (LTP; 100 Hz; panel a) or at a low frequency that normally induces long-term depression (LTD, 1 Hz; panel b) are shown. $^*p < 0.01$ compared to each of the other values.

blastoma cells suggest that FK506 can have multiple effects on ER Ca^{2+} homeostasis, enhancing Ca^{2+} release through ryanodine receptors and inhibiting Ca^{2+} uptake into ER by inhibiting the ER Ca^{2+}–ATPase (61). Finally, another FK506-binding protein called FKBP13 is located in the lumen of the ER and may share properties of molecular chaperones including their ability to be upregulated at the transcriptional level in response to ER stress (62).

Very recent findings, emerging from studies of the physiological and pathological actions of PS1, lend further support to a role for perturbed ER calcium homeostasis in the pathogenesis of AD. Cultured neural cell lines stably overexpressing mutant forms of PS1 linked to AD (L286V and M146V mutations) exhibit enhanced calcium release from IP3-sensitive stores (51) and ryanodine-sensitive stores (11) when stimulated with selective agonists. Levels of ryanodine receptor mRNA and protein are increased in cultured cells overexpressing mutant PS1 and in neurons from mice expressing mutant PS1, and PS1 may interact directly with ryanodine receptors (11). Because cells expressing mutant PS1 also respond to thapsigargin (an inhibitor of the ER calcium ATPase) with enhanced calcium release (51), it appears that PS1 mutations somehow result in an overfilling of ER calcium stores. Similar alterations in ER calcium signaling are observed in fibroblasts from PS1 mutant knockin mice, suggesting that overfilling of calcium stores is a fundamental cellular defect conferred by PS1 mutations (63). Dantrolene, an agent that selectively inhibits calcium release from ryanodine-sensitive stores, protects neurons against the death-promoting effect of PS1 mutations emphasizing the centrality of calcium release to the pathogenic action of the mutations (23). When taken together with data showing that levels of radiolabeled ryanodine binding are increased in subiculum and region CA1 of hippocampus during early stages of AD, but are decreased in patients with late-stage disease (9), the data suggest that increases in levels of ryanodine receptors may precede neuronal degeneration in vulnerable neuronal populations in AD.

As is the case with PS1, PS2 is an integral membrane protein localized in the ER. Recent findings suggest a role for PS2 in modulating calcium release from ER. For example, IP_3-induced calcium signals are potentiated in oocytes expressing mutant PS2 compared to oocytes expressing wild-type PS2 (64). In addition, PS2 interacts with sorcin, a calcium-binding protein known to modulate ryanodine receptor channel activity (65). The interaction of sorcin with PS2 is enhanced under conditions in which intracellular calcium levels are increased, suggesting the possibility that sorcin might modulate neuronal calcium homeostasis via a presenilin-mediated mechanism. Whether alterations in immunophilins contribute to the pathogenesis of AD remains to be established. However, it has been shown that cyclosporin A can protect neurons expressing mutant PS1 against various metabolic and oxidative insults relevant to the pathogenesis of AD *(24)*.

IMMUNOSUPPRESSANTS, GLIAL CELLS, AND AD

Inflammatory processes involving the activation of microglia, brain-resident macrophages, have been implicated in the pathogenesis of AD, based upon their association with amyloid plaques, and epidemiological data suggesting that antiinflammatory drugs can reduce risk for AD *(66)*. Aβ can stimulate microglia to produce neurotoxic agents such as nitric oxide and excitotoxins *(67,68)*. Both FK506 and cyclosporin A can suppress activation of microglia *(69)*. Stimulation of prostaglandin E2 receptors induces increased levels of APP mRNA and protein in primary cortical astrocyte cultures, and this effect of the prostaglandin is inhibited by cyclosporin A and FK506 *(70)*. The latter findings are consistent with a role for prostaglandins produced in response to brain injury in promoting amyloid deposition, and suggest the possibility that immunosuppressants will inhibit this process.

IMPLICATIONS FOR PREVENTION AND TREATMENT OF AD

How might the information gathered on immunosuppressants and neuronal degeneration in experimental models of AD described above be translated into the development of treatments for AD patients? The considerable data demonstrating neuroprotective effects of cyclosporin A in experimental models relevant to AD and other neurodegenerative conditions, suggest that agents that suppress the mitochondrial membrane permeability transition may prevent or slow the neurodegenerative process. Because serious side-effects can result from chronic immunosuppressant treatment, it would be desirable to develop approaches for delivery of the drugs to the brain. The blood–brain barrier is normally impermeable to immunosuppressants such as FK506 and cyclosporin A. However, the penetrability of cyclosporin A into the brain may be increased by modulating levels and/or activity of P-glycoprotein, a protein that influences blood–brain permeability to many different drugs *(71)*. Other approaches are also being used to facilitate penetration of immunosuppressants, including encapsulation of the drugs in lipophilic delivery vectors *(72)*.

Considerable evidence suggests that, in many cases, it is inhibition of mitochondrial PTP pore formation that is responsible for the neuroprotective effects of cyclosporin A. With this thought in mind, several groups have been developing analogs of cyclosporin A that retain their ability to inhibit the PTP, but lack immunosuppressant (calcineurin-inhibiting) activity. One such analog, N-Me-Val-4-cyclosporin A, has proven effective in preventing neuronal degeneration in cell culture and in vivo models of ischemic brain injury *(47,73)*. In addition to the potential application of cyclosporin A and related antiapoptotic agents to prevention of neuronal degeneration in AD patients, such agents may prove useful in transplantation therapy. Animal studies have shown that cyclosporin A can significantly enhance survival of mouse embryonic cholinergic neurons after transplantation into the forebrain of adult rats *(74)*.

Although research into the functions of immunophilins associated with the ER is still in its infancy, the evidence suggesting that alterations in ER calcium regulation and protein processing are central to the pathogenesis of AD has implications for novel therapeutic approaches for AD. One such approach is to inhibit calcium release from the ER by using drugs such as dantrolene that inhibit ryanodine receptors *(10,23)*, or FK506 and related compounds that reduce calcium release by virtue of their interactions with immunophilins associated with ryanodine receptors *(58)*.

REFERENCES

1. Cummings JL, Vinters HV, Cole GM, Khachaturian ZS. Alzheimer's disease: etiologies, pathophysiology, cognitive reserve, and treatment opportunities. Neurology 1998;51:S2–S17.
2. Mattson MP. Cellular actions of β-amyloid precursor protein, and its soluble and fibrillogenic peptide derivatives. Physiol Rev 1997;77:1081–1132.
3. Hardy, J. (1997) Amyloid, the presenilins and Alzheimer's disease. Trends Neurosci 1997;20:154–159.
4. Mattson MP, Guo Q, Furukawa K, Pedersen WA. Presenilins, the endoplasmic reticulum, and neuronal apoptosis in Alzheimer's disease. J Neurochem 1998;70:1–14.
5. Haass C, De Strooper B. The presenilins in Alzheimer's disease—proteolysis holds the key. Science 1999;286:916–919.
6. Mattson MP, Pedersen WA, Duan W, et al. Cellular and molecular mechanisms underlying perturbed energy metabolism and neuronal degeneration in Alzheimer's and Parkinson's diseases. Ann NY Acad Sci 1999;893:154–175.
7. Gibson GE, Park LC, Zhang H, et al. Oxidative stress and a key metabolic enzyme in Alzheimer brains, cultured cells, and an animal model of chronic oxidative deficits. Ann NY Acad Sci 1999;893:79–94.
8. Grynspan F, Griffin WR, Cataldo A, et al. Active site-directed antibodies identify calpain II as an early-appearing and pervasive component of neurofibrillary pathology in Alzheimer's disease. Brain Res 1997;763:145–158.
9. Kelliher M, Fastbom J, Cowburn RF, et al. Alterations in the ryanodine receptor calcium release channel correlate with Alzheimer's disease neurofibrillary and beta-amyloid pathologies. Neuroscience 1999;92:499–513.

10. Mattson MP, LaFerla FM, Chan SL, et al. Calcium signaling in the ER: its role in neuronal plasticity and neurodegenerative disorders. Trends Neurosci 2000;23:222–229.

11. Chan SL, Mayne M, Holden CP, et al. Presenilin-1 mutations increase levels of ryanodine receptors and calcium release in PC12 cells and cortical neurons. J Biol Chem 2000;275:18,195–18,200.

12. Mattson MP, Cheng B, Davis D, et al. β-Amyloid peptides destabilize calcium homeostasis and render human cortical neurons vulnerable to excitotoxicity. J Neurosci 1992;12:376–389.

13. Guo Q, Fu W, Sopher BL, et al. Increased vulnerability of hippocampal neurons to excitotoxic necrosis in presenilin-1 mutant knockin mice. Nature Med 1999;5:101–106.

14. Lee VM. Disruption of the cytoskeleton in Alzheimer's disease. Curr Opin Neurobiol 1995;5:663–668.

15. Delacourte A, Buee L. Normal and pathological au proteins as factores for microtubule assembly. Int Rev Cytol 1997;171:167–224.

16. Mattson MP, Fu W, Waeg G, Uchida K. 4-hydroxynonenal, a product of lipid peroxidation, inhibits dephosphorylation of the microtubule-associated protein tau. NeuroReport 1997;8:2275–2281.

17. Mattson MP. Antigenic changes similar to those seen in neurofibrillary tangles are elicited by glutamate and calcium influx in cultured hippocampal neurons. Neuron 1990;4:105–117.

18. Goedert M, Crowther RA, Spillantini MG. Tau mutations cause frontotemporal dementias. Neuron 1998;21:955–958.

19. Mattson MP, Duan W. "Apoptotic" biochemical cascades in synaptic compartments: roles in adaptive plasticity and neurodegenerative disorders. J. Neurosci. Res. 1999;58:152–166.

20. Duan W, Rangnekar VM, Mattson MP. Prostate apoptosis response-4 production in synaptic compartments following apoptotic and excitotoxic insults: evidence for a pivotal role in mitochondrial dysfunction and neuronal degeneration. J Neurochem 1999;72:2312–2322.

21. Guo Q, Fu W, Xie J, et al. Par-4 is a mediator of neuronal degeneration associated with the pathogenesis of Alzheimer disease. Nat Med 1998;4:957–962.

22. Begley JG, Duan W, Chan S, et al. Altered calcium homeostasis and mitochondrial dysfunction in cortical synaptic compartments of presenilin-1 mutant mice. J Neurochem 1999;72:1030–1039.

23. Guo Q, Sopher BL, Furukawa K, et al. Alzheimer's presenilin mutation sensitizes neural cells to apoptosis induced by trophic factor withdrawal and amylid beta-peptide: involvement of calcium and oxyradicals. J Neurosci 1997; 17:4212–4222.

24. Keller JN, Guo Q, Holtsberg FW, et al. Increased sensitivity to mitochondrial toxin-induced apoptosis in neural cells expressing mutant presenilin-1 is linked to perturbed calcium homeostasis and enhanced oxyradical production. J Neurosci 1998;18:4439–4450.

25. Hemenway CS, Heitman J. Calcineurin. Structure, function, and inhibition. Cell Biochem Biophys 1999;30:115–151.

26. Gong CX, Singh TJ, Grundke-Iqbal I, Iqbal K. Alzheimer's disease abnormally phosphorylated tau is dephosphorylated by protein phosphatase-2B (calcineurin). J Neurochem 1994;62:803–806.

27. Garver TD, Kincaid RL, Conn RA, Billingsley ML. Reduction of calcineurin activity in brain by antisense oligonucleotides leads to persistent phosphorylation of tau protein at Thr181 and Thr231. Mol Pharmacol 1999;55:632–641.

28. Kayyali US, Zhang W, Yee AG, et al. Cytoskeletal changes in the brains of mice lacking calcineurin A alpha. J Neurochem 1997;68:1668–1678.

29. Xie HQ, Johnson GV. Calcineurin inhibition prevents calpain-mediated proteolysis of tau in differentiated PC12 cells. J Neurosci Res 1998;53:153–164.

30. Ladner CJ, Czech J, Maurice J, et al. Reduction of calcineurin enzymatic activity in Alzheimer's disease: correlation with neuropathologic changes. J Neuropathol Exp Neurol 1996;55:924–931.

31. Billingsley ML, Ellis C, Kincaid RL, et al. Calcineurin immunoreactivity in Alzheimer's disease. Exp Neurol 1994;126:178–184.

32. Brion JP, Couck AM, Conreur JL. Calcineurin (phosphatase 2B) is present in neurons containing neurofibrillary tangles and in a subset of senile plaques in Alzheimer's disease. Neurodegeneration 1995;4:13–21.

33. Asai A, Qiu J, Narita Y, et al. High level calcineurin activity predisposes neuronal cells to apoptosis. J Biol Chem 1999;274:34,450–34,458.

34. Alexanian AR, Bamburg JR. Neuronal survival activity of s100betabeta is enhanced by calcineurin inhibitors and requires activation of NF-kappaB. FASEB J 1999;13:1611–1620.

35. Desdouits F, Buxbaum JD, Desdouits-Magnen J, et al. Amyloid beta peptide formation in cell-free preparations: regulation by protein kinase C, calmodulin, and calcineurin. J Biol Chem 1996;271:24,670–24,674.

36. Ankarcrona M, Dypbukt JM, Orrenius S, Nicotera P. Calcineurin and mitochondrial function in glutamate-induced neuronal cell death. FEBS Lett 1996;394:321–324.

37. Stein-Behrens BA, Lin WJ, Sapolsky RM. Physiological elevations of glucocorticoids potentiate glutamate accumulation in the hippocampus. J Neurochem 1994;63:596–602.

38. Mattson MP. Apoptosis in neurodegenerative disorders. Nat Rev Mol Cell Biol 2000;1:120–129.

39. Su J H, Anderson AJ, Cummings B, Cotman CW. Immunocytochemical evidence for apoptosis in Alzheimer's disease. NeuroReport 1994;5:2529–2533.

40. Masliah E, Mallory M, Alford M, et al. Caspase dependent DNA fragmentation might be associated with excitotoxicity in Alzheimer disease. J Neuropathol Exp Neurol 1998;57:1041–1052.

41. Chan SL, Griffin WS, Mattson MP. Evidence for caspase-mediated cleavage of AMPA receptor subunits in neuronal apoptosis and Alzheimer's disease. J Neurosci Res 1999;57:315–323.

42. Su JH, Deng G, Cotman CW. Bax protein expression is increased in Alzheimer's brain: correlations with DNA damage, Bcl-2 expression, and brain pathology. J Neuropathol Exp Neurol 1997;56:86–93.

43. Vincent I, Rosado M, Davies P. Mitotic mechanisms in Alzheimer's disease? J Cell Biol. 1996;132:413–425.
44. Keller JN, Kindy MS, Holtsberg FW, et al. Mitochondrial MnSOD prevents neural apoptosis and reduces ischemic brain injury: suppression of peroxynitrite production, lipid peroxidation and mitochondrial dysfunction. J Neurosci 1998;18:687–697.
45. Lemasters JJ, Nieminen AL, Qian T, et al. The mitochondrial permeability transition in cell death: a common mechanism in necrosis, apoptosis and autophagy. Biochim Biophys Acta 1998;1366:177–196.
46. Friberg H, Ferrand-Drake M, Bengstsson F, et al. Cyclosporin A, but not FK 506, protects mitochondria and neurons against hypoglycemic damage and implicates the mitochondrial permeability transition in cell death. J Neurosci 1998;18:5151–159.
47. Matsumoto S, Friberg H, Ferrand-Drake M, Wieloch T. (1999) Blocade of mitochondrial permeability transition pore diminishes infarct size in the rat after transient middle cerebral artery occlusion. J Cereb Blood Flow Metab 1999;19:736–741.
48. Sheehan JP, Swerdlow RH, Miller SW, et al. Calcium homeostasis and reactive oxygen species production in cells transformed by mitochondria from individuals with sporadic Alzheimer's disease. J Neurosci 1997;17:4612–4622.
49. Cassarino DS, Swerdlow RH, Parks JK, et al. Cyclosporin A increases resting mitochondrial membrane potential in SY5Y cells and reverses the depressed mitochondrial membrane potential of Alzheimer's disease cybrids. Biochem Biophys Res Commun 1998;248:168–173.
50. Kruman II, Mattson MP. Pivotal role of mitochondrial calcium uptake in neural cell apoptosis and necrosis. J Neurochem 1999;72:529–540.
51. Guo Q, Furukawa K, Sopher BL, et al. Alzheimer's PS-1 mutation perturbs calcium homeostasis and sensitizes PC12 cells to death induced by amyloid beta-peptide. Neuroreport 1996;8:379–383.
52. Chapman PF, White GL, Jones MW, et al. Impaired synaptic plasticity and learning in aged amyloid precursor protein transgenic mice. Nat Neurosci 1999;2:271–276.
53. Parent A, Linden DJ, Sisodia SS, Borchelt DR. Synaptic transmission and hippocampal long-term potentiation in transgenic mice expressing FAD-linked presenilin 1. Neurobiol Dis 1999;6:56–62.
54. Zaman SH., Parent A, Laskey A, et al. Enhanced synaptic potentiation in transgenic mice expressing presenilin 1 familial Alzheimer's disease mutation is normalized with a benzodiazepine. Neurobiol Dis 2000;7:54–63.
55. Mark J, Hensley K, Butterfield DA, Mattson MP. Amyloid beta-peptide impairs ion-motive ATPase activities: evidence for a role in loss of neuronal Ca^{2+} homeostasis and cell death. J Neurosci 1995;15:6329–6249.
56. Albensi BC, Sullivan PG, Thompson MB, et al. Cyclosporin ameliorates traumatic brain-injury-induced alterations of hippocampal synaptic plasticity. Exp Neurol 2000;162:385–389.
57. Scheff SW, Sullivan PG. Cyclosporin A significantly ameliorates cortical damage following experimental traumatic brain injury in rodents. J Neurotrauma 1999;16:783–792.

58. Marks R. Immunophilin Modulation of Calcium Channel Gating. Methods 1996;9:177–187.

59. Dawson TM, Steiner JP, Dawson VL, et al. Immunosuppressant FK506 enhances phosphorylation of nitric oxide synthase and protects against glutamate neurotoxicity. Proc Natl Acad Sci USA 1993;90:9808–9812.

60. Cameron AM, Steiner JP, Sabatini DM, et al. Immunophilin FK506 binding protein associated with inositol 1,4,5-trisphosphate receptor modulates calcium flux. Proc Natl Acad Sci USA 1995;92:1784–1788.

61. Bultynck G, Smet PD, Weidema AF, et al. Effects of the immunosuppressant FK506 on intracellular Ca^{2+} release and Ca^{2+} accumulation mechanisms. J Physiol (Lond) 2000;525:681–693.

62. Bush KT, Hendrickson BA, Nigam SK. Induction of the FK506-binding protein, FKBP13, under conditions which misfold proteins in the endoplasmic reticulum. Biochem J 1994;303:705–708.

63 Leissring MA, Akbari Y, Fanger CM, et al. Capacitative calcium entry deficits and elevated luminal calcium content in mutant presenilin-1 knockin mice. J Cell Biol 2000;149:793–798.

64. Leissring MA, Parker I, LaFerla FM. Presenilin-2 mutations modulate amplitude and kinetics of inositol 1, 4,5-trisphosphate-mediated calcium signals. J Biol Chem 1999;274:32,535–32,538.

65. Pack-Chung E, Meyers MB, Pettingell WP, et al. Presenilin 2 interacts with sorcin, a modulator of the ryanodine receptor. J Biol Chem 2000;275: 14,440–14,445.

66. McGeer EG, McGeer PL. Brain inflammation in Alzheimer disease and the therapeutic implications. Curr Pharm Des 1999;5:821–836.

67. Meda L, Cassatella MA, Szendrei GI, et al. Activation of microglial cells by beta-amyloid protein and interferon-gamma. Nature 1995;374:647–650.

68. Tan J, Town T, Paris D, et al. Microglial activation resulting from CD40-CD40L interaction after beta-amyloid stimulation. Science 1999;286: 2352–2355.

69. Sawada M, Suzumura A, Marunouchi T. Down regulation of CD4 expression in cultured microglia by immunosuppressants and lipopolysaccharide. Biochem Biophys Res Commun 1992;189:869–876.

70. Lee RK, Knapp S, Wurtman RJ Prostaglandin E2 stimulates amyloid precursor protein gene expression: inhibition by immunosuppressants. J Neurosci 1999;19:940–947.

71. Schinkel AH, Wagenaar E, Mol CA, van Deemter L. P-glycoprotein in the blood-brain barrier of mice influences the brain penetration and pharmacological activity of many drugs. J Clin Invest 1996;97:2517–2524.

72. Uno T, Kazui T, Suzuki Y, et al. Pharmacokinetic advantages of a newly developed tacrolimus oil-in-water-type emulsion via the enteral route. Lipids 1999;34:249–254.

73. Khaspekov L, Friberg H, Halestrap A, et al. Cyclosporin A and its nonimmunosuppressive analogue N-Me-Val-4-cyclosporin A mitigate glucose/oxygen deprivation-induced damage to rat cultured hippocampal neurons. Eur J Neurosci 1999;11:3194–3198.

74. Howard MA 3d, Dacey RG Jr, Winn HR. Brain xenografts: the effect of cyclosporin A on graft survival. J Neurosurg 1988;69:121–126.

8

Cyclosporin A Protects Striatal Neurons from Mitochondrial Dysfunction

Implications for Huntington's Disease

Liza Leventhal and Jeffrey H. Kordower

HUNTINGTON'S DISEASE

Huntington's disease (HD) is a devastating neurodegenerative disease characterized by involuntary choreiform movements, psychiatric disturbances, behavioral changes, cognitive abnormalities of the frontal-type, as well as dementia *(1)*. The age of onset is usually between the third and fifth decade of life, although juvenile (<20 yr of age) and late-onset (>65 yr of age) cases do occur *(2)*. HD is an autosomal dominant, fully penetrant, genetic defect on the short arm of chromosome 4, specifically at the IT15 gene locus *(3)*. The genetic defect on chromosome 4 results in an increased number of repeats (>39) encoding polyglutamine tracts (CAG). The gene encodes for the protein huntingtin. Intranuclear inclusions are found in cortical and striatal neurons in postmortem tissue of HD patients as a result of the polyglutamine-expanded N-terminal region of mutant huntingtin suggesting that aggregation of this protein may be involved in the pathogenesis of HD *(4)*. Recently, CAG expansion has been shown to activate caspase-8, a known trigger of apoptotic cell death *(5)*. However, the specific mechanism(s) by which the polyglutamine expansion damages and ultimately destroys neurons remains to be established.

Pathologically, HD can be defined as a genetic disorder characterized by a programmed, premature death of a specific population of vulnerable neurons. The most striking changes occur in the caudate nucleus and putamen. Within these striatal regions, medium-sized spiny neurons are particularly vulnerable *(6–10)*. By contrast, large aspiny interneurons and medium aspiny neurons are less affected. Neurochemically, HD involves an impairment and loss of γ-aminobutyric acid (GABA)-containing neurons, which provide inhibitory innervation to the globus pallidus and substantia nigra

From: *Immunosuppressant Analogs in Neuroprotection*
Edited by: C. V. Borlongan, O. Isacson, and P. R. Sanberg © Humana Press Inc., Totowa, NJ

pars reticulata *(6–10)*. Early in the disease, GABAergic/enkephalinergic projections to the external globus pallidus appear preferentially affected *(11,12)*. Furthermore, levels of choline striatal acetyltransferase, substance P, cholecystokinin, and angiotensin-converting enzyme are also reduced *(1)*. Neurons containing NADPH-diaphorase and neurotensin are unaffected in HD *(13)* and a number of peptides that colocalize with NADPH–diaphorase and such as somatostatin and neuropeptide Y are also relatively spared *(2)*. Other nonstriatal brain regions such as the cerebral cortex, globus pallidus, and substantia nigra may also be affected in HD *(6–10)*. Neurodegeneration observed in non-striatal regions is variable and does not correlate with disease severity *(1,3,6–8,10)*. There are currently no effective treatments for the individuals that suffer from HD.

In contrast to other neurodegenerative diseases such as Parkinson's or Alzheimer's disease, genetic testing can positively identify individuals who are destined to have HD. When a patient with PD is first diagnosed clinically, there has already been an extensive loss of striatal dopamine and severe degeneration of dopaminergic neurons within the substantia nigra pars compacta *(14)*. Similarly, in patients with AD, within the first year of diagnosis significant decreases in cortical markers of acetylcholine can be observed, and there is already a considerable accumulation of neuritic plaques and neurofibrillary tangles *(14)*. Thus, in PD and AD extensive neurological damage sufficient to produce clinical symptoms must occur in order to make a diagnosis. Thus even with the development of novel and potent new therapies, a neuropathological process has already begun at the time of diagnosis and this ongoing cascade may be difficult to slow or reverse. HD is one clear exception in that detection can occur very early in life, even *in utero*. Hence individuals who will ultimately become HD patients can unequivocally be identified before onset of neural degeneration or clinical symptoms. If a therapeutic intervention were made available, it could be used well before the onset of the cellular degenerative processes providing an opportunity to delay or prevent clinical symptoms. If neuroprotection is the ultimate goal for treating HD patients, the focus of ongoing therapeutic strategies research should target the GABAergic medium-sized spiny striatal neurons that are severely impaired in HD by attempting to prevent or slow the loss of these vulnerable neurons.

RODENT MODELS OF HD

The ability to develop therapeutic strategies for HD depends in part on the accuracy of animal models in mimicking the disease process. Early models of HD used either nonspecific mechanical/electrolytic lesions of the striatum or pharmacological induction of dyskinesia-like behaviors in rodents (for review, *see* ref. *15*). These models lacked both anatomical and behavioral specificity. Initially, it was suggested that cell death in HD resulted from a slow endogenous excitotoxic process *(1,16)*. Accordingly, intrastriatally administrated excitatory amino acids were employed as animal models of HD *(15)*. Quinolinic acid lesions of the striatum reproduce the pattern of degeneration observed in HD patients with a preferential loss of medium spiny GABAergic neurons and sparing of both medium spiny neurons that stain for NADPH-diaphorase and large aspiny cholinergic neurons *(7)*. Excitotoxic lesions of the striatum also mimic motor and cognitive changes observed in HD *(17,18)*.

It has also been suggested that neuronal death occurring in HD is related to mitochondrial dysfunction *(19)*. The mitochondrial toxin 3-nitropropionic acid (3NP) produces striatal lesions similar to those observed in HD *(19)*. Systemic administration of 3NP, an irreversible inhibitor of succinate dehydrogenase and complex II, selectively damages medium-sized spiny neurons in the striatum of rats and nonhuman primates reproducing some of HD's neuropathological and behavioral sequelae *(19–22)*. Initial animal studies employing 3NP were difficult to perform because of high mortality rates and disparate lesion sizes under identical dosing regimens. However, a recent investigation has demonstrated that there are strain differences in 3NP sensitivity in rodents, such that more uniform dosing and consistent lesions are observed in the Lewis rat strain *(23)*. This important finding allows for an improved means to evaluate novel therapeutic strategies.

While QA and 3NP lesions can replicate the pattern of degeneration and many behavioral features of HD, the mechanisms of cell death are clearly different from what occurs in the disease. Since HD is a genetic disorder and the gene responsible for HD is known, transgenic technology allowed for the creation of genetic models of HD that duplicated the genetic defect seen in HD. Several HD models have been generated to date with a wide spectrum of biological phenomena due to differing promoters, amount of the coding sequence included in the transgene, or the mouse strain used. The demonstration by gene targeting that HD knockouts were lethal embryologically suggested that the HD mutation likely acted via a gain of function rather by a dominant-negative mechanism. Thus, the introduction of the HD mutation into the mouse germline could be expected to generate a mouse model of HD. For the most part, transgenic HD animals that express mutated huntingtin display an overt behavioral phenotype that is observed independent of substantial pathological changes. The first HD mice were described by Bates and coworkers *(24)* who initially created four R6 mouse lines with CAG repeats between 115 and 156 in length. Three of these lines displayed both transgene expression and a behavioral phenotype with a behavioral onset between 2 and 4–5 mo depending on repeat length. These mice displayed an irregular gait, stereotypic grooming behavior, shuddering, tremor, myoclonus, and a tendency to clasp hindlimbs. Detailed motor analyses revealed that the timing of motor deficits as measured by rotorod, beam walking, swimming, and footprint analyses differed depending upon the nature and difficulty of the task being measured with deficits being found as early as 5 wk of age *(24)*. Subsequent reports using one of the mouse lines revealed cognitive deficits on the Morris water maze as well as alterations in synaptic plasticity within the CA1 hippocampal region and the dentate gyrus *(25)*. Initial reports revealed that, although significant behavioral abnormalities were present early on, no evidence of cell death was seen at 12 wk of age. However, fibrillar intranuclear inclusions could be seen in the cortex, striatum, and cingulate gyrus in these animals *(26,27)*. More recent studies revealed degeneration within the dorsal striatum, anterior cingulate gyrus, and purkinje cells of the cerebellum late in the disease process *(28)*. Hayden and coworkers *(29)*created a YAC transgenic mouse model of HD that recapitulates many of the features of HD. The YAC mice are transgenic for the entire huntingtin gene, including all its regulatory sequences. YAC mice with 46 or 72 polyglutamine repeats developed a progressive neurodegenerative phenotype characterized by behavioral, electrophysiological, and molecular abnormalities similar to those observed in HD patients. YAC72 mice displayed hyperkinetic behavior and a loss of long-term potentiation. YAC72 mice had a 40–80% loss of medium spiny neurons within the lateral striatum, an effect that occurred independent of neuronal aggregate formation. The morphology of striatal cells in these mice was consistent with apoptosis. A third group led by Dan Tagle created a transgenic mouse model using full-length huntingtin. These animals display motor deficits beginning at 2 mo of age. Neuronal loss occurs in the striatum, but not until the end-stage of the disease process. We have found that dendritic changes precede neuronal loss and that mitochondrial impairment appears to be a consequence, and not a cause, of the neuropathological changes. The pathological changes seen in transgenic HD mice are not immutable as both creatine *(31)* and caspase-inhibitors *(32)* have been shown to be neuroprotective in these models. These studies demonstrate that the pathogenic cascade mediated by polyglutamine tract expansion can be prevented by novel experimental therapeutic strategies.

More recently, a novel model incorporating the genetic mutation involved in HD has been developed. This model employs intrastriatal transfection of an adeno-associated viral vector encoding for exon 1 of the polyglutamine expansion observed in HD *(33)*. This novel method has advantages to most transgenic techniques in that it allows for direct targeting of expanded polyglutamine expression to striatal neurons that are most affected in HD. Histological evaluation of the striatum in animals injected with AAV encoding for an expanded 97 polyglutamine repeats revealed rapid formation of intracellular cyctoplasmic aggregates similar to those observed in HD *(33)*. Within the striatum, these animals also developed many ubiquitinated nuclear inclusion bodies that induced cell loss via an apoptotic pathway *(33)*. The potential of this model to extend beyond rodent to nonhuman primate models has important implications for future testing of novel therapeutic strategies.

MITOCHONDRIAL DYSFUNCTION AND HD

The role mitochondria play in cell death and neurodegeneration is an area of intense investigation. The degree of mitochondrial calcium buffering during excitotoxic events is critical not only in determining neuronal viability, but also establishing whether the cell undergoes a necrotic or apoptotic fate. It has been suggested that necrotic cell death following acute neuronal injury results from deficient mitochondrial and glycolytic ATP production causing loss of ionic homeostasis and osmotic cell lysis *(34)*. However, the role of mitochondria-induced necrosis in chronic neurodegenerative disorders is unclear. In contrast to necrotic cell death, the role of mitochondria in apoptotic death is better understood. Exposure to high levels of calcium or oxidative stress causes the mitochondria megachannel to open resulting in subsequent disruption of mitochondrial potential termed mitochondrial permeability transition (MPT) *(35,36)*. MPT occurs during many types of neuronal injury and often leads to the release of procaspases, cytochrome *c*, and apoptosis inducing factor, all early triggers of apoptotic cell death *(37–39)*. Thus, MPT is considered an early event in some forms of apoptotic cell death *(37–39)*.

In some neurodegenerative diseases mitochondrial aberrations are associated with primary mitochondrial DNA abnormalities but in others mitochondrial irregularities result in secondary dysfunction of the mitochondrial respiratory chain. This precipitates a cascade of events ultimately leading to cell death *(34)*. It has been suggested that inherited mitochondrial defects could be the cause of neuronal degeneration resulting from energy defects and oxidative damage since mitochondrial metabolism is the primary source of high-energy intermediates and free radicals *(34)*.

Despite the discovery of the genetic abnormality in HD located in chromosome 4 *(3)*, and the related mutant protein huntingtin, the mechanism by which neurodegeneration occurs in HD patients is still unclear. A growing body of evidence indicates that mitochondrial dysfunction may play an important role in the pathogenesis of HD and this mitochondrial dysfunction may be mediated by the genetic mutation *(16,19,40)*. This concept is supported by the selectivity and susceptibility of rodent and primate medium-sized spiny striatal neurons to mitochondrial toxins *(19–22)* as well as data from transgenic mouse studies. HD transgenic mice have impaired energy metabolism secondary to the genetic deficit that may contribute to cell death including mitochondrial complex IV deficiency and elevated nitric oxide and superoxide radical generation *(41)*. Further, marked reductions in *N*-acetylaspartate concentrations *(42)* and increased sensitivity to mitochondrial toxins *(43)* have also been reported in HD mice.

Postmortem studies in human brain tissue also suggest that mitochondrial dysfunction may be a primary pathological event in HD. HD brains have biochemical defects in the mitochondrial respiratory chain *(44,45)* as well as reductions in the activity of mitochondrial complex II–III in caudate *(44–46)* and putamen *(45)*. Recently, repeat length-dependent mitochondrial impairment in lymphoblasts obtained from HD patients has also been reported *(40)*. Therefore, prevention of mitochondrial dysfunction maybe an important neuroprotective strategy for HD regardless of whether dysfunction involves primary or secondary mitochondrial impairment.

CYCLOSPORINE AND MITOCHONDRIA
PERMEABILITY TRANSITION

The linkage between mitochondrial dysfunction, neuronal death, and HD suggests that blockade of MPT might be neuroprotective in this patient population. Indeed, compounds that block MPT and the initiation of cell death have proved protective in numerous models of neuronal injury (e.g., *47–50*). One such drug is the immunosuppressant agent cyclosporin A (CsA). CsA is an immunophilin, defined as a group of proteins including FK506 and rapamycin that serve as receptors for immunosuppressant drugs. Unlike other immunophilin compounds, CsA is unique in that it has the ability to inhibit MPT *(51)*. These actions are mediated by CsA's ability to inhibit translocation of the mitochondrial matrix-specific cyclophilin D to the inner mitochondrial membrane resulting in decreased sensitivity of the mitochondrial megachannel to calcium ions *(51)*. Based upon this property, CsA has been investigated for its potential use as a neuroprotective agent.

Studies in vitro have demonstrated that CsA attenuates apoptosis induced by mitochondrial complex 1 toxins, such as 1-methyl-4-phenyl-1,2,3,6-tetrahydropyridine, rotenone, tetrahydroisoquinoline *(47)*, and calcium ionophore A2317 *(52)*. CsA also prevents delayed mitochondrial depolarization resulting from exposure to *N*-methyl-D-aspartate (NMDA: *48*), or ion-induced mitochondrial swelling secondary to calcium withdrawal *(49)*. The ability of CsA to cross the blood–brain barrier (BBB) is limited in vivo, requiring high doses or disruption of the BBB for CsA to reach vulnerable neuronal systems *(53)*. Employing procedures to penetrate the brain parenchyma, CsA protection has been observed following ischemia–reperfusion *(50)*, transient forebrain ischemia *(53)*, hypoglycemia *(49)*, or traumatic brain injury *(54)*. Thus, based on the previous studies, CsA might have therapeutic potential in attenuating cell death in neurodegenerative diseases such as HD in which cell death may result from mitochondrial impairment.

CYCLOSPORIN A TREATMENT AND 3-NITROPRIOPONIC ACID

Given the ability of CsA to prevent cell death in models of neuronal injury involving mitochondrial impairment and the evidence that mitochondrial dysfunction may play an important role in the pathogenesis of HD, our laboratory recently investigated whether CsA could protect striatal cells from the mitochondrial toxin 3NP.

We initially examined the ability of CsA to protect striatal neurons from 3NP-induced cell death in vitro *(55)*. Striatal cultures were derived from the lateral ganglionic eminence, the developmental primordia of the striatum *(56)*, and were used in a microisland preparation *(57,58)*. In the first experiment, cultures were pretreated once with 0, 0.2, 1, or 5 *M* concentrations of CsA and exposed to either 0 or 5 m*M* 3NP. All cultures were fixed for quantification of glutamate acid decarboxylase immunoreactive (GAD-ir), a marker of medium sized spiny striatal neurons. Significant differences in GAD-ir were observed between treatment groups. Analysis of GAD-ir neuronal counts revealed that 3NP treatment significantly decreased GAD-ir neurons to 20% of control levels. Relative to control cultures, neurons in these cultures appeared degenerative, displaying shrunken cell bodies and stunted processes (Fig. 1A,B). Pretreatment with a 0.2 *M* and 1.0 *M*, but not 5.0 *M* dose of CsA significantly attenuated the 3NP-induced loss of GAD-ir cells. Importantly, CsA-treated cultures displayed a sparing of GAD-ir neurons and neuronal processes (Fig. 1C) compared to 3NP alone (Fig. 1B).

In the second in vitro experiment, cultures were pretreated twice with 0, 0.2, 1, or 5 *M* concentrations of CsA beginning 1 d prior to, and on the day of, exposure to either 0 or 5 m*M* 3NP. All cultures were fixed for quantification of GAD-ir neurons. Significant differences in GAD-ir neurons were again observed between treatment groups. Analysis of GAD-ir neuronal counts revealed that 3NP treatment significantly decreased GAD-ir neurons to 30% of control levels. Pretreating the cultures twice with 0.2 μM or 5.0 μM CsA significantly attenuated the 3NP-induced loss of GAD-ir cells.

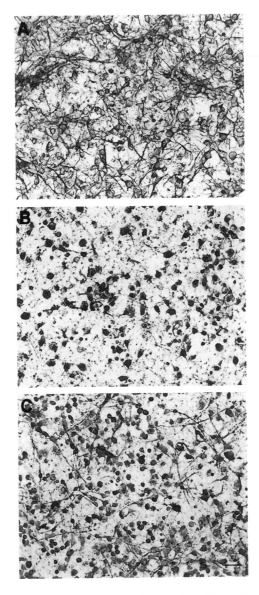

Fig. 1. GAD-ir staining of striatal cultures. **(A)** Control cultures displayed numerous GAD-ir neurons with extensive processes. **(B)** In contrast, 3NP-treated cultures appeared devastated with a dramatic decrease in number of GAD-ir cells. The remaining cells displayed shrunked cell bodies and stunted processes. **(C)** In striatal cultures treated once with 1 μ*M* CsA, there was an attenuation of 3NP-induced loss of GAD-ir neurons as well as a sparing of neuronal processes. Scale bar = 35 μm. (Leventhal et al., 2000; reprinted with permission from *Journal of Comparative Neurology*)

In contrast, the 1.0 μM dose of CsA failed to protect GAD-ir cells. Thus, in vitro, CsA produced neuroprotective effects upon GABAergic neurons with a single administration of the lower 0.2 and 1.0 μM doses, but not at the higher 5.0 μM dose. When treated twice, a similar level of neuroprotection was observed, but this treatment did not appear additive relative to singly treated cultures.

Based on the in vitro data, we examined whether CsA would protect striatal neurons from 3NP neurotoxicity in vivo. For reasons described above, we employed the Lewis rat model of HD—a model that causes bilateral striatal degeneration of medium-sized spiny neurons *(55)*. Since CsA purportedly has limited access to the brain, the first experiment examined whether CsA could provide protection from 3NP toxicity with and without BBB disruption. In this experiment, rats received a saline injection into the striatum unilaterally to disrupt the BBB on one side. Rats were also simultaneously implanted with an osmotic minipump containing 3NP (40 mg/kg/d) into the subcutaneous space for 6 d *(23)*. Animals received daily intraperitoneal injections of CsA (15 mg/kg) or vehicle commencing 1 d prior to surgery and continuing daily throughout the 3NP treatment period. After sacrifice all tissue was fixed for immunohistochemical visualization of dopamine- and adenosine-3',5'-monophosphate-regulated phosphoprotein (DARPP32), a marker for medium sized spiny striatal neurons *(59,60)* and stereological analysis *(61)*.

Stereological analysis of DARPP32 immunostained sections through the striatum following 3NP and CsA treatment revealed a significant difference between hemispheres. Specifically, 3NP-treated rats receiving CsA with unilateral BBB disruption displayed protection only in the striatum ipsilateral to the disruption. The number of striatal DARPP32-ir neurons contralateral to BBB disruption was similar to that observed in nondisrupted vehicle-treated 3NP rats. These data clarify an important issue. The protection was not likely due to CsA degrading 3NP in the periphery since a sparing of neurons was significantly greater in the striatum for which CsA could gain access. It is possible that unilateral disruption of BBB may cause a slight disruption of the contralateral hemisphere resulting in CsA increased penetration. However, previous studies do not support this contention *(62)*.

The second experiment examined whether CsA (0, 5, 15, 20 mg/kg) could protect striatal neurons from 3NP toxicity in rats in a dose-dependent manner following bilateral disruption of the BBB. In this experiment, rats received bilateral intrastriatal saline injections to facilitate CsA crossing the BBB. Rats were simultaneously implanted with an osmotic minipump containing 3NP (40 mg/kg/d) into the subcutaneous space for 6 d *(23)*. Animals then received daily intraperitoneal injections of CsA or vehicle commencing 1 d prior to surgery and continuing throughout the 3NP treatment period. After sacrifice, all tissue was fixed for immunohistochemical visualization DARPP32 and choline-acetyltransferase (ChAT), a marker for cholinergic striatal interneurons.

Stereological counts of striatal DARPP32-ir cells revealed significant differences between treatment groups. DARPP32-ir cells counts were significantly decreased in vehicle-treated 3NP rats compared to nonlesioned vehicle controls. Rats receiving 3NP lesioned treatment and vehicle displayed large areas of degeneration within the striatum characterized by a comprehensive loss of DARPP32-ir neurons (Fig. 2B,D). Similarly, 3NP lesioned rats treated with CsA 5 mg/kg displayed similar numbers of DARPP32-ir neurons as 3NP-lesioned vehicle-treated animals. By contrast, rats treated with 15 or 20 mg/kg CsA displayed a robust protection of DARPP32-ir neurons within the striatum (Fig. 2A,C). In fact, DARPP32-ir cell counts for 3NP rats treated with 15 or 20 mg/kg CsA were indistinguishable from nonlesioned vehicle controls. Also 3NP-lesioned rats treated with the higher 15 or 20 mg/kg dose of CsA had a significantly greater number of DARPP32-ir neurons compared to rats treated with the lower 5 mg/kg dose of CsA illustrating the dose dependency of this effect. Furthermore, within the lesion area, all treatment groups displayed large cell bodies that were positive for ChAT-ir confirming the selectivity of the toxin (Fig. 2E,F).

These present data show that CsA protects striatal neurons from 3NP-toxicity. Other researchers have recently reported preliminary data suggest that CsA reduces functional impairments in 3NP-treated rats *(63)*. In this experiment attenuation of hindlimb paralysis was observed in CsA-treated 3NP rats compared to control 3NP-treated rats. Importantly, behavioral protection was observed at 20 mg/kg ip an identical dose in which neuropathological protection was observed *(55)*.

CONCLUSION AND IMPLICATIONS

Although it is known that CsA prevents MPT and ensuing mitochondrial dysfunction within the brain, the specific mechanism(s) by which CsA protects medium-sized spiny neurons from 3NP toxicity remains unknown. Studies in vitro demonstrated that 3NP results in dose-dependent cell death a delayed apoptosis at lower doses and an acute excitotoxic necrosis at higher doses *(64)*. The present in vitro data employed a dose that is known to result in apoptotic cell death. Thus it is likely that CsA protection in vitro is mediated by inhibiting this apoptotic cell death initi-

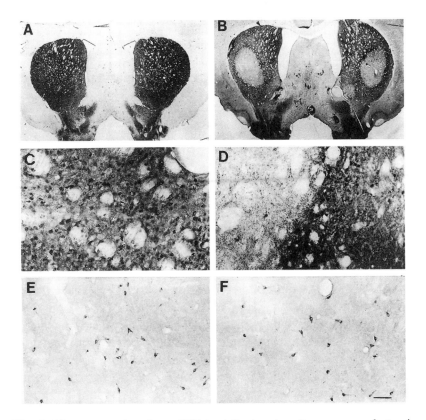

Fig. 2. Neuroprotection from 3NP toxicity in vivo. Low-power photomicrographs of DARPP32-ir. (**A**) 3NP rats treated with 15 mg/kg CsA displayed a protection of DARPP32-ir neurons within the precommisural striatum. (**B**) In contrast, vehicle-treated 3NP rats displayed large areas of decreased DARPP-32-ir. Higher-power photomicrographs of striatal DARPP32-ir in the same section as **A** and **B**. (**C**) CsA/3NP-treated rats had numerous medium-sized DARPP32-ir positive neurons throughout the striatum. (**D**) Conversely, within the lesion area **B** of veh/3NP-treated rats there was a marked loss in the number of DARPP32-ir cells. High-power photomicrograph of ChAT-ir. (**E**) CsA/3NP-treated rats had equally distributed ChAT-ir neurons throughout the striatum. (**F**) Similarly, in the lesion area **B** and surrounding regions of veh/3NP-treated rats ChAT-ir neurons were spared. Scale bar = 1000 μm (**A** and **B**) and 50 μm (**C–F**). (Leventhal et al., 2000; reprinted with permission from *Journal of Comparative Neurology.*)

ated by mitochondrial impairment *(39)*. Similarly, 3NP studies in vivo have demonstrated strain differences, method of toxin delivery, and dosing can affect the magnitude and form of striatal cell death *(23)*. The Lewis rat model accurately reproduced the pattern of cell loss observed in HD including the preferential degeneration of GABAergic projection neurons with a relative sparing of interneurons *(23)*. Furthermore, the Lewis rat model also used a dosing regimen that produces many TUNEL-positive cells and apoptotic bodies *(23)*. Therefore, it is likely that CsA protection in vivo is preventing apoptosis resulting from mitochondrial impairment. Research also indicates a potential role for CsA in abating some of the pathological features of HD. Specifically, this occurs by reducing repeat length-dependent mitochondrial impairment in lymphoblasts obtained from HD patients *(40)* and by protecting striatal neurons from calcium ionophore-induced toxicity in vitro *(52)*. However, additional studies are necessary to confirm the specific mechanisms by which CsA protects against cell death produced by 3NP toxicity.

In summary, CsA treatment protects medium-sized spiny neurons from 3NP, a toxin that mimics the primary neuropathological features seen in HD. Our laboratory's data support previous experiments indicating that in order for systemically administered CsA to reach maximal therapeutic levels within the parenchyma the BBB must be compromised *(53)*. This issue is meaningful as it relates to potential clinical benefits. By disrupting the BBB, lower doses of CsA could potentially be used to provide striatal protection, avoiding the toxicity associated with higher doses *(65,66)*. Furthermore, it indicates the need for novel compounds with better access to the brain and lacking the negative side effects associated with CsA treatment. Thus, CsA or more lipophilic analogs of this compound may be of potential therapeutic benefit by protecting this vulnerable population of neurons from the primary pathological event observed in HD.

ACKNOWLEDGMENTS

We thank Drs. Stephane Palfi, Caryl Sortwell, Timothy Collier, and Rose Hanbury for their collaboration in this project as well as Bridget Gavin-Terraova for expert technical assistance. In addition, we are grateful to Dr. Paul Greengard for the gift of the DARPP32 antibody. This work was funded by T32A600257 (L.L), AG00844, and NS35078 (J.H.K).

REFERENCES

1. Greenamyre JT, Shoulson I. (1994) Huntington's disease. In: Calne D, ed. Neurodegenerative Diseases, Saunders, Philadelphia, PA, pp. 685–704.
2. Conneally PM. Huntington disease: genetics and epidemiology. Am J Hum Genet 1984;36:506–526.
3. Huntington's Disease Collaborative Research Group. A novel gene containing a trinucleotide repeat that is expanded and unstable on Huntington's disease chromosomes. Cell 1993;72:971–978.

4. DiFiglia M, Sapp E, Chase KO, et al. Aggregation of huntingtin in neuronal intranuclear inclusions and dystrophic neurites in brain. Science 1997;277: 1990–1993.

5. Sanchez I, Xu OU, Juo P, et al. Caspase-8 is required for cell death induced by expanded polyglutamine repeats. Neuron 1999;22:623–633.

6. Ferrante RJ, Kowall NW, Beal MF, et al. Selective sparing of a class of striatal neurons in Huntington's disease. Science 1985;230:561–563.

7. Ferrante RJ, Beal MF, Kowall NW, et al. Sparing of acetylcholinesterase-containing striatal neurons in Huntington's disease. Brain Res 1987;411: 162–166.

8. Graveland GA, Williams RS, DiFiglia M. Evidence for degenerative and regenerative changes in neostriatal spiny neurons in Huntington's disease. Science 1985;227:770–773.

9. Kowall NW, Ferrante RJ, Martin JB. Pattern of cell loss in Huntington's disease. Trends Neurosci 1987;10:24–29.

10. Vonsattel JP, Myers RH, Stevens TJ, et al. Neuropathological classification of Huntington's disease. J Neuropathol Exp Neurol 1985;44:559–577.

11. Albin RL, Young AB, Penney JB, et al. Abnormalities of striatal projection neurons and N-methyl-D-aspartate receptors in presymptomatic Huntington's disease [see comments]. N Engl J Med 1990;322:1293–1298.

12. Albin RL, Reiner A, Anderson KD, et al. Preferential loss of striato-external pallidal projection neurons in presymptomatic Huntington's disease. Ann Neurol 1992;31:425–430.

13. Martin JB, Gusella JF. Huntington's disease. Pathogenesis and management. N Engl J Med 1986;315:1267–1276.

14. Bjorklund A, Campbell K, Sirinathsinghji DJ, et al. Functional capacity of striatal transplants in the rat Huntington model. In: Dunnett SB, Bjorklund A, eds. Functional Neural Transplantation. Raven Press, New York, pp. 157–195.

15. Emerich DF, Sanberg PR. Animal models in Huntington's disease. In: Boulton AA, Baker GB, Butterworth RF, eds., Neuromethods, vol. 17. Humana Press, Totowa, NJ, pp. 65–134.

16. Albin RL, Greenamyre JT. Alternative excitotoxic hypotheses. Neurology 1992;42:733–738.

17. Isacson O, Brundin P, Kelly PA, et al. Functional neuronal replacement by grafted striatal neurones in the ibotenic acid-lesioned rat striatum. Nature 1984;311:458–460.

18. Emerich DF, Winn SR, Hantraye PM, et al. Protective effect of encapsulated cells producing neurotrophic factor CNTF in a monkey model of Huntington's disease. Nature 1997;386:395–399.

19. Beal MF, Brouillet E, Jenkins BG, et al. Neurochemical and histologic characterization of striatal excitotoxic lesions produced by the mitochondrial toxin 3-nitropropionic acid. J Neurosci 1993;13:4181–4192.

20. Brouillet E, Hantraye P, Ferrante RJ, et al. Chronic mitochondrial energy impairment produces selective striatal degeneration and abnormal choreiform movements in primates. Proc Nat Acad Sci USA 1995;92:7105–7109.

21. Guyot MC, Hantraye P, Dolan R, et al. Quantifiable bradykinesia, gait abnormalities and Huntington's disease-like striatal lesions in rats chronically treated with 3-Nitropropionic acid. Neuroscience 1997;79:45–56.
22. Palfi S, Ferrante RJ, Brouillet E, et al.Chronic 3-nitropropionic acid treatment in baboons replicates the cognitive and motor deficits of Huntington's disease. J Neurosci 1996;16:3019–3025.
23. Ouary S, Bizat N, Altairac S, et al. Major strain differences in response to chronic 3-Nitropriopionic acid in rats: Implications for neuroprotection studies. Neuroscience 2000;97:521–530.
24. Mangiarini L, Sathasivam K, Seller M, et al. Exon 1 of the HD gene with an expanded CAG repeat is sufficient to cause a progressive neurological phenotype in transgenic mice. Cell 1996;87:493–506.
25. Murphy K, Carter P, Lione RJ, et al. Abnormal synaptic plasticity and impaired spatial cognition in mice transgenic for exon 1 of the human Huntington's disease mutation. J Neurosci 2000;20;5115–5123.
26. Becher MW, Kotzuk JA, Sharp AH, et al. Intranuclear neuronal inclusions in Huntington's disease and dentatorubral and pallidoluysian atrophy: correlation between the density of inclusions and IT15 CAG triplet repeat length. Neurobiol Dis 1997;4:387–397.
27. Davies SW, Turmaine M, Cozens BA, et al. Formation of neuronal intranuclear inclusions underlies the neurological dysfunction in mice transgenic for the HD mutation. Cell 1997;90;537–548.
28. Davies SW, Turmaine M, Cozens BA, et al. From neuronal includions to neurodegeneration: neuropathological investigation of a transgenic mouse model of Huntington's disease. Proc Trans R Soc Lond 1999;354:971–979.
29. Hodgson JG, Agopyan N, Gutekunst CA, et al. A YAC mouse model for Huntington's disease with full-length mutant huntingtin, cytoplasmic toxicity, and selective striatal neurodegeneration. Neuron 1999;23:181–192.
30. Reddy PH, Williams M, Charles V, et al. Behavioural abnormalities and selective neuronal loss in HD transgenic mice expressing mutated full-length HD cDNA. Nat Genet 1998;20:198–202.
31. Ferrante RJ, Andreassen OA, Jenkins BG, et al. Neuroprotective effects of creatine in a transgenic mouse model of Huntington's disease. J Neurosci 2000;20:4389–4397.
32. Ona VO, Li M, Vonsattel JP, et al. Inhibition of caspase-1 slows disease progression in a mouse model of Huntington's disease. Nature 1999;399:263–267.
33. Senut MC, Suhr ST, Kaspar B, Gage FH. Intraneuronal aggregate formation and cell death after viral expression of expanded polyglutamine tracts in the adult rat brain. J Neurosci 2000;20:219–229.
34. Fiskum G, Murphy AN, Beal MF. Mitochondria in neurodegeneration: acute ischemia and chronic neurodegenerative diseases. J Cereb Blood Flow Metab 1999;4:351–369.
35. Crompton M, Costi A, Hayat L. Evidence for the presence of a reversible Ca^{2+}-dependent pore activated by oxidative stress in heart mitochondria. Biochem J 1987;245:915–918.

36. Gunther TE, Pfeiffer DR. Mechanisms by which mitochondria transport calcium. Am J Physiol 1990;258:C755–786.
37. Marchetti P, Castedo M, Susin SA, et al. Mitochondrial permeability transition is a central coordinating event of apoptosis. J Exp Med 1996;184:1155–1160.
38. Kroemer G. The proto-oncogene Bcl-2 and its role in regulating apoptosis. Nat Med 1997;3:614–620.
39. Green DR, Reed JC. Mitochondria and apoptosis. Science 1998;281:1309–1312.
40. Sawa A, Wiegand GW, Cooper J, et al. Increased apoptosis of Huntington disease lymphoblasts associated with repeat length-dependent mitochondrial depolarization. Nat Med 1999;10:1194–1198.
41. Tabrizi SJ, Workman J, Hart PE, et al. Mitochondrial dysfunction and free radical damage in the Huntington R6/2 transgenic mouse. Ann Neurol 2000;47:80–86.
42. Jenkins BG, Klivenyi P, Kustermann E, et al. Nonlinear decrease over time in N-acetyl aspartate levels in the absence of neuronal loss and increases in glutamine and glucose in transgenic Huntington's disease mice. J Neurochem 2000;74:2108–2119.
43. Bogdanov MB, Ferrante RJ, Kuemmerle S, et al. Increased vulnerabilityto 3-nitropropionic acid in an animal model of Huntington's disease. J Neurochem 1998;71:2642–2644.
44. Brennan WA Jr, Bird ED, Aprille JR. Regional mitochondrial respiratory activity in Huntington's disease brain. J Neurochem 1985;44:1948–1950.
45. Browne SE, Bowling AC, MacGarvey U, et al. Oxidative damage and metabolic dysfunction in Huntington's disease: selective vulnerability of the basal ganglia. Ann Neurol 1997;41:646–653.
46. Gu M, Gash MT, Mann VM, et al. Mitochondrial defect in Huntington's disease caudate nucleus. Ann Neurol 1996;39:385–389.
47. Seaton TA, Cooper JM, Schapira AH. Cyclosporin inhibition of apoptosis induced by mitochondrial complex I toxins. Brain Res 1998;809:12–17.
48. Nieminen AL, Petrie TG, Lemasters JJ, Selman WR. Cyclosporin A delays mitochondrial depolarization induced by *N*-methyl-D-aspartate in cortical neurons: evidence of the mitochondrial permeability transition. Neuroscience 1996;75:993–997.
49. Friberg H, Ferrand-Drake M, Bengtsson F, et al. A, but not FK 506, protects mitochondria and neurons against hypoglycemic damage and implicates the mitochondrial permeability transition in cell death. J Neurosci 1998; 18:5151–5159.
50. Shiga Y, Onodera H, Matsuo Y, Kogure K. Cyclosporin A protects against ischemia-reperfusion injury in the brain. Brain Res 1992;595:145–148.
51. Connern CP, Halestrap AP. Recruitment of mitochondrial cyclophilin to the mitochondrial inner-membrane under conditions of oxidative stress that enhance opening of a calcium-sensitive non-specific channel. Biochem J 1994;302:321–324.
52. Petersen A, Castilho PF, Hansson O, et al. Oxidative stress, mitochodrial permeability transition and activation of caspases in calium ionophore A23187-induced death of cultured striatal neurons. Brain Res 2000;857:20–29.

53. Uchino H, Elmer E, Uchino K, et al. Amelioration by cyclosporin A of brain damage in transient forebrain ischemia in the rat. Brain Res 1998;812:216–226.

54. Okonkwo DO, Povlishock JT. An intrathecal bolus of cyclosporin A before injury preserves mitochondrial integrity and attenuates axonal disruption in traumatic brain injury. J Cereb Blood Flow Metab 1999;4:443–451.

55. Leventhal L, Sortwell CE, Hanbury R, et al. Cyclosporin A protects striatal neurons in vitro and in vivo from 3-nitropropionic acid toxicity. J Comp Neurol 2000;425:471–478.

56. Pakzaban A, Deacon TW, Burns LH, Isacson O. Increased proportion of acetylcholiineserase-rich zones and improved morphological integration in host striatum of fetal grafts derived from lateral but not medial ganglionic eminence. Exp Brain Res 1993;97:13–22.

57. Sortwell CE, Collier TJ, Sladek JR. Co-grafted embyronic striatum increases the survival of grafted embyronic dopamine neurons. J Comp Neurol 1998;399:530–540.

58. Takeshima T, Shimoda K, Johnston JM, Commissiong JW. Standardized methods to bioassay neurotrophic factors for dopaminergic neurons. J Neurosci Methods 1996;67:27–41.

59. Hemmings HC Jr, Nairn AC, Aswad DW, Greengard P. (1984) DARPP-32, a dopamine- and adenosine 3':5'-monophosphate-regulated phosphoprotein enriched in dopamine-innervated brain regions. II. Purification and characterization of the phosphoprotein from bovine caudate nucleus. J Neurosci 1984;4:99–110.

60. Hsu SM, Raine L. Protein A, avidin, and biotin in immunohistochemistry. J Histochem Cytochem 1981;29:1349–1353.

61. Ma SY. The subtantia nigra in Parkinson's disease: a morphometric study on neuronal changes. Doctoral thesis, University of Turku, Finland.

62. Kordower JH, Chen EY, Winkler C, et al. Grafts of EGF-responsive neural stem cells derived from GFAP-hNGF transgenic mice: Trophic and tropic effects in a rodent model of Huntington's disease. J Comp Neurol 1997;387:96–113.

63. Watanabe S, Park LCH, Gibson GE, Borlongan CV. Acute effects of 3-Nitroproprionic acid and cyclosporine-A in adult rats. Soc Neurosci Abstr 2000;579:1558.

64. Pang Z, Geddes PW. Mechanisms of cell death induced by the mitochondrial toxin 3-Nitropropionic acid: acute excitotoxic necrosis and delayed apoptosis. J Neurosci 1997;17:3064–3073.

65. Gijtenbeek JM, van den Bent MJ, Vecht CJ. Cyclosporine neurotoxicity: a review. J Neurol 1999;246:339–346.

IV

Immunosuppressants, Stroke, and Traumatic Brain Injury

9

Cyclosporin A Protects Mitochondria in an In Vitro Model of Hypoxia/Reperfusion Injury

Vladimir Gogvadze and Christoph Richter

INTRODUCTION

A major problem in organ infarct or transplantation is hypoxia–reperfusion injury (HRI), where an initial, rather innocuous deprivation of oxygen and energy is followed upon reoxygenation by major damage *(1–3)*.

Many experimental data indicate that mitochondria are one of the most important targets in HRI. Ischemia is accompanied by mitochondrial dysfunction, as assessed by measurements of mitochondrial respiratory activities in vitro and/or release of mitochondrial constituents (enzymes, adenine nucleotides) in vitro and in vivo *(4,5)*. Following brief periods of ischemia, mitochondrial function is usually normalized during reperfusion. However, particularly after ischemia of longer duration, reperfusion may be accompanied by secondary mitochondrial failure. After short periods of ischemia, this is observed in selectively vulnerable areas and, after intermediate to prolonged periods of ischemia, in other areas as well *(6)*.

It has remained unsettled if the mitochondrial dysfunction is the result or the cause of cell death. Although it has commonly been assumed that such failure is secondary to cell injury by other mechanisms, recent results suggest that mitochondrial dysfunction may be the cause of cell death. In many models of HRI the immunosuppressive agent cyclosporin A (CsA), when allowed to cross the blood–brain barrier, was a potent neuroprotectant. It should be mentioned that the ability of CsA to protect cells during ischemia and reperfusion apparently is not conditioned by its immunosuppresive properties. Treatment with CsA (50 mg/kg, iv) showed a robust reduction of brain damage when administered 30 min before insulin-induced hypoglycemic brain damage in vivo. Ultrastructural examination of the dentate gyrus revealed a marked swelling of dendrites and mitochondria during the hypoglycemic insult. In CsA-treated animals, mitochondria resumed a nor-

From: *Immunosuppressant Analogs in Neuroprotection*
Edited by: C. V. Borlongan, O. Isacson, and P. R. Sanberg © Humana Press Inc., Totowa, NJ

mal and contracted appearance during and after the hypoglycemic insult. However, treatment with FK506 (2 mg/kg, iv), a compound with immuno-suppressive action similar to that of CsA, was not protective *(7)*. Moreover, nonimmunosuppressive cyclosporin A analog N-methyl-Val-4-cyclosporin A (10 mg/kg, ip), administered during reperfusion and at 24 h of reperfusion, diminished infarct size in a rat model of transient focal ischemia of 2 h duration *(8)*. Because CsA is a specific blocker of the mitochondrial permeability transition (MPT) pore, a voltage-gated channel allowing molecules and ions with a mass <1500 Da to pass the inner mitochondrial membrane, this provides indirect evidence that damage of mitochondria is the main cause of cell death *(9,10)*.

It is well known that mitochondria can take up and retain cytosolic Ca^{2+} when its concentration increases to levels that allow operation of the low-affinity uptake system. Since the influx of Ca^{2+} across a damaged plasma membrane is a frequent cause of cell death, it can be supposed that mito-chondria may act as a "safety device" against toxic increases of cytoplasmic Ca^{2+} *(11)*. However, this function is not limitless, and Ca^{2+} overload leads to mitochondrial damage. Mitochondria swell and become leaky, membrane potential drops, and accumulated Ca^{2+} is released. This phenomenon is called the mitochondrial permeability transition *(12)*. It is well established that Ca^{2+} is obligatory for MPT induction. The sensitivity of MPT to Ca^{2+} can be greatly increased by an elevated phosphate concentration, oxidative stress, depletion of adenine nucleotides and oxidation of pyridine nucleotides *(13)*. Experiments on isolated cells in vitro demonstrate that cell calcium accumulation or oxidative stress triggers MPT pore opening, which leads to collapse of the mitochondrial membrane potential, ATP hydrolysis, enhanced production of reactive oxygen species (ROS), and cell death *(14)*.

A hallmark of HRI is an increased cytosolic Ca^{2+} content caused by hypoxia, followed by an increased generation of ROS in the cytosol and in mitochondria subsequent to reoxygenation, conditions that favor the activation of the MPT pore *(15,16)*. Thus, the beneficial effect of CsA could be related to its ability to block the MPT pore. Probably, though, the mitochondrial dysfunction involves not only the assembly of an MPT pore and subsequent deenergization of cells but also other mechanisms. Because reperfusion is associated with release of mitochondrial proteins, it is likely that such proteins, for example, cytochrome *c*, trigger cascades of events leading to cell death. It is suggested that cytochrome *c* is a specific marker for damage to mitochondria caused by hypoxia, and its loss may affect respiratory chain function *(17)*.

The analysis of the mechanisms of ROS-induced mitochondrial damage revealed that release of accumulated Ca^{2+} is not accompanied by stimulation of sucrose entry into, K^+ release from, and swelling of mitochondria provided reuptake of the released Ca^{2+} is prevented *(13)*. Therefore it was concluded that *(18–20)*:

1. Prooxidant-induced Ca^{2+} release from rat liver mitochondria does not require "pore" formation in the mitochondrial inner membrane.
2. This release occurs via a specific pathway from intact mitochondria.
3. An ongoing release of Ca^{2+}, which can be induced by prooxidants, followed by Ca^{2+} reuptake (Ca^{2+} "cycling"), damages mitochondria and can lead to cell death.
4. A nonspecific permeability transition ("pore" formation) is likely to be secondary to Ca^{2+} cycling by mitochondria.

Previous work has documented a role of glutathione peroxidase in regulating hydrogen peroxide- or organic hydroperoxide-induced Ca^{2+} release from energized mitochondria *(21)*. Peroxides added to mitochondria undergo reduction by glutathione peroxidase at the expense of glutathione, whose product, glutathione disulfide, can in turn be reduced by NADPH-dependent glutathione reductase. Regeneration of the NADP+ is catalyzed by the energy-linked NADH-dependent transhydrogenase giving rise to NAD+. In the presence of Ca^{2+} NAD+ is hydrolyzed in mitochondria to nicotinamide and ADPribose. The formation of ADPribose can lead to ADP-ribosylation of mitochondrial membrane protein(s), some of which regulate Ca^{2+} release from the organelle. Inhibition of NAD+ hydrolysis by cyclosporin A (CSA) completely prevents Ca^{2+} release *(22)*.

The pyridine nucleotide-dependent mechanism of Ca^{2+} release from mitochondria plays an important role in the regulation of intramitochondrial Ca^{2+} homeostasis. Owing to their high capacity for storing Ca^{2+}, mitochondria are considered a "safety device" against Ca^{2+} overload in the cytoplasm under pathological conditions when uncontrolled influx of Ca^{2+} occurs across the plasma membrane *(11)*. When the cytosolic level of Ca^{2+} is high, mitochondrial Ca^{2+} accumulation increases, thus preventing a toxic Ca^{2+} overload of the cytoplasm. However, for normal mitochondrial functioning, the intramitochondrial concentration of Ca^{2+} must be maintained at a certain physiological level, since at least three mitochondrial dehydrogenases are Ca^{2+}-dependent: pyruvate, β-ketoglutarate, and isocitrate dehydrogenase *(23)*. Release of Ca^{2+} from intact mitochondria via the NAD^+ hydrolysis-dependent mechanism with subsequent export from the cytoplasm by plasma membrane Ca^{2+} ATPases should normalize intramitochondrial Ca^{2+} homeostasis and keep the dehydrogenases functionally active. However, if plasma membrane ATPases are impaired, Ca^{2+} released from mitochondria will reaccumulate, thereby stimulating the cycling of Ca^{2+} with subsequent collapse of the mitochondrial membrane potential and induction of MPT *(12,24)*.

In this in vitro study we investigate the response of mitochondria to conditions that prevail in HRI, that is, relatively high Ca^{2+} concentrations in combination with extra- and intramitochondrially acting prooxidants. We find that under these conditions mitochondria are damaged in a Ca^{2+}-dependent manner, and that the extent and site(s) of damage depend on both the kind of respiratory substrate and of prooxidants used; the major damage is due to hydrolysis of oxidized pyridine nucleotides followed by Ca^{2+} cycling; and this damage is effectively prevented by a therapeutically relevant concentration of cyclosporin A (CsA).

MATERIALS AND METHODS

Isolation of Mitochondria

The isolation of rat liver mitochondria was achieved by differential centrifugation. Briefly, livers were homogenized in ice-cold buffer [210 mM mannitol, 70 mM sucrose, and 5 mM 4-(2-hydroxyethyl)-1-piperazinesulfonic acid containing the chelator 1 mM ethylenediaminetetraacetic acid (EDTA)]. The mitochondrial pellet obtained after the high-speed centrifugation was washed once in the same buffer without the chelator. The protein content was determined by the Biuret method with BSA as standard.

Labeling of Mitochondrial Pyridine Nucleotides In Vivo

Overnight-fasted rats were injected intravenously with (*carboxyl-*^{14}C)nicotinic acid (12.5 μCi, 0.223 μmol) *(25)* in phosphate-buffered saline. After 3 h, the animals were killed, and liver mitochondria were isolated.

Standard Incubation Procedure

Mitochondria were incubated at 25°C with continuous stirring, and in the case of nicotinamide release measurements with oxygenation, in 100 mM KCl, 100 mM sucrose, 5 mM Tris-HCl, pH 7.4 containing 1 mM KH$_2$PO$_4$ with 5 mM β-hydroxybutyrate or 5 mM succinate as respiratory substrates.

Mitochondrial Respiration

Mitochondrial respiration was measured with a Clark-type electrode. Mitochondria were incubated according to the standard procedure with a protein content of 1.5 mg/mL. The respiratory control index (RCR) was calculated as the ratio of the rate of oxygen consumption during (state 3) and after (state 4) ADP-stimulated respiration. The statistical analysis was done by Student's *t*-test.

Ca^{2+} Uptake and release

Mitochondria were preincubated according to the standard procedure in the presence of 50 μM arsenazo III and 30 μM Ca^{2+}. Ca movements across the inner mitochondrial membrane were followed spectrophotometrically at 675–685 nm.

Redox State of Pyridine Nucleotides

The redox state of the mitochondrial pyridine nucleotides was measured spectrophotometrically at 340–370 nm in mitochondria incubated in the presence of 30 μM Ca^{2+}.

Pyridine Nucleotide Hydrolysis

Mitochondrial pyridine nuleotides were labeled in vivo, mitochondria were isolated and incubated at 1 mg of protein/ml according to the standard procedure. Nicotinamide release was analyzed by Millipore filtration as described.

RESULTS

Effect of Cyclosporin A on Mitochondrial Respiration

Figure 1 reports mitochondrial oxygen consumption supported by the site I respiratory substrate β-hydroxybutyrate. Mitochondria in the presence of EGTA are tightly coupled (Fig. 1, trace A). Exposure of these mitochondria to the prooxidant *t*-butylhydroperoxide (tbh) (Fig. 1, trace B), which is metabolized intramitochondrially *(25)*, or to Ca^{2+} (Fig. 1, trace C) leaves their degree of coupling and maximal respiration essentially unaffected. By contrast, tbh and Ca^{2+} together uncouple mitochondria and decrease their maximal respiration (Fig. 1, trace D). CSA prevents the mitochondrial deterioration induced by the combined presence of tbh and Ca^{2+} (Fig. 1, trace E). Similar results are obtained when tbh is replaced by an extramitochondrial generator of oxygen radicals and hydrogen peroxide, xanthine oxidase–hypoxanthine–iron ions (XO–HX–Fe) (not shown in Fig. 1), except that the damage observed under these conditions is more pronounced. Figure 2 compiles the respiratory rates and values obtained under the various conditions.

With respiration supported by the site II substrate succinate mitochondria had a respiratory control ratio (RCR) of 4.0. tbh and Ca^{2+} by itself or in combination at concentrations that were used in the experiments with β-hydroxybutyrate as a respiratory substrate neither affected the degree of coupling nor the maximal respiration (results not shown in Fig. 2).

Prooxidant-induced Ca^{2+} release from mitochondria, followed by Ca^{2+} cycling, causes selective damage of site I of the respiratory chain (Fig. 3).

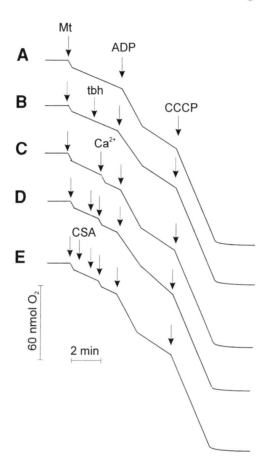

Fig. 1. Mitochondrial respiration supported by 5 mM β-hydroxybutyrate in the presence of prooxidants. Mitochondria (Mt) were incubated according to the standard procedure. Respiration was measured with a Clark-type electrode (*see* the section Materials and Methods). EGTA (5 mM), ADP (150 μM), and the uncoupler CCCP were added as indicated by the arrows. Trace **(A)**, control; trace **(B)**, as trace A + tbh; trace **(C)**, as trace A + Ca^{2+} (20 nmol/mg of protein); trace **(D)**, as trace A + tbh and Ca^{2+}; trace **(E)**, as trace D + CSA.

Thus, when tbh is added to Ca^{2+}-loaded mitochondria, β-hydroxybutyrate-supported respiration initially increases, then decreases and becomes unresponsive to the uncoupler; however, these mitochondria remain fully responsive to succinate (Fig. 3, trace A). CSA (Fig. 3, trace B) or EGTA (not shown) protect mitochondria from the prooxidant plus Ca^{2+}-induced, site I-specific damage. The same results were obtained with XO–HX–Fe instead of tbh (not shown).

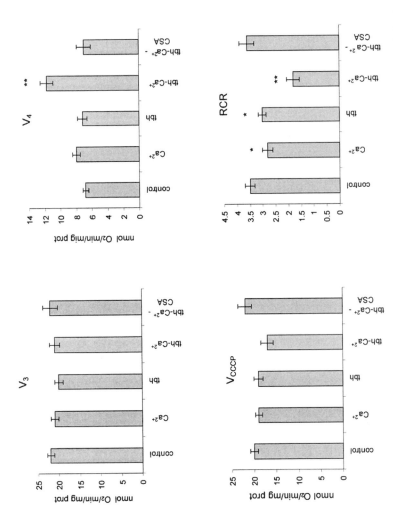

Fig. 2. Respiration rate and respiratory control index. Mitochondrial respiration supported by 5 m*M* β-hydroxybutyrate was measured as in Fig. 1. Respiratory control indices were calculated as described in the Materials and Methods section. Data are expressed as mean +SEM ($n = 4 - 6$); *$p < .05$; **$p < .005$. V_3, respiration rate in state 3; V_4, respiration rate in state 4; V_{CCCP}, respiration rate in the presence of uncoupler; RCR, respiratory control index.

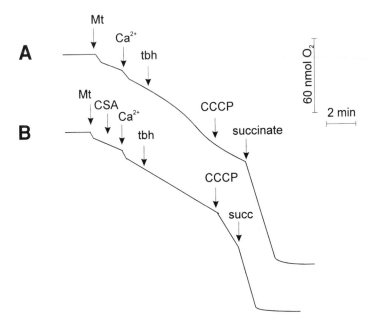

Fig. 3. *t*-Butylhydroperoxide-induced uncoupling and inhibition of mitochondrial respiration. Mitochondria were incubated according to the standard procedure in the presence of 5 m*M* β-hydroxybutyrate. Respiration was measured with a Clark-type electrode (*see* the section Materials and Methods). Ca^{2+} (20 nmol/mg of protein), tbh, the uncoupler CCCP, and succinate were added as indicated by the arrows and triangles. Trace **(A)**, control; trace **(B)**, as trace A + CSA; or EGTA. Succ, 5 m*M* succinate; tbh, 30 µ*M* *t*-butylhydroperoxide; 0.5 µ*M* carbonyl cyanide *m*-chlorophenylhydrazone (CCCP); 1 µ*M* cyclosporin A (CSA); 5 m*M* EGTA.

Effect of Cyclosporin A on Mitochondrial Retention of Ca^{2+}

Figure 4, panel A reports the tbh-induced Ca^{2+} release from mitochondria. Addition of prooxidant to Ca^{2+}-loaded mitochondria resulted in time-dependent release of Ca^{2+} from mitochondria. The response of mitochondria to the joint presence of Ca^{2+} and prooxidant depends on which substrate is available. Mitochondria are more sensitive when they oxidize NAD-dependent substrates such as β-hydroxybutyrate or pyruvate *plus* malate, compared to succinate. Estimation of the ability of mitochondria to accumulate and retain Ca^{2+} in the presence of prooxidants revealed that tbh induced release of Ca^{2+} soon after addition to Ca^{2+}-loaded mitochondria oxidizing β-hydroxybutyrate (Fig. 4, panel A). Release is very much delayed when mitochondria respire on succinate (Fig. 4, panel B). Inhibition of electron flow at site I by rotenone shortens considerably the time of Ca^{2+} retention by

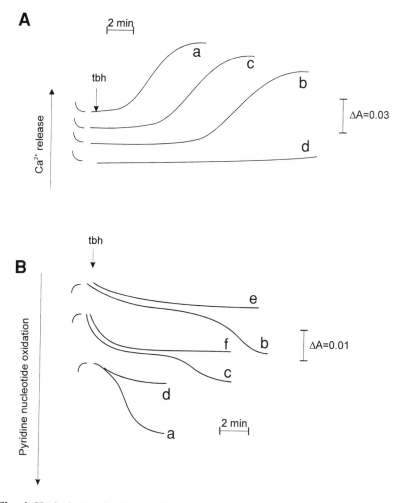

Fig. 4. Hydrolysis of mitochondrial pyridine nucleotides. Mitochondria labeled at the nicotinamide moiety were incubated (time: 0 min) according to the standard procedure. After 30 s they were exposed to 20 nmol of Ca^{2+}/mg of protein (panel **A**, traces a–d), or 30 nmol of Ca^{2+}/mg of protein (panel **B**, traces a–f), and 2 min later the prooxidant was added as indicated below. Pyridine nucleotide hydrolysis was analyzed by determination of nicotinamide release with Millipore filtration. Panel **A**, 5 mM β-hydroxybutirate (trace a) 5 mM succinate (trace b), 5 mM succinate + rotenone (trace c), or 5 mM β-hydroxybutirate in the presence of cyclosporin A (trace d) were used as respiratory substrates. Mitochondria were loaded with 30 nmol of Ca^{2+}. Panel **B**, 5 mM β-hydroxybutyrate as respiratory substrate; trace a, Ca^{2+} (20 nmol/mg of protein); trace b, as trace a + XO–HX–Fe; trace c, as trace a + tbh; trace d, as trace b + CSA; trace e, as trace c + CSA; trace f, mitochondria were depleted of Ca^{2+} with 5 mM EGTA prior to addition β-hydroxybutyrate and at time 2 min 15 s exposed to XO–HX–Fe or tbh.

mitochondria oxidizing succinate (Fig. 4, panel B, trace C). CSA, which inhibits pyridine nucleotide hydrolysis, completely prevents the tbh-induced Ca^{2+} release from mitochondria oxidizing β-hydroxybutyrate or succinate (panel B, trace d).

Effect of Prooxidant on the Redox State of Mitochondrial Pyridine Nucleotides

Figure 4, panel B shows the tbh-induced oxidation of pyridine nucleotides in mitochondria respiring on β-hydroxybutyrate or succinate. Oxidation of pyridine nucleotides on addition of tbh in mitochondria energized by β-hydroxybutyrate (Fig. 4, panel B, trace a) is much faster than in mitochondria energized by succinate (Fig. 4, panel B, trace b). Rotenone enhances the extent of tbh-induced pyridine nucleotide oxidation in succinate-energized mitochondria (Fig. 4, panel B, trace c). CSA does not affect the initial phase of pyridine nucleotide oxidation, but prevents the second phase of oxidation in mitochondria oxidizing both β-hydroxybutyrate or succinate in the presence or absence of rotenone (Fig. 4, panel B, traces d–f). This second phase of the disappearance of reduced pyridine nucleotides is most likely caused by prooxidant-stimulated hydrolysis of pyridine nucleotides, followed by oxidation of reduced pyridine nucleotides in response to thermodynamic equilibration *(26,27)*.

Cyclosporin A Prevents Prooxidant-Induced Hydrolysis of Pyridine Nucleotides

In Ca^{2+}-loaded mitochondria respiring on β-hydroxybutyrate extensive hydrolysis of pyridine nucleotides occurs, as judged from nicotinamide release (Fig. 4, panel A, traces a–c). Even without added prooxidant hydrolysis takes place (Fig. 4, panel A, trace a) because in β-hydroxy-butyrate-energized mitochondria Ca^{2+} uptake causes extensive pyridine nucleotide oxidation (result not shown), a prerequisite for their hydrolysis. Hydrolysis is stimulated by prooxidants, either generated extramitochondrially (Fig. 4, panel A, trace b), or being metabolized intramitochondrially (Fig. 4, panel A, trace c). CSA completely prevents pyridine nucleotide hydrolysis induced by either prooxidant (Fig. 4, panel A, traces d and e). No hydrolysis takes place in Ca^{2+}-depleted mitochondria exposed to the prooxidants (Fig. 4, panel A, traces a–d).

The substrate dependence of pyridine nucleotide hydrolysis is shown in Fig. 4, panel B. In Ca^{2+} loaded mitochondria (30 nmol/mg protein) respiring on β-hydroxybutirate, extensive hydrolysis of pyridine nucleotides occurs (trace a), which is completely prevented by CSA (trace d). With succinate as respiratory substrate (trace b) pyridine nucleotide hydrolysis is very limited, but facilitated in the presence of rotenone (trace c).

DISCUSSION

The oxidation–reduction state of mitochondrial pyridine nucleotides regulates Ca^{2+} release from succinate-energized mitochondria in the presence of rotenone. It has been shown previously that in the presence of prooxidant hydrolysis of oxidized pyridine nucleotides and subsequent ADP-ribosylation of (a) membrane protein(s) stimulates Ca^{2+} efflux from intact mitochondria (for review, *see* ref. *28*). This may be followed by mitochondrial damage if cyclic Ca^{2+} uptake and release ("Ca^{2+} cycling") across the inner mitochondrial membrane is allowed *(13)*. Accordingly, inhibitors that prevent pyridine nucleotide hydrolysis or (mono)ADP-ribosylation, such as CSA *(29)*, ATP *(30)*, 4-hydroxynonenal *(31)*, or *m*-iodobenzyl guanidine *(32)* prevent Ca^{2+} release and also protect mitochondria from Ca^{2+} cycling-induced damage.

To mimic in an in vitro model the conditions prevailing upon reperfusion after hypoxia, in the present study isolated rat liver mitochondria were energized and exposed to Ca^{2+} and prooxidants which act intra- or extramitochondrially. Several conclusions can be drawn from the results obtained:

1. Not simply the exposure to prooxidants and Ca^{2+} is deleterious to mitochondria, but the prooxidant-induced stimulation of the Ca^{2+} release pathway, which requires pyridine nucleotide hydrolysis, followed by Ca^{2+} cycling. This is evident from the transient increase of β-hydroxybutyrate-supported respiration due to increased Ca^{2+} cycling followed by inhibition of respiration, and from the protection by CSA or EGTA, compounds which prevent pyridine nucleotide hydrolysis and/or Ca^{2+} cycling, respectively.
2. When mitochondria contain oxidized pyridine nucleotides and Ca^{2+} they experience specific damage at site I of the respiratory chain. When tbh is added to Ca^{2+}-loaded mitochondria oxidizing β-hydroxybutyrate, the respiration rate initially increases (Fig. 3). This initial rise is explained by activation of Ca^{2+} cycling and dissipation of $\Delta\Psi$. Acceleration of respiration is followed by its suppression, and finally respiration becomes unresponsive to the uncoupler. This can be explained by deterioration of complex I of respiratory chain, due to hydrolysis of NAD+. However, these mitochondria remain fully responsive to succinate (Fig. 3, trace a). CSA (Fig. 3, trace b) or EGTA (not shown) protect mitochondria from the prooxidant *plus* Ca^{2+}-induced, site I-specific damage.
3. CSA at a therapeutically relevant concentration *(33)* completely protects mitochondria in this in vitro model of HRI.

Mitochondrial Ca^{2+} release studies have so far mainly employed succinate as respiratory substrate in combination with rotenone, an inhibitor of site I of the respiratory chain. Here we show that respiratory substrates can control a prooxidant-dependent release of Ca^{2+} from mitochondria. Because prooxidant-induced Ca^{2+} efflux is conditioned upon the hydrolysis of oxidized pyridine nucleotides, this efflux is prevented by CSA, which inhibits NAD+ hydrolysis. However Ca^{2+} efflux can be significantly delayed when reversed electron flow from succinate to NAD+ is allowed. Therefore, CSA protects mitochondria by inhibiting the hydrolysis of oxidized pyridine nucleotides, an obligatory step in the sequence of events leading to Ca^{2+} release and subsequent Ca^{2+} cycling (19), whereas succinate protects by keeping mitochondrial pyridine nucleotides largely reduced (34). Pyridine nucleotide hydrolysis is also the cause of the site I-specific inhibition of respiration in the presence of prooxidants and Ca^{2+}, as is evident from protection by CSA or succinate.

A disturbance of the cellular Ca^{2+} homeostasis is responsible for the toxicity of various agents (35) and contributes to some pathological states, such as HRI or inflammation (36). Under conditions of uncontrolled Ca^{2+} entry into the cell, mitochondrial damage due to calcium cycling is often considered the final trigger of cell death (37). In such a situation activation of succinate oxidation can delay mitochondria damage and hence may protect cells. Thus, enhanced succinate oxidation can be considered to protect against Ca^{2+} cycling-induced cell killing. This correlates well with the concept that under situations of increased physiological activity or stress succinate is predominantly formed and oxidized (38).

The ability of succinate to keep mitochondrial pyridine nucleotides reduced and hence protect mitochondria in an HRI model explains early experimental results showing that after 60 min ischemia, 30 min of reperfusion resulted in partial restoration of mitochondrial function with succinate but not α-ketoglutarate as a substrate (39). Lactate accumulation was also partially reversed with reperfusion. Histological examination subsequent to the ischemic episode revealed development of partial necrosis in 9 of 10 ischemic lobes. α-Ketoglutarate oxidation is more sensitive to injury than succinate oxidation. The authors conclude that with proper choice of substrate, measurement of mitochondrial function just after an ischemic insult may predict subsequent hepatic failure due to cellular necrosis.

Our findings confirm and extent previous reports. Thus, CSA prevents prooxidant-induced Ca^{2+} release from isolated heart (40), liver (22,41), and kidney (42) mitochondria. The drug also protects hepatocytes against prooxidant-induced mitochondrial Ca^{2+} cycling and cell killing (43). Specific loss of site I activity of kidney mitochondria exposed to the oxygen radical generator XO–HX–Fe and Ca^{2+} has been reported (44), but the underlying mechanism was not elucidated. It has also been shown that CSA restores ATP synthesis and coupling in mitochondria not before but after reperfusion of previously hypoxic rat liver *(45)*. It therefore appears that CSA, in addition to its immunosuppressive properties, is useful to mitigate HRI-related organelle, cell, and organ damage caused by prooxidant-induced mitochondrial Ca^{2+} cycling.

REFERENCES

1. Fan C, Zwacka RM, Engelhardt JF. Therapeutic approaches for ischemia/ reperfusion injury in the liver. J Mol Med 1999;77:577–592.
2. Hancock WW. Current trends in transplant immunology. Curr Opin Nephrol Hypertens 1999;8:317–324.
3. Kurokawa T, Takagi H. Mechanism and prevention of ischemia-reperfusion injury. Transplant Proc 1999;31:1775–1776.
4. Duchen MR, McGuinness O, Brown LA, Crompton M. On the involvement of a cyclosporin A sensitive mitochondrial pore in myocardial reperfusion injury. Cardiovasc Res 1993;27:1790–1794.
5. Shimizu S, Kamiike W, Hatanaka N, et al. Enzyme release from mitochondria during reoxygenation of rat liver. Transplantation 1994;57:144–148.
6. Siesjo BK, Elmer E, Janelidze S, et al. Role and mechanisms of secondary mitochondrial failure. Acta Neurochir Suppl 1999;73:7–13.
7. Friberg H, Ferrand-Drake M, Bengtsson F, et al. Cyclosporin A, but not FK 506, protects mitochondria and neurons against hypoglycemic damage and implicates the mitochondrial permeability transition in cell death. J Neurosci 1998;18:5151–5159.
8. Matsumoto S, Friberg H, Ferrand-Drake M, Wieloch T. Blockade of the mitochondrial permeability transition pore diminishes infarct size in the rat after transient middle cerebral artery occlusion. J Cereb Blood Flow Metab 1999;19:736–741.
9. Arteaga D, Odor A, Lopez RM, et al. Impairment by cyclosporin A of reperfusion-induced arrhythmias. Life Sci 1992;51:1127–1134.
10. Griffiths EJ, Halestrap AP. Protection by Cyclosporin A of ischemia/ reperfusion-induced damage in isolated rat hearts. J Mol Cell Cardiol 1993;25:1461–1469.
11. Carafoli E. Intracellular calcium homeostasis. Annu Rev Biochem 1987; 56:395–433.
12. Halestrap AP. (1994) Interaction between oxidative stress and calcium overload on mitochondrial function. In: Darley-Usmar V, Schapira AHV, eds. Mitochondria: DNA, Proteins and Disease. Portland Press, London, pp. 113–142.
13. Schlegel J, Schweizer M, Richter C. "Pore" formation is not required for the hydroperoxide-induced Ca^{2+} release from rat liver mitochondria. Biochem J 1992;285:65–69.
14. Lemasters JJ, Qian T, Bradham CA, et al. Mitochondrial dysfunction in the pathogenesis of necrotic and apoptotic cell death. J Bioenerg Biomembr 1999;31:305–319.

15. Braunwald E, Kloner RA. Myocardial reperfusion: a double-edged sword? J Clin Invest 1985;76:1713–1719.
16. Bolli R. Oxygen-derived free radicals and myocardial reperfusion injury: an overview. Cardiovasc Drugs Ther 1991;5:249–268.
17. Naro F, Fazzini A, Grappone C, et al. Release of cytochromes from hypoxic and reoxygenated guinea pig heart. Cardioscience 1993;4:177–184.
18. Nicotera P, Bellomo G, Orrenius S. The role of Ca^{2+} in cell killing. Chem Res Toxicol 1990;3: 484–494.
19. Richter C, Kass GEN. Oxidative stress in mitochondria: its relationship to cellular Ca^{2+} homeostasis, cell death, proliferation, and differentiation. Chem Biol Interact 1991;77:1–23.
20. Hennet T, Richter C, Peterhans E. Tumour necrosis factor-alpha induces superoxide anion generation in mitochondria of L929 cells. Biochem J 1993;289:587–592.
21. Richter C, Frei B. Ca^{2+} release from mitochondria induced by prooxidants. Free Radical Biol Med 1988;4:365–375.
22. Richter C, Theus M, Schlegel J. Cyclosporin A inhibits mitochondrial pyridine nucleotide hydrolysis and calcium release. Biochem Pharmacol 1990;40: 779–782.
23. Denton RM, McCormack JG. On the role of the calcium transport cycle in heart and other mammalian mitochondria. FEBS Lett 1980;119:1–8.
24. Zoratti M, Szabo I. The mitochondrial permeability transition. Biochem Biophys Acta 1995;1241:139–176.
25. Lötscher HR, Winterhalter KH, Carafoli E, Richter, C. Hydroperoxide-induced loss of pyridine nucleotides and release of calcium from rat liver mitochondria. J Biol Chem 1980;255:9325–9330.
26. Schweizer M, Richter C. Gliotoxin stimulates Ca^{2+} release from intact rat liver mitochondria. Biochemistry 1994;33:13,401–13,405.
27. Schweizer M, Durrer P, Richter C. Phenylarsine oxide stimulates pyridine nucleotide-linked Ca^{2+} release from rat liver mitochondria. Biochem Pharmacol 1994;48:967–973.
28. Richter C. Mitochondrial calcium transport. In: Ernster L, ed. Molecular Mechanisms in Bionergetics. Elsevier, Amsterdam, pp. 349–358.
29. Richter C, Theus M, Schlegel J. Cyclosporin A inhibits mitochondrial pyridine nucleotide hydrolysis and Ca^{2+} release. Biochem Pharmacol 1990;40: 779–782.
30. Hofstetter W, Muhlebach T, Lotscher HR, et al. ATP prevents both hydroperoxide-induced hydrolysis of pyridine nucleotides and release of calcium in rat liver mitochondria. Eur J Biochem 1981;117:361–367.
31. Richter C, Meier P. Inhibition of pro-oxidant-induced mitochondrial pyridine nucleotide hydrolysis and calcium release by 4-hydroxynonenal. Biochem J 1990;269:735–737.
32. Richter C. The prooxidant-induced and spontaneous mitochondrial calcium release: inhibition by meta-iodo-benzylguanidine (MIBG), a substrate for mono(ADP-ribosylation). Free Radic Res Commun 1990;8:329–334.

33. Kahan BD. Cyclosporin: the base for immunosuppressive therapy: present and future. Transplant Proc 1993;25:508–510.
34. Chance B, Hollunger G. The interaction of energy and electron transfer reaction in mitochondria. I. General properties and nature of the products of succinate-linked reduction of pyridine nucleotides. J Biol Chem 1961;236:1534–1543.
35. Nicotera P, Bellomo G, Orrenius S. Calcium mediated mechanisms in chemically-induced cell death. Annu Rev Pharmacol Toxicol 1992;32:449–470.
36. Allen SP, Stone D. (1994) Mitochondrial function in ischemia/reperfusion in the heart. In: Darley-Usmar V, Schapira AHV, eds. Mitochondria: DNA, Proteins and Disease. Portland Press, London, pp. 143–155.
37. Orrenius S, Nicotera P. The calcium ion and cell death. J Neural Transm Suppl 1994;43:1–11.
38. Kondrashova MN. Biochemical cycle of excitation. In: Chance B, ed. Biological and Biochemical Oscillators. Academic Press, New York, pp. 373–387.
39. Rhodes RS, DePalma RG, Druet RL. Reversibility of ischemically induced mitochondrial dysfunction with reperfusion. Surg Gynecol Obstet 1977; 145:719–724.
40. Crompton M, Costi A. Kinetic evidence for a heart mitochondrial pore activated by Ca^{2+}, inorganic phosphate and oxidative stress: a potential mechanism for mitochondrial dysfunction during cellular Ca^{2+} overload. Eur J Biochem 1988;178:489–501.
41. Schweizer M, Schlegel J, Baumgartner D, Richter C. Sensitivity of mitochondrial peptidyl-prolyl cis-trans isomerase, pyridine nucleotide hydrolysis and Ca^{2+} release to cyclosporin A and related compounds. Biochem Pharmacol 1993;45:641–646.
42. Schlegel J, Meier P, Kass GEN, Richter C. Inhibition by cyclosporin A of the prooxidant-induced but not of the sodium-induced calcium release from rat kidney mitochondria. Biochem Pharmacol 1991;42:2193–2197.
43. Kass GEN, Juedes MJ, Orrenius S. Cyclosporin A protects hepatocytes against prooxidant-induced cell killing. A study on the role of mitochondrial Ca^{2+} cycling in cytotoxicity. Biochem Pharmacol 1992;44:1995–2003.
44. Malis CD, Bonventre JV. Mechanism of calcium potentiation of oxygen free radical injury to renal mitochondria. A model for post-ischemic and toxic mitochondrial damage. J Biol Chem 1986;261:14,201–14,208.
45. Kurokawa T, Kobayashi H, Harada A, et al. Beneficial effects of cyclosporin on postischemic liver injury in rats. Transplantation 1992;53:308–311.

10

Protective Effect of Cyclosporin A on Glial Activation and White Matter Alterations Induced by Chronic Cerebral Hypoperfusion

Hideaki Wakita, Hidekazu Tomimoto and Ichiro Akiguchi

INTRODUCTION

Cerebral white matter (WM) lesions are frequent correspondents in ischemic cerebrovascular disease (CVD) and constitute the core pathology in Binswanger's disease, a form of vascular dementia. These cerebrovascular WM lesions have been thought to result from chronic cerebral ischemia, and may be responsible for the cognitive impairments [1–3] and gait disorders of the elderly [4,5]. These lesions are characterized pathologically by diffuse axonal loss, demyelination and gliosis in the WM [6–12].

Cerebrovascular WM lesions can be experimentally induced in the rat brain as a result of chronic cerebral hypoperfusion created by the permanent occlusion of both common carotid arteries [13]. In this model, the cerebral blood flow (CBF) decreases, with values ranging from 40 to 82% of normal, over a prolonged period [14–16]. These animals with a decreased CBF exhibit a significant learning impairment [17–19]. Microglia and astroglia are also activated briefly after ischemia in a manner that predicts the extent and severity of the subsequent WM lesions [13].

Recent investigations suggest that a variety of inflammatory and immunological responses ensue after cerebral ischemia [20–22]. Microglia, the immune effector cells of the central nervous system [23–25], are activated in acute cerebral ischemia and express major histocompatibility complex (MHC) antigens [26,27]. These activated microglia secrete cytotoxic substances such as inflammatory cytokines, reactive oxygen species, nitric oxide, and prostanoids [28–39]. This activation of the microglia can also be detected in the cerebrovascular WM lesions from patients with ischemic CVD and Binswanger's disease [11,12,40,41].

From: *Immunosuppressant Analogs in Neuroprotection*
Edited by: C. V. Borlongan, O. Isacson, and P. R. Sanberg © Humana Press Inc., Totowa, NJ

Cyclosporin A (CsA), a widely used immunosuppressant *(42)*, binds cyclophillin and inhibits calcineurin activity, thereby suppressing cytokine gene expression and inhibiting T lymphocytes *(43–46)*. Recent studies have demonstrated that CsA has a neuroprotective effect in cerebral ischemia *(47–54)*, although the underlying pathomechanism remains unclear.

In this chapter, we focus on the effects of CsA on the activation of glial cells and WM rarefaction observed in a rat model of chronic cerebral hypoperfusion *(13)*. The pharmacological suppression of these glia attenuated the WM lesions *(55–57)*, suggesting that immunological responses may be involved in the pathogenesis of these cerebrovascular WM lesions. Furthermore, the therapeutic window and the safety of CsA have been assessed for its potential therapeutic application in cerebrovascular WM lesions in CVD patients.

EXPERIMENTAL PROCEDURES

Animal Preparation

Male Wistar rats (purchased from the Shimizu Experimental Supply Co. Ltd., Japan), weighing 150–200 g, were used. The animals were anesthetized with sodium pentobarbital (25 mg/kg, ip), and were allowed spontaneous respiration throughout the surgical procedure. Through an anterior midline cervical incision, both common carotid arteries were exposed and double-ligated with silk sutures. The rectal temperature was monitored and maintained between 36.5 and 37.5°C during the surgical procedure. After the operation, the rats were kept in animal quarters with food and water *ad libitum*.

Administration of CsA

The rats received a daily intraperitoneal injection of CsA (10 mg/kg) diluted in vehicle solution from 1 d before the operation to 14 d afterward, and thereafter on every third day beyond the 14 d. Six to nine animals were used at each postischemic period in the CsA-treated groups. As a control, six animals underwent the same surgery but received an intraperitoneal administration of vehicle only (130 mg/kg polyoxyethylated castor oil and 6.6% ethanol in saline) in the same manner at each postischemic period. Five animals were subjected to a sham operation (the same surgery except for occlusion), but were killed immediately.

Other groups of rats received different amounts of CsA (5 mg/kg in eight rats and 15 mg/kg CsA in nine rats) in the same manner as the 10 mg/kg CsA-treated group. These animals were then killed at 14 d after the operation, thus enabling a dose-response investigation. In addition, the effects of posttreatment with CsA was examined. Five rats received a daily intraperitoneal injection of 10 mg/kg CsA beyond 7 d, and were sacrificed on d 14 after the operation.

To assess the safety of CsA, the erythrocyte, leukocyte, and thrombocyte count, serum glutamic oxaloacetic transaminase (GOT), glutamic pyruvic transaminase (GPT), blood urea nitrogen (BUN), and creatinine levels were monitored for 30 d after the ligation in these animals, which received either 10 mg/kg CsA or vehicle from 1 d before the operation. The kidney tissues were examined by hematoxylin-eosin staining in those animals receiving either 10 mg/kg CsA or vehicle for 7 d, from 1 d before the operation.

Assessment of the WM Lesions

At 7, 14, and 30 d after the ligation of the carotid arteries, the animals were deeply anesthetized with sodium pentobarbital (80 mg/kg ip), perfused transcardially with 0.01 M phosphate-buffered saline (PBS), and then perfused with a fixative containing 4% paraformaldehyde and 0.2% picric acid in 0.1 M phosphate buffer (PB, pH 7.4). The brains and optic nerves were then immersed for 12 h in 4% paraformaldehyde in 0.1 M PB (pH 7.4), and coronal brain blocks including the caudoputamen and hippocampus were embedded in paraffin. Then 2-μm-thick paraffin sections were cut on a microtome, and stained with Klüver-Barrera and Bielschowsky stains. The severity of the WM lesions was graded as normal (grade 0), disarrangement of the nerve fibers (grade 1), formation of marked vacuoles (grade 2), and the disappearance of myelinated fibers (grade 3) *(13,16,40,55–57)*. Four animals were used for the grading of the WM lesions.

Immunohistochemistry for Glial Cell Markers

The rest of the coronal blocks were stored in 15% sucrose in 0.1 M PB (pH 7.4) until used for immunohistochemistry. Serial sections (20 μm thick) were cut in a cryostat. The sections were incubated overnight with the following monoclonal antibodies (dilutions in parentheses): OX18 (Sera Lab, 1:400) against MHC class I antigen, OX6 (Sera Lab, 1:100) against MHC class II (Ia) antigen, and OX1 (Sera Lab, 1:100) against leukocyte common antigen (LCA).

A polyclonal antiserum directed against glial fibrillary acidic protein (GFAP; Dako, 1:20,000) was used to identify the astroglia. The sections were subsequently immunostained with the avidin–biotin–peroxidase complex (ABC) method, and were then counterstained with hematoxylin. The number of nuclei with immunoreactive perikarya and processes were counted in four animals. The numerical density of the immunoreactive cells was expressed as the number of cells per 0.3 mm^2 in the region of interest *(13,55–57)*.

Statistical Analysis

Values were expressed as means ± SD. Differences in the laboratory blood data were determined by a one-factor ANOVA between each group. The mortality rates between each group were compared by Fisher's exact probability test. Differences in the numerical densities of the immunoreactive cells and the grading scores between each group were determined by a two-factor factorial ANOVA followed by Fisher's protected least significant difference procedure. A $p < 0.05$ was considered to be statistically significant.

RESULTS

Mortality Rate and Side Effects Caused by CsA

Of the 22 rats that received 10 mg/kg CsA from 1 d before the operation, one animal (4.5%) died within 7 d after the operation and three more rats (13.6%) died beyond 7 d. Of the eight animals that received 5 mg/kg CsA, two (25%) died within 7 d after the operation and none died beyond 7 d. Of the nine animals that received 15 mg/kg CsA, two (22.2%) died within 7 d and one more (11.1%) died beyond 7 d. Of the five rats that started their 10 mg/kg CsA injection 8 d after the operation, one (20.0%) died after 8 d. Of the 18 animals that received the vehicle, four (22.2%) died within 7 d, and none died beyond 7 d. There were no significant differences in the mortality rates between the CsA-treated versus the vehicle-treated groups. In all groups, the surviving animals occasionally showed ptosis and transient difficulties in feeding.

The erythrocyte, leukocyte, and thrombocyte count, serum GOT, GPT, BUN, and creatinine levels did not differ significantly between the vehicle-treated versus the CsA-treated animals (Table 1). There were no obvious histological abnormalities in the kidneys of the animals that received 10 mg/kg CsA.

Effect of CsA on WM Lesions

In the sham-operated animals, there were no detectable WM lesions. Large infarcts were not observed in the vehicle-treated animals. In the 10 mg/kg CsA-treated group, two rats showed a large infarct in the gray matter and were excluded from the statistical analysis.

After 7 d of ligation, the most severe WM lesions (vacuole formation, disarrangement, and loss of the myelinated fibers) were observed in the optic nerve and the optic tract of the vehicle-treated animals. Less intense changes

Table 1
Summary of the Laboratory Blood Data in Rats Receiving Either Vehicle or 10 mg/kg CsA from 1 d Before the Operation to 30 d After

	Erythrocyte ($\times10^4$/mm3)	Leukocyte ($\times10^2$/mm3)	Thrombocyte ($\times10^3$/mm3)	GOT (IU/L)	GPT (IU/L)	BUN (mg/dL)	Creatinine (mg/dL)
Vehicle							
($n = 4$)	809.3 ± 60.5	63.3 ± 16.2	736.0 ± 91.0	94.3 ± 8.2	21.8 ± 6.1	23.0 ± 2.5	0.47 ± 0.04
CsA							
($n = 4$)	887.0 ± 38.0	58.8 ± 9.7	878.0 ± 83.6	99.0 ± 9.5	32.3 ± 11.9	21.3 ± 3.0	0.47 ± 0.05

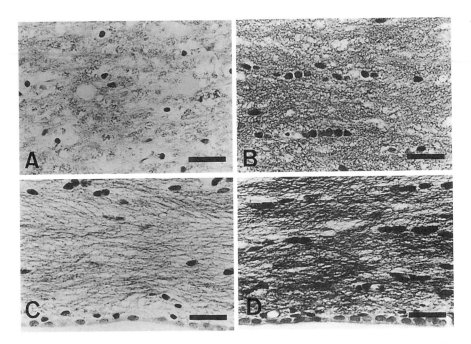

Fig. 1. Photomicrographs of Klüver-Barrera staining of the optic nerve **(A,B)** and the medial part of the corpus callosum **(C,D)**. The animals received an intraperitoneal administration of vehicle (A,C) or 10 mg/kg CsA (B,D) for 30 d. Note that the extent of the WM rarefaction was less severe in the CsA-treated rats. Bars indicate 30 μm.

were observed in the medial part of the corpus callosum adjoining the lateral ventricle, the anterior commissure, the internal capsule, and the fiber bundles of the caudoputamen. After 14 and 30 d, the grading scores remained the same as the scores at 7 d of postligation in the vehicle-treated animals (Figs. 1A,C and 2). In the 10 mg/kg CsA-treated animals, the severity of the WM lesions was reduced ($p < 0.01$) between 7 and 30 d, as compared with the vehicle-treated animals (Figs. 1B,D and 2).

The number of axons also decreased on the Bielschowsky staining in the above WM regions in the vehicle-treated animals from 7 to 30 d after ligation. With 10 mg/kg CsA administration, this axonal loss was less severe.

The grading scores of the WM lesions were then compared between varying amounts of CsA after 14 d of ligation (Fig. 3). All doses of CsA significantly reduced the grading score as compared with the vehicle-treated animals ($p < 0.05$ in 5 mg/kg CsA group and $p < 0.01$ in 10 and 15 mg/kg CsA groups). Furthermore, these scores were lower in the 10 and 15 mg/kg

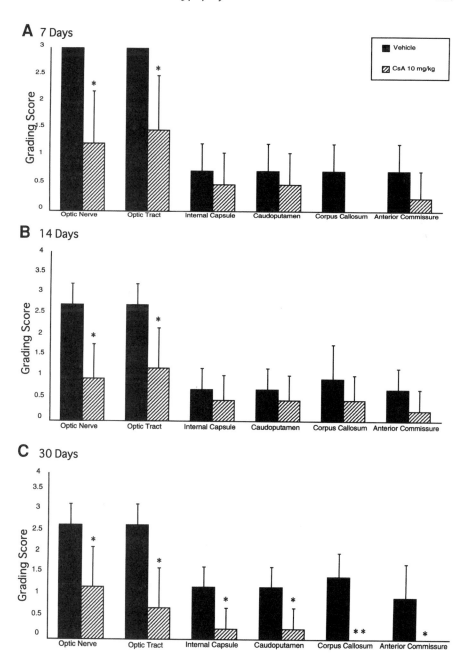

Fig. 2. Histograms of the grading scores for the WM lesions in rats receiving either vehicle or 10 mg/kg CsA from 1 d before the operation to 7 (**A**), 14 (**B**), and 30 (**C**) d after the operation. *$p < 0.05$ and **$p < 0.01$ by Fisher's protected least significant difference procedure as compared to the vehicle-treated animals.

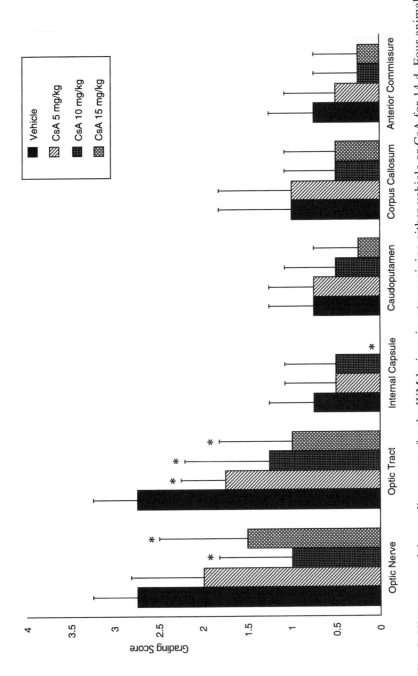

Fig. 3. Histograms of the grading scores for the WM lesions in rats receiving either vehicle or CsA for 14 d. Four animals were used in each group. *$p < 0.05$ by Fisher's protected least significant difference procedure as compared to the vehicle-treated animals.

CsA-treated animals than in the 5 mg/kg treated ones ($p < 0.05$), indicating a dose-related protective effect for CsA. However, there were no significant differences between the 10 and 15 mg/kg CsA-treated groups. Posttreatment with 10 mg/kg CsA alleviated the WM lesions as compared to the vehicle-treated group ($p < 0.05$), but the suppression was more obvious in the pretreated animals than in the posttreated ones ($p < 0.05$, Fig. 4).

Effects of CsA on Glial Cells

In the WM of the sham-operated animals, there was positive immunostaining for the MHC class I and II (Ia) antigens and LCA in only a few glial cells. GFAP-immunopositive astroglia were distributed predominantly in the WM. From 7 to 30 d after the ligation, the brains of the vehicle-treated animals showed an increase in the number of microglia/macrophages that were immunoreactive for the MHC class I and II antigens and LCA in various WM regions such as the optic nerve, optic tract, corpus callosum, internal capsule, anterior commissure, and traversing fiber bundles of the caudoputamen (Fig. 5A).

Microglia/macrophages immunoreactive for the MHC antigens and LCA were most numerous at 14 d in these regions (Fig. 6). The number of astroglia immunoreactive for GFAP increased from 7 to 30 d after the ligation (Fig. 5C). In the CsA-treated animals, microglia/macrophages immunolabeled for the MHC antigens and LCA were fewer in number than in the vehicle-treated animals, from 7 to 30 d ($p < 0.01$, Figs. 5B and 6). The number of GFAP-immunopositive astroglia was also reduced in the CsA-treated animals in the corresponding regions (Fig. 5D).

All doses of CsA resulted in a significant reduction in the number of MHC class II immunopositive microglia/macrophages ($p < 0.01$), as compared with vehicle-only treatment (Fig. 7). However, the 10 and 15 mg/kg CsA treatment groups showed a greater numerical decrease in the MHC class II immunopositive microglia/ macrophages ($p < 0.05$ for 10 mg/kg and $p < 0.01$ for 15 mg/kg) than the 5 mg/kg CsA treatment group.

Posttreatment with 10 mg/kg CsA was also effective in suppressing the numerical increase of MHC class II immunopositive microglia/ macrophages in the WM ($p < 0.01$). However, the number of these cells decreased more prominently in the animals pretreated with 10 mg /kg CsA than in the animals posttreated with the same dose ($p < 0.05$, Fig. 8).

DISCUSSION

Recent investigations have demonstrated that the immunosupressants CsA and FK506 have a neuroprotective effect in cerebral ischemia *(47–54,58–64)*.

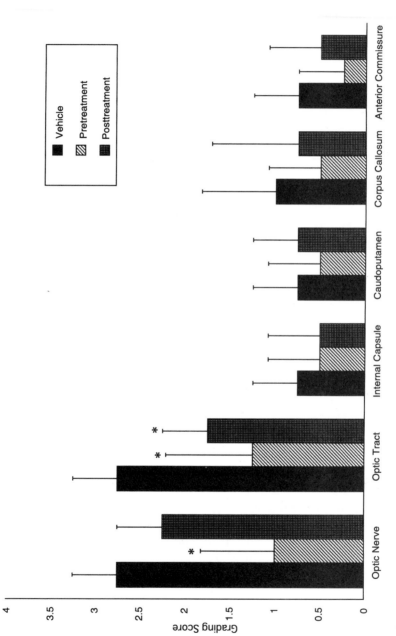

Fig. 4. Histograms of the grading scores for the WM lesions in rats receiving either vehicle, 10 mg/kg CsA from one day before the operation to 14 d after the operation (pretreatment), or 10 mg/kg CsA from 8 to 14 d after the operation (posttreatment). *$p < 0.05$ by Fisher's protected least significant difference procedure as compared to the vehicle-treated animals.

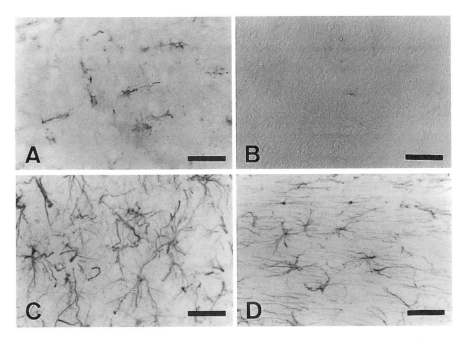

Fig. 5. Photomicrographs of the immunohistochemical staining for MHC class II antigen in the internal capsule (**A, B**) and GFAP in the optic tract (**C, D**). The animals received an intraperitoneal administration of vehicle (**A, C**) or 10 mg/kg CsA (**B, D**) for 14 d. In the CsA-treated animals, microglia/macrophages immunoreactive for MHC class II antigen and astroglia immunoreactive for GFAP were much less prominent as compared to the vehicle-treated animals. Bars indicate 60 μm in **A, B,** and 30 μm in **C, D**.

In this chapter, we showed that CsA attenuated the glial activation and WM lesions induced by chronic cerebral hypoperfusion. A similar neuroprotective role has also been shown for FK506 using the same model *(56)*.

Although FK506 and CsA are structurally unrelated to each other, these drugs both bind immunophyllins (FKBP and cyclophyllin, respectively). The drug/immunophyllin complex then inhibits calcineurin, a calcium/calmodulin-dependent phosphatase. Calcineurin affects a diverse number of cellular actions related to both immunologic and non-immunologic mechanisms by regulating protein phosporylation and Ca^{2+} homeostasis. Although the exact mechanisms underlying these neuroprotective effects in the present study remain uncertain, some aspects of the above-mentioned actions may be involved.

First, CsA may have prevented the ischemic WM damage mediated by immunologic mechanisms. In a previous study using a chronic cerebral

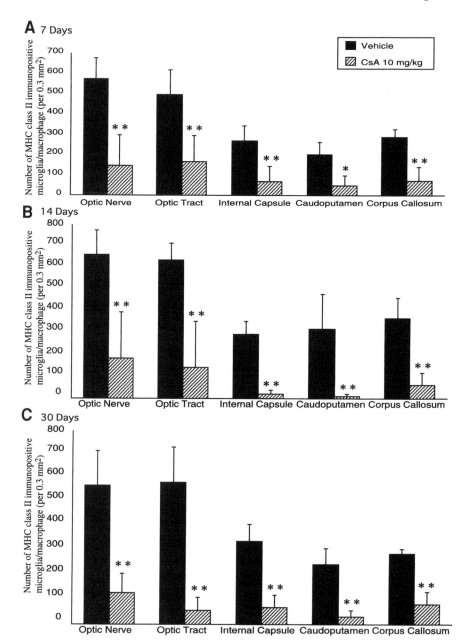

Fig. 6. Histograms of the numerical density of MHC class II immunopositive microglia/macrophages in the WM of rats receiving either vehicle or 10 mg/kg CsA from 1 d before the operation to 7 **(A)**, 14 **(B)**, and 30 **(C)** d after the operation. $*p < 0.05$ and $**p < 0.01$ by Fisher's protected least significant difference procedure as compared to the vehicle-treated animals.

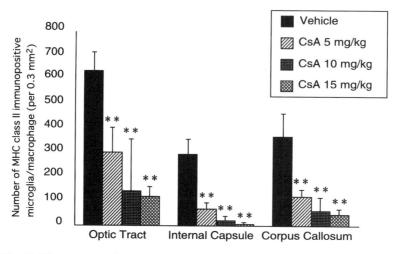

Fig. 7. Histograms of the numerical density of MHC class II immunopositive microglia/macrophages in the WM of rats receiving either vehicle or CsA for 14 d. $*p < 0.05$, $**p < 0.01$ by Fisher's protected least significant difference procedure as compared to the vehicle-treated animals.

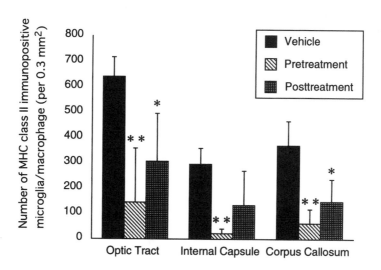

Fig. 8. Histograms of the numerical density of MHC class II immunopositive microglia/macrophages in the WM of rats receiving either vehicle or 10 mg/kg CsA from 1 d before the operation to 14 d after the operation (pretreatment), or 10 mg/kg CsA from 8 to 14 d after the operation (posttreatment). $*p < 0.05$, $**p < 0.01$ by Fisher's protected least significant difference procedure as compared to the vehicle-treated animals.

hypoperfusion model, the microglia were activated in parallel with the extent and severity of the rarefaction of the WM *(13)*. The suppression of both the microglial activation and the subsequent development of the WM lesions by CsA raises the possibility that a CsA-mediated suppression of the microglia resulted in the prevention of the WM lesions.

Microglia are key mediators of the immune response, and produce a variety of cytokines such as interleukin (IL)-1, IL-6 and tumor necrosis factor (TNF)-α *(28,29,38)*. Microglia also release cytotoxins such as inflammatory prostanoids, reactive oxygen species and nitrogen intermediates *(30–37,39)*. Because several cytokines such as IL-1β *(65–67)*, TNF-α *(68)* and transforming growth factor-β *(67)* are upregulated after cerebral ischemia, some of these cytokines may be involved in the pathogenesis of the WM lesions. Indeed, interferon-γ induces MHC antigen expression on the microglia *(69)* and potentiates demyelination *(70)*. TNF-α and lymphotoxin mediate the degeneration of the myelin *(71,72)*, and apoptosis of oligodendroglia *(73,74)*. CsA also has the potential to suppress the release of IL-1α, IL-2, and TNF-α from macrophages *(75–77)*.

In addition, CsA may have alleviated the WM lesions by acting on T cells. In pathologic conditions of the WM such as multiple sclerosis *(78)* and experimental allergic encephalomyelitis *(79)*, MHC-restricted antigen presentation by the microglia/macrophages and the subsequent T-cell activation is a central pathological event. T cells are another major source of cytokine production, and T-cell-derived cytokines could enhance the production of cytokines and cytotoxins by the microglia *(80,81)*. In chronic cerebral hypoperfusion model, the infiltration of CD4$^+$ and CD8$^+$ lymphocytes was suppressed in the WM after the administration of CsA *(55)*. Because CsA inhibits Ca^{2+}-dependent T cell activation *(82)*, the WM lesions may have been attenuated along this pathway.

Second, a large body of evidence suggests that mitochondrial dysfunction may contribute to ischemic neuronal death *(83–90)*. CsA is known to block the Ca^{2+}-induced mitochondrial permeability transition (MPT) by inhibiting the opening of the permeability transition pores under conditions of oxidative stress *(91,92)*. Therefore, the protective effects of CsA on the WM may be attributable to the maintenance and/or restoration of mitochondrial function. Indeed, Ca^{2+}-induced MPT is provoked by CsA but not FK506 *(93)*, and the nonimmunosuppressive CsA analog *N*-methyl-Val-4-cyclosporin A, which blocks the MPT pore, also diminished the infarct size in rats after a transient occlusion of the middle cerebral artery *(94)*. Similarly, in traumatic brain injury, the inhibition of the MPT by CsA preserved mitochondrial integrity in the axons and attenuated axonal damage *(95–98)*.

Third, CsA may have protected against the WM lesions by inhibiting NMDA-mediated neurotoxicity. CsA inhibits calcineurin activity, and this suppression of calcineurin activity leads to the phosphorylation of NOS and a decrease in NO synthesis *(99,100)*. Because NMDA neurotoxicity is mediated at least in part by NO *(101)*, the suppression of NOS may play a role in alleviating NMDA receptor-mediated ischemic damage. However, this possibility has become more unlikely because a recent study showed that ischemia-evoked NO production was not affected by FK506 *(102)*.

Finally, the apoptotic cell death of the oligodendroglia and its inhibition by CsA may contribute to the protective effects of CsA on the WM *(103)*. There is a paradigm that suggests that apoptosis represents a physiological mode of superfluous cell deletion with minimal tissue reaction, or even with an active inhibition of inflammation. However, apoptosis seems to be a crucial step that initiates ischemia-induced inflammation and the subsequent tissue damage, since antiapoptotic agents have been reported to suppress inflammation and tissue injury in a recent study *(104)*. The oligodendroglia undergo apoptosis in both the white and gray matter, with a concomitant activation of caspase-3 in this model *(105)*. Therefore, CsA may alleviate oligodendroglial apoptosis by suppressing calcineurin, which in turn dephosphorylates BAD, a proapoptotic member of the Bcl-2 family that promotes apoptosis.

CONCLUSIONS

This study shows that both pretreatment and posttreatment with a clinically relevant dosage of CsA is beneficial in suppressing the microglial activation and the subsequent development of WM lesions in a chronic cerebral hypoperfusion model. This suggests an involvement of immunological pathomechanisms in these cerebrovascular WM lesions, and may support the applicability of immunosuppressive agents in the treatment of patients with cerebrovascular WM lesions and cognitive impairment. However, there are several problems to be resolved such as nephrotoxicity, which has been encountered occasionally with the use of CsA *(106,107)*. Another perplexing problem is the considerable neurotoxicity of CsA itself, which may manifest as a cerebral WM lesion in nonneurologic patients *(108)*. In addition, these patients may be particularly susceptible to side effects such as infection because cerebrovascular disease patients with cognitive impairments generally tend to be of advanced age.

Finally, this chronic cerebral hypoperfusion model is a useful tool to investigate the pathophysiology of cerebrovascular WM lesions, and it may also be useful in screening drugs which may prevent the WM lesions in patients with cerebrovascular disease and vascular dementia.

REFERENCES

1. Kawamura J, Meyer JS, Terayama Y, Weathers S. Leukoaraiosis correlates with cerebral hypoperfusion in vascular dementia. Stroke 1991;22:609–614.
2. Awad IA, Masaryk T, Magdinec M. Pathogenesis of subcortical hyperintense lesions on magnetic resonance imaging of the brain. Observations in patients undergoing controlled therapeutic internal carotid artery occlusion. Stroke 1993;24:1339–1346.
3. Pantoni L, Garcia JH. Pathogenesis of leukoaraiosis: a review. Stroke 1997;28:652–659.
4. Roman GC. Senile dementia of the Binswanger type: a vascular form of dementia in the elderly. JAMA 1987;258:1782–1788
5. Baloh RW, Yue Q, Socotch TM, Jacobson KM. White matter lesions and disequilibrium in older people. I. Case-control comparison. Arch Neurol 1995;52:970–974
6. Goto K, Ishii N, Fukasawa H. Diffuse white-matter disease in the geriatric population. A clinical, neuropathological, and CT study. Radiology 1981; 141:687–953.
7. Awad IA, Johnson PC, Spetzler RF, Hodak JA. Incidental subcortical lesions identified on magnetic resonance imaging in the elderly, II: postmortem pathological correlations. Stroke 1986;17:1090–1097.
8. Fisher CM, Binswanger's encephalopathy: a review. J. Neurol. 1989;236: 65–79.
9. Janota I, Mirsen TR, Hachinski VC, et al. Neuropathologic correlates of leukoaraiosis. Arch Neurol 1989;46:1124–1128.
10. Révész T, Hawkins CP, Boulay EPGH, Barnard RO, McDonald WI. Pathological findings correlated with magnetic resonance imaging in subcortical arteriosclerotic encephalopathy (Binswanger's disease). J Neurol Neurosurg Psychiatr 1989;52:1337–1344.
11. Tomimoto H, Akiguchi I, Akiyama H, et al. T cell infiltration and expression of MHC class II antigen by macrophage/microglia in a heterogeneous group of leukoencephalopathy. Am J Pathol 1993;143:579–586.
12. Akiguchi I, Tomimoto H, Wakita H, et al. Cytopathological alterations and therapeutic approaches in Binswanger's disease. Neuropathology 1999; 19:119–128.
13. Wakita H, Tomimoto H, Akiguchi I, Kimura J. Glial activation and white matter changes in the rat brain induced by chronic cerebral hypoperfusion: An immunohistochemical study. Acta Neuropathol (Berl) 1994;87:484–492.
14. Tsuchiya M, Sako K, Yura S, Yonemasu Y. Cerebral blood flow and histopathological changes following permanent bilateral carotid artery ligation in Wistar rats. Exp Brain Res 1992;89:87–92.
15. Otori T, Katsumata T, Kashiwagi F, et al. Measurement of regional cerebral blood flow (rCBF) and glucose utilization (rCGU) in rat brain under chronic hypoperfusion following bilateral carotid occlusion. Cerebrovasc. Dis 1996; 6(Suppl):71.
16. Tomimoto H, Akiguchi I, Wakita H, Kimura J. White matter lesions after occlusion of the bilateral carotid arteries in the rat: temporal profile of cere-

bral blood flow (CBF), oligodendroglia and myelin. Brain Nerve 1997;49:639–644.

17. de la Torre JC, Fortin T, Parks GAS, et al. Chronic cerebrovascular insufficiency induces dementia-like deficits in aged rats. Brain Res 1992; 582:186–195.

18. Ni J, Ohta H, Matsumoto K, Watanabe H. Progressive cognitive impairment following chronic cerebral hypoperfusion induced by permanent occlusion of bilateral carotid arteries in rats. Brain Res 1994;653:231–236.

19. Ohta H, Nishikawa H, Kimura H, et al. Chronic cerebral hypoperfusion by permanent internal carotid ligation produces learning impairment without brain damage in rats. Neuroscience 1997;79:1039–1050.

20. Perry VH, Andersson P, Gordon S. Macrophages and inflammation in the central nervous system. Trends Neurosci 1993;16:268–273.

21. Lucchesi BR. Complement activation, neutrophils, and active oxygen radicals in reperfusion injury. Stroke 1993;24(Suppl I):141–147

22. Barone FC, Feuerstein GZ. Inflammatory mediators and stroke: new opportunities for novel therapeutics. J Cereb Blood Flow Metab 1999;19:819–834.

23. Giulian D. (1987) Ameboid microglia as effectors of inflammation in the C.N.S. J Neurosci Res 1987;18:155.

24. Gehrmann J, Matsumoto Y, Kreutzberg GW. Microglia: intrinsic immunoeffector cell of the brain. Brain Res Rev 1995;20:269–287.

25. Kreutzberg GW. Microglia: a sensor for pathological event in the C.N.S. Trends Neurosci 1996;8:312–318

26. Morioka T, Kalehua AN, Streit WJ. The microglial reaction in the rat dorsal hippocampus following transient cerebral ischemia. J Cereb Blood Flow Metab 1991;11:966–973.

27. Gehrmann J, Bonnekoh P, Miyazawa T, et al. Immunocytochemical study of an early microglial activation in ischemia. J Cereb Blood Flow Metab 1992;12:257–269.

28. Giulian D, Baker TJ, Shih LN, Lachman LB. Interleukin 1 of the central nervous system is produced by ameboid microglia. J Exp Med 1986;164: 594–604.

29. Sawada M, Kondo N, Suzumura A, Marunouchi T. Production of tumor necrosis factor-alpha by microglia and astrocytes in culture. Brain Res 1989;491:394–397.

30. Righi M, Mori L, de Libero G, et al. Monokine production by microglial cell clones. Eur J Immunol 1989;19:1443–1448.

31. Théry C, Chamak B, Mallat M. Cytotoxic effect of brain macrophages on developing neurons. Eur J Neurosci 1991;3:1155–1164.

32. Chao CC, Hu S, Molitor TW, et al. Activated microglia mediate neuronal cell injury via a nitric oxide mechanism. J Immunol 1992;149:2736–2741.

33. Banati RB, Germann J, Schubert P, Kreutzberg GW. Cytotoxicity of microglia. Glia 1993;7:111–118.

34. Corradin SB, Mauel J, Denis-Donini S, et al. Inducible NOS activity of cloned murine microglial cells. Glia 1993;7:255–262.

35. Dickson DW, Lee SC, Mattiace LA, et al. Microglia and cytokines in neurological disease, with special reference to AIDS and Alzheimer's disease. Glia 1993;7:75–83.

36. Giulian D, Vaca K. Inflammatory glia mediate delayed neuronal damage after ischemia in the central nervous system. Stroke 1993;24(Suppl I): 184–190.

37. Lees GJ. The possible contribution of microglia and macrophages to delayed neuronal death after ischemia. J Neurol Sci 1993;114:119–122.

38. Lee SC, Liu W, Dickson DW, et al. Cytokine production by human microglia and astrocytes: differential production of lipopolysaccharide and IL-1β. J Immunol 1993;150:2659–2667.

39. Meda L, Cassatella MA, Szendrei GI, et al. Activation of microglial cells by β-amyloid protein and IFN-γ. Nature 1995;374:647–652.

40. Tomimoto H, Akiguchi I, Wakita H, Kimura J. Changes in glial cells in Binswanger's type infarction. Brain Nerve 1994;468:771–779.

41. Akiguchi I, Tomimoto H, Suenaga T, et al. Alterations in glia and axons in the brains of Binswanger's disease patients. Stroke 1997;28:1423–1429.

42. Faulds DF, Goa KL, Benfield P. Cyclosporin: a review of its pharmacodynamic and pharmacokinetic properties, and therapeutic use in immunoregulatory disorders. Drugs 1993;45:953–1040.

43. Ryffel B. Pharmacology of cyclosporine. VI. Cellular activation: regulation of intracellular events by cyclosporine. Pharmacol Rev 1990;41:407–422.

44. Schreiber SL. Chemistry and biology of the immunophillins and their immunosuppressive ligands. Science 1991;251:283–287.

45. Schreiber SL, Crabtree GR. The mechanism of action of cyclosporin A and FK506. Immunol Today 1992;13:136–142.

46. Schumacher A, Nordheim A. Progress towards a molecular understanding of cyclosporin A-mediated immunosuppression. Clin Investig 1992;70: 773–779.

47. Shiga Y, Onodera H, Matsuo Y, Kogure K. Cyclosporin A protects against ischemia-reperfusion injury in the brain. Brain Res 1992;595:145–148.

48. Ogawa N, Tanaka K, Kondo Y, et al. The preventive effect of cyclosporin A, an immunosuppressant, on the late onset reduction of muscarinic acetylcholine receptors in gerbil hippocampus after transient forebrain ischemia. Neurosci Lett 1993;152:173–176.

49. Uchino H, Elmer E, Uchino K, et al. Cyclosporin A dramatically ameliorates CA1 hippocampal damage following transient forebrain ischaemia in the rat. Acta Physiol Scand 1995;155:469–471.

50. Li PA, Uchino H, Elmer E, Siesjo BK. Amelioration by cyclosporin A of brain damage following 5 or 10 min of ischemia in rats subjected to preischemic hyperglycemia. Brain Res 1997;753:133–140.

51. Kuroda S, Siesjo BK. Reperfusion damage following focal ischemia: pathophysiology and therapeutic windows. Clin Neurosci 1997;4:199–212.

52. Uchino H, Elmer E, Uchino K, et al. Amelioration by cyclosporin A of brain damage in transient forebrain ischemia in the rat. Brain Res 1998;812: 216–226.

53. Kuroda S, Janelidze S, Siesjo BK. The immunosuppressants cyclosporin A and FK506 equally ameliorate brain damage due to 30-min middle cerebral artery occlusion in hyperglycemic rats. Brain Res 1999;835:148–153.
54. Yoshimoto T, Siesjo BK. Posttreatment with the immunosuppressant cyclosporin A in transient focal ischemia. Brain Res 1999;839:283–291.
55. Wakita H, Tomimoto H, Akiguchi I, Kimura J. Protective effect of cyclosporin A on the white matter changes in the rat brain after chronic cerebral hypoperfusion. Stroke 1995;26:1415–1422.
56. Wakita H, Tomimoto H, Akiguchi I, Kimura J. Dose-dependent, protective effect of FK506 against white matter changes in the rat brain after chronic cerebral ischemia. Brain Res 1998;792:105–113
57. Wakita H, Tomimoto H, Akiguchi I, et al. A cyclooxygenase-2 inhibitor attenuates white matter damage in chronic cerebral ischemia. NeurorReport 1999;14:1461–1465
58. Sharkey J, Butcher SP. Immunophilins mediate the neuroprotective effects of FK506 in focal cerebral ischaemia. Nature 1994;371:336–339.
59. Sharkey J, Crawford JH, Butcher SP, Marston HM. Tacrolimus (FK506) ameliorates skilled motor deficits produced by middle cerebral artery occlusion in rats. Stroke 1996;27:2282–2286.
60. Ide T, Morikawa E, Kirino T. An immunosuppressant, FK506, protects hippocampal neurons from forebrain ischemia in the mongolian gerbil. Neurosci Lett 1996;204:157–160.
61. Tokime T, Nozaki K, Kikuchi H. Neuroprotective effect of FK506, an immunosuppressant, on transient global ischemia in gerbil. Neurosci Lett 1996;206:81–84.
62. Yagita Y, Kitagawa K, Matsushita K, et al. Effect of immunosuppressant FK506 on ischemia-induced degeneration of hippocampal neurons in gerbils. Life Sci 1996;59:1643–1650.
63. Drake M, Friberg H, Boris-Möller F, et al. The immunosuppressant FK506 ameliorates ischaemic damage in the rat brain. Acta Physiol Scand 1996;158:155–159.
64. Butcher SP, Henshall DC, Teramura Y, et al. Neuroprotective actions of FK506 in experimental stroke: in vivo evidence against an antiexcitotoxic mechanism. J Neurosci 1997;17:6939–6946
65. Minami M, Kuraishi Y, Yabuuchi K, et al. Induction of interleukin-1β mRNA in rat brain after transient forebrain ischemia. J Neurochem 1992;58:390–392.
66. Liu T, McDonnell PC, Young PR, et al. Interleukin-1 beta mRNA expression in ischemic rat cortex. Stroke 1993;24:1746–1750.
67. Wießner C, Gehrmann J, Lindholm D., et al. Expression of transforming growth factor-β1 and interleukin-1β mRNA in rat brain following transient cerebral ischemia. Acta Neuropathol 1993;(Berl);86:439–446.
68. Liu T, Clark RK, McDonnell PC, et al. Tumor necrosis factor-α expression in neurons. Stroke 1994;25:1481–1488.
69. Steininger B, van der Meide PH. Rat ependyma and microglia cells express class II MHC antigens after interavenous infusion of recombinant gamma interferon. J Neuroimmunol 1988;19:111–118.

70. Vass K, Heininger K, Schäfer B, et al. Interferon-γ potentiates antibody-mediated demyelination in vivo. Ann Neurol 1992;32:198–206.

71. Selmaj KW, Raine CS. Tumor necrosis factor mediates myelin and oligodendrocyte damage in vitro. Ann Neurol 1988;23:339–346

72. Selmaj K, Raine CS, Farooq M, et al. Cytokine cytotoxicity against oligodendrocytes. Apoptosis induced by lymphotoxin. J Immunol 1991;147: 1522–1529.

73. Hisahara S, Shoji S, Okano H, Miura M. ICE/CED-3 family executes oligodendrocyte apoptosis by tumor necrosis factor. J Neurochem 1997;69: 10–20.

74. Akassoglou K, Bauer J, Kassiotis G, et al. Oligodendrocyte apoptosis and primary demyelination induced by local TNF/p55TNF receptor signaling in the central nervous system of transgenic mice: models for multiple sclerosis with primary oligodendrogliopathy. Am J Pathol 1998;153:801–813

75. Benson A, Ziegler K. Macrophage as targets for inhibition by cyclosporine. Transplantation 1989;47:696–703.

76. Espevik T, Figari IS, Shalaby MR, et al. Inhibition of cytokine production by cyclosporin A and transforming growth factor beta. J Exp Med 1987;166: 571–576.

77. Keicho N, Sawada S, Kitamura K, et al. Effects of an immunosuppressant, FK506, on interleukin 1 alpha production by human macrophages and a macrophage-like cell line, U937. Cell Immunol 1991;132:285–294.

78. Bo L, Mork S, Kong PA, et al. Detection of MHC class II-antigens on macrophages and microglia, but not on astrocytes and endothelia in active multiple sclerosis lesions. J Neuroimmunol 1994;51:135–146.

79. McCombe PA, Fordyce BW, de Jersey J, et al. Expression of CD45RC and Ia antigen in the spinal cord in acute experimental allergic encephalomyelitis: an immunocytochemical and flow cytometric study. J Neurol Sci 1992; 113:177–186.

80. Conde M, Andrade J, Bedoya FJ, et al. Inhibitory effect of cyclosporin A and FK506 on nitric oxide production by cultured macrophages. Evidence of a direct effect on nitric oxide synthase activity. Immunology 1995; 84:476–481.

81. Hellendall RP, Ting JPY. Differential regulation of cytokine-induced major histocompatibility complex class II expression and nitric oxide release in rat microglia and astrocytes by effectors of tyrosine kinase, protein kinase C, and cAMP. J Neuroimmunol 1997;74:19–29.

82. Kronke M, Leonard WJ, Depper JM., et al. Cyclosporin A inhibits T-cell growth factor gene expression at the level of mRNA transcription. Proc Natl Acad Sci USA 1984;81:5214–5218.

83. Dux E, Mies G, Hossmann KA, Siklos L. Calcium in the mitochondria following brief ischemia of gerbil brain. Neurosci Lett 1987;78:295–300.

84. Silver IA, Erecinska M. Ion homeostasis in rat brain in vivo: intra- and extra-cellular (Ca^{2+}) and (H^+) in the hippocampus during recovery from short-term, transient ischemia. J Cereb Blood Flow Metab 1992;12:759–772.

85. Zaidan E, Sims NR. The calcium content of mitochondria from brain subregions following short-term forebrain ischemia and recirculation in the rat. J Neurochem 1994;63:1812–1819.

86. Abe K, Aoki M, Kawagoe J, et al. Ischemic delayed neuronal death. A mitochondrial hypothesis. Stroke 1995;26:1478–1489.

87. Siesjo BK, Siesjo P. Mechanisms of secondary brain injury. Eur J Anaesthesiol 1996;13:247–268.

88. Kristal BS, Dubinsky JM. Mitochondrial permeability transition in the central nervous system: induction by calcium cycling-dependent and -independent pathways. J Neurochem 1997;69:524–538.

89. Kristian T, Siesjo BK. Calcium in ischemic cell death. Stroke 1998;29: 705–718.

90. Friberg H, Connern C, Halestrap AP, Wieloch T. Differences in the activation of the mitochondrial permeability transition among brain regions in the rat correlate with selective vulnerability. J Neurochem 1999;72:2488–2497.

91. Zoratti M, Szabo I The mitochondrial permeability transition. Biochim Biophys Acta 1995;1241:139–176.

92. Gunter TE, Pfeiffer DR. Mechanisms by which mitochondria transport calcium. Am J Physiol 1990;258:755–786.

93. Friberg H, Ferrand-Drake1 M, Bengtsson F, et al. Cyclosporin A, but not FK 506, protects mitochondria and neurons against hypoglycemic damage and implicates the mitochondrial permeability transition in cell death. J Neurosci 1998;18:5151–5159.

94. Matsumoto S, Friberg H, Ferrand-Drake M, Wieloch T. Blockade of the mitochondrial permeability transition pore diminishes infarct size in the rat after transient middle cerebral artery occlusion. J Cereb Blood Flow Metab 1999;19:736–741.

95. Okonkwo DO, Povlishock JT. An intrathecal bolus of cyclosporin A before injury preserves mitochondrial integrity and attenuates axonal disruption in traumatic brain injury. J Cereb Blood Flow Metab 1999;19:443–451.

96. Okonkwo DO, Buki A, Siman R, Povlishock JT. Cyclosporin A limits calcium-induced axonal damage following traumatic brain injury. Neuroreport 1999;10:353–358.

97. Buki A, Okonkwo DO, Povlishock JT. Postinjury cyclosporin A administration limits axonal damage and disconnection in traumatic brain injury. J Neurotrauma 1999;16:511–521.

98. Sullivan PG, Thompson MB, Scheff SW. Cyclosporin A attenuates acute mitochondrial dysfunction following traumatic brain injury. Exp Neurol 1999; 160:226–234.

99. Conde M, Andrade J, Bedoya FJ, et al. Inhibitory effect of cyclosporin A and FK506 on nitric oxide production by cultured macrophages. Evidence of a direct effect on nitric oxide synthase activity. Immunology 1995;84:476–481.

100. Dawson TM, Steiner JP, Dawson VL, et al. Immunosuppressant FK506 enhances phosphorylation of nitric oxide synthase and protects against glutamate neurotoxicity. Proc Natl Acad Sci USA 1993;90:9808–9812.

101. Dawson VL, Dawsom TM, Bartley DA, et al. Mechanisms of nitric oxide-mediated neurotoxicity in primary brain cultures. J Neurosci 1993;13: 2651–2661.
102. Toung TJ, Bhardwaj A, Dawson VL, et al. Neuroprotective FK506 does not alter in vivo nitric oxide production during ischemia and early reperfusion in rats. Stroke 1999;30:1279–1285.
103. Wang HG, Pathan N, Ethell IM, et al. Ca^{2+}-induced apoptosis through calcineurin dephosphorylation of BAD. Science 1999;284:339–343.
104. Daemen MARC, van't Veer C, Denecker G, et al. Inhibition of apoptosis induced by ischemia-reperfusion prevents inflammation. J Clin Invest 1999;104:541–549.
105. Tomimoto H, Ihara M, Kinoshita M, et al. Capase mediated apoptosis of oligodendroglia in leukoaraisosis. 1st International Workshop of the White Matter Study Group, p. 25.
106. Shulman H, Striker G, Deeg HJ, et al. Nephrotoxicity of cyclosporin A after allogeneic marrow transplantation: glomerular thromboses and tubular injury. N Engl J Med 1981;305:1392–1395.
107. Klintmalm GB, Iwatsuki S, Starzl TE. Nephrotoxicity of cyclosporin A in liver and kidney transplant patients. Lancet 1981;1:470–471.
108. Gijtenbeek JM, van den Bent MJ, Vecht CJ. Cyclosporine neurotoxicity: a review. J Neurol 1999;246:339–346.

11

Blockade of Late-Onset Reduction of Muscarinic Acetylcholine Receptors by Immunosuppressants in Forebrain Ischemia

Ken-ichi Tanaka, M. Asanuma, and Norio Ogawa

INTRODUCTION

Five minutes of transient ischemia induces an almost complete loss of neurons in the CA1 regions of the gerbil hippocampus within a few days; this phenomenon is known as "delayed neuronal death" *(1)*. However, pyramidal neurons in the CA3 regions usually survive after transient cerebral ischemia. The ischemia-induced pyramidal cell changes in the hippocampal CA1 regions suggest that synaptic connections between pyramidal cells and their afferent nerve endings may be transiently or persistently destroyed. Although the molecular basis for the permanent neuronal destruction induced by transient ischemia has not been fully determined, there are several plausible hypotheses. Ischemic neuronal damage may be induced by several factors, including the following mechanisms:

1. Hypoxia and energy failure *(2)*.
2. Oxidative stress *(3–5)*.
3. Immune mechanisms *(6–10)*.
4. Apoptosis *(5,11,12)*.

LATE-ONSET REDUCTION OF MUSCARINIC ACETYLCHOLINE RECEPTORS (LORMAR)

Ischemia-Induced Cholinergic Dysfunction in the Hippocampus

Electron-microscopic examination has indicated that most of the postsynaptic neurons in gerbil hippocampal CA1 regions are destroyed and removed by ischemic insult *(13,14)*, and thereafter presynaptic structures are maintained for many months *(1,15)*. Although presynaptic terminals contain numerous synaptic vesicles that appear to be capable of releasing neurotrans-

From: *Immunosuppressant Analogs in Neuroprotection*
Edited by: C. V. Borlongan, O. Isacson, and P. R. Sanberg © Humana Press Inc., Totowa, NJ

mitters, acetylcholine (ACh) concentrations markedly fluctuate just after recirculation and then remain below control levels from 60 min to 7 d of recirculation, and by 14 d, ACh concentrations eventually return to normal levels *(16,17)*.

This result indicates that presynaptic terminals that seem to be morphologically intact after ischemic insult are functionally damaged.

LORMAR in Transient Cerebral Ischemia

When transient cerebral ischemia is induced in gerbils for 5 min, selective delayed neuronal death occurs over about 1 wk in the hippocampal CA1 area, beginning after 2 or 3 d in the same way as in rats. Muscarinic acetylcholine receptors (mACh-Rs) decrease in the transient ischemic gerbil hippocampus *(6,18,19)* and several brain regions of middle cerebral artery-occluded Wistar rats *(20,21)*. In gerbils, mACh-Rs are unchanged for the first 4 d postischemia, and then gradually decrease and show a 90% loss compared to the sham-operated group after 21 d. Moreover, the large loss of mACh-Rs after transient ischemia occurs later and more gradually than that of N-methyl-D-aspartate binding sites *(16,22)*. Although delayed neuronal death does not progress further, a late-onset reduction of mACh-Rs (LORMAR) in the hippocampus progresses further from d 7, or does lipid peroxidation *(16)*. These findings indicate that even 5 min ischemia causes late-onset and progressive degeneration of mACh-Rs.

Effects of Immunophilin Ligands on LORMAR

Daily administration of CsA for 7 d beginning just after recirculation has no significant influence on mACh-Rs and muscarinic M1 receptors (M1-Rs) in terms of either affinity (K_d) or binding capacity (B_{max}) in sham-operated gerbils. In ischemic gerbils, the B_{max} is markedly decreased as compared with that in the sham-operated gerbils. However, this reduction can clearly be prevented by a postischemic daily administration of CsA *(6)*.

On the other hand, CsA, when administrated three times early on the day of ischemia, 2 and 6 h after recirculation, has also been observed to significantly restore LORMAR in a CsA-treated ischemia group at d 14 compared with time-matched controls *(23)*. Neither ischemic insult nor CsA treatment significantly influences the K_d value for mACh-Rs *(23)*. Therefore, it seems that long-term continuous administration of CsA is not always necessary to induce a neuroprotective action against transient cerebral ischemia. Rather, an early administration of CsA appears to be more important than chronic administration.

In the case of FK506, there is no significant change in the K_d values for mACh-Rs among all four groups, which includes sham-operated or ischemic gerbils with or without FK506, respectively. In the sham-operated groups, neither FK506 nor vehicle shows any effects on the B_{max} value. Although the B_{max} value of the vehicle-treated ischemic group is significantly decreased, that of the FK506-treated ischemic group is recovered to sham-operated levels *(24)*.

Thus, immunophilin ligands prevent LORMAR induced by transient ischemia. However, the protective effects of immunophilin ligands, at least CsA, against LORMAR may have no relation to its immunosuppressive action *(6,23–25)*. Because CsA prevents glial activation in the hippocampal CA1 regions, glial cells play a central role in the immune responses of the central nervous system (CNS) *(26,27)*.

Another possible explanation for the protective effects of immunophilin ligands on LORMAR is a direct influence on the interaction between interleukin (IL)-2 and the cholinergic system. CsA exerts its protective effects on cholinergic neurons via some immunosuppressive properties by modulating cytokines in the CNS. IL-2 reduces the amount of ACh released from rat hippocampal slices *(28)* and enhances the amnesia and hyperactivity induced by the anticholinergic drug scopolamine in mice *(29)*, suggesting that IL-2 has an anticholinergic effect on the CNS. Thus, the inhibition of IL-2 production by CsA administration could have a protective effect on the cholinergic system after the ischemic insult.

These results therefore suggest that LORMAR might be associated with not only immune responses mediated by glia cells but also unknown mechanisms unrelated to the central immune system.

ISCHEMIC NEURONAL CELL DEATH CONSISTS OF IMMUNE RESPONSE AND APOPTOSIS

Immune Responses Mediated by Glia Cells in the Brain

The brain has been believed for a long time to be an immunologically privileged site that is isolated from the peripheral immune system by the blood–brain barrier (BBB). However, it is now evident that there is an immune network consisting primarily of glial cells and cytokines in the brain *(27)*, especially in the presence of several neurological diseases *(30)*. Experimental data on brain ischemia have also suggested the importance of immune mechanisms in the brain. In the case of transient forebrain ischemia in rodents, glia cells begin to accumulate before completion of delayed neuronal death of the hippocampal CA1 pyramidal cells at d 4 after reperfusion of cerebral blood flow. Astrocytes immunostained by antiglial fibrillary acidic protein (GFAP) show hypertrophy and hyperplasia in the CA1 regions, starting from d 1 or d 2 and lasting for several weeks after ischemia

(31–34). Compared with the astrocytic reaction, the microglial response is very early, since microglial cells are activated within a few hours after ischemia–reperfusion *(35).* For example, microglias in the rat cerebral cortex are activated 3 h after transient focal ischemia *(36),* indicating that signal transduction mediated by tyrosine phosphorylation is involved in the early activation of microglias. Microglias immunolabeled with major histocompatibility complex (MHC) class I antigens and MHC class II antigens are occasionally seen in normal rat brain *(37).* However, in the hippocampal CA1 regions, these immunoreactivities are rarely seen *(37).* One day after transient forebrain ischemia, MHC class I + microglias begin to be expressed in the pyramidal layer of the hippocampal CA1. MHC class II + microglias seem to appear somewhat later, exhibiting a phagocytic form with spheroid or ameboid morphology *(37).* MHC class I and II immunoreactivities also continue for approx 8 wk after transient ischemia but gradually disappear during the course of hippocampal sclerosis *(37).* As a consequence, microglias are activated by signals from the cells damaged by ischemia, releasing cytokines, and activated astrocytes *(38).* Incidentally, microglias and astrocytes also produce IL-1, IL-6, tumor necrosis factor (TNF)-α, and other cytokines. These cytokines play a major role in neurological disorders by mutual regulation of glial function and proliferation, as well as by regulation of neuronal function, regeneration, and growth. Moreover, activated microglias are well known to generate free radicals, with the conventional hypothesis being that immunosuppressants can be used to inhibit activated microglias. Thus, it seems that glia cells, particularly microglias and astrocytes, might play an important role in the ischemic cell death mediated by transient ischemia-induced immune responses.

On the other hand, interactions with the peripheral immune system may also occur. Adhesion molecules such as intercellular adhesion molecule-1 (ICAM-1) and leukocyte function-associated antigen-3 (LFA-3) serve as receptors for binding with peripheral leukocytes in various states, including inflammation and ischemia, suggesting that the brain is also influenced by a peripheral immune mechanism *(39).*

Effects of Immunophilin Ligands on Glial Activation in Transient Ischemia

In 5-min transient-ischemic gerbils, CsA treatment cannot prevent delayed neuronal death in the hippocampal CA1 pyramidal neurons nor can vehicle treatment *(6).* However, CsA prevents increases in the number of GFAP+ astrocytes induced by transient ischemia in the hippocampal CA1 regions *(6).* By contrast, MHC class II positive cells include both resting and reactive microglias. In sham-operated groups, MHC class II+ resting microglias have sporadically been seen in all examined brain regions *(25)*. In ischemia groups, the number of MHC class II+ microglias (both resting and reactive) increases in hippocampal CA1 regions on d 3 after transient ischemia, and MHC class II immunoreactivities remain intensely on d 10. However, CsA ameliorates MHC class II immunoreactivities in the hippocampal CA1 regions compared with the vehicle-treated ischemic group on d 10. Regions other than the hippocampal CA1 regions have shown only sporadic MHC class II positive microglias (resting form) in all groups *(25)*. Some studies have reported a reduced expression of MHC class II antigen on T cells, monocytes, and endothelial cells by CsA *(40)*. Thus, it seems that CsA ameliorates altered microglial functions *(25)*. In addition, early and single-day administration of CsA does not affect ischemia-induced delayed neuronal death in the hippocampal CA1 regions, although both early and chronic administration of CsA prevents LORMAR *(6,23,25)*.

FK506 administration induces no pathological change in sham-operated groups. Delayed neuronal death is seen in the pyramidal neurons in the hippocampal CA1 regions on d 10 after transient forebrain ischemia in both FK506- and vehicle-treated groups; therefore, consecutive administration of FK506 cannot prevent delayed neuronal death, although FK506 prevents LORMAR *(24)*. Since delayed neuronal death is inhibited by the administration of FK506 within 1 h after transient ischemia, it seems that the inhibition of calcineurin (CaN) activity in hippocampal CA1 pyramidal cells during the initial period is related to the neuroprotective action of FK506.

According to our histopathological study in this gerbil model, FK506 cannot prevent the accumulation of GFAP+ astroglia in the ischemic hippocampus, although CsA prevents both the astroglial *(6)* and microglial activation *(25)* induced by transient ischemia in gerbils. Furthermore, early treatment with CsA only in the initial stages of ischemia–reperfusion similarly restores LORMAR with astroglial and microglial activation in ischemic gerbils *(23)*. The possibility of a discrepancy between immunophilin ligands CsA and FK506 may be due to the difference in the action mechanisms of neuroprotection and/or neurorestoration.

Anti-Apoptosis Properties of Immunophilin Ligands

Because the binding of immunosuppressants with immunophilins is considered to lead to an inhibition of CaN activity *(41)*, many studies have been conducted on the relationship between cerebral ischemia and CaN. CaN is found at high concentrations in hippocampal CA1 pyramidal cells, and its levels decrease in response to delayed neuronal death. However, there have been reports that an upregulation of CaN occurs in afferent fibers to the CA1 regions and in astrocytes *(42)*. Recent studies have shown that anti-CD3-induced apoptosis is mediated by Fas-ligand production, which is regulated by the CaN-activated nuclear factor of activated T-cells (NF-AT) *(43)* and the interaction between Fas and Fas-ligand *(44–46)*. CaN has also been found to be activated by the dephosphorylation of Bad and nitric oxide synthase *(47,48)*. Furthermore, CaN-induced apoptosis is due to activation of the cytochrome *c*/caspase-3 pathway in neurons *(49)*. Therefore, CaN appears to participate in apoptosis in various ways, and ischemic neuronal cell death is known to involve apoptosis at least to some extent *(50)*.

In contrast, the mitochondrial permeability transition (MPT) causes subsequent mitochondrial dysfunction and cell death via mitochondrial swelling, depolarization, and uncoupling of oxidative phosphorylation *(51–53)*. Moreover, MPT is regulated by Bax in mitochondrial dysfunction, with a resultant release of cytochrome *c* to the cytosol *(54,55)*. It is well known that Bax, as one of proapoptotic factors in the Bcl-2 family *(56)*, has been shown to induce the characteristic features of apoptosis, which include cell death, DNA fragmentation, and caspase activation *(54,55)*. CsA, but not FK506, inhibits Ca^{2+}-dependent MPT *(57–59)* and prevents the apoptotic cell death induced by the overexpression of Bax to inhibit MPT *(54)*. Nakatsuka and associates *(49)* also have reported that the release of cytochrome *c* from mitochondria to the cytosol is recognized in the early stages of delayed neuronal death in the gerbil hippocampus. FK506 also protects against apoptotic cell death after transient focal cerebral ischemia by means of an amelioration of mitochondrial dysfunction *(60)*, which is a crucial event in the cellular commitment to the apoptotic program *(61)*.

In addition, apoptotic cell death is also induced by a withdrawal of neurotrophic factor. In the case of cerebral ischemia, it seems that NGF produced by astrocytes acts on nearby neurons to rescue them from ischemic cell damage *(62)*. Immunophilin ligands are also considered to be neurotrophic in every neurotransmission system including cholinergic-, dopaminergic-, and serotonergic-systems *(63)*. In studies PC12 cells and sensory ganglia, CsA or FK506 have shown neurotrophiclike activity *(64)*.

As a consequence, CsA and FK506 may have antiapoptotic effects to protect against ischemic neuronal cell death. Moreover, transient ischemia-induced LORMAR might be caused or influenced by apoptotic cell death.

Multiple Neuroprotective Properties of Immunophilin Ligands

Immunophilins are receptor proteins for immunophilin ligands, with CsA binding specifically to cyclophilin (CyP) and FK506 to FK506 binding protein (FKBP). Immunophilins in the brain are considered to be related to a release of intracellular Ca^{2+}, control of NO toxicity, control of the release of neurotransmitters, and neurotrophiclike activity *(63)*. The mechanism of action is believed to involve binding of the immunophilin ligands– immunophilin complex with CaN to inhibit the dephosphorylating effects of CaN. However, the neurotrophic effects of CsA and FK506 can be functionally dissociated from their immunosuppressive properties, as nonimmunosuppressive derivatives of CsA or FK506 have potent neurotrophic effects comparable to their mother compounds *(63,65–72)*. Furthermore, the neurotrophic actions of immunophilin ligands are restricted to damaged neurons, in contrast to neurotrophic factors, which also elicit neurite outgrowth in naive neurons *(63)*. This property of immunophilin ligands may be advantageous, as neuroprotective drugs, in contrast to neurotrophic factors, act on not only damaged neurons but also naive neurons, thus causing undesirable effects. Therefore, several properties of immunophilin ligands, including their neurotrophic activities, are mediated by an inhibition of rotamase activity rather than by an inhibition of CaN activity *(66,68)*, although inhibition of both CaN and rotamase could contribute to the neuroprotective effects of CsA or FK506 *(63,65,68,73)*. Besides their CaN and rotamase activity, immunophilin ligands are also thought to exert chaperone activity in, for example, the folding of carbonic anhydrase *(74)*. Moreover, chaperone proteins prevent the formation of functionless aggregates that appear to induce neurodegenerated disease by means of random adhesion to other proteins *(74,75)*, and this property of immunophilin ligands may also have relevance to the neurotrophic effects.

CHRONIC CEREBRAL ISCHEMIA AND VASCULAR DEMENTIA

Chronic Cerebral Hypoperfusion as an Animal Model of Vascular Dementia

Central cholinergic function is closely linked to intellectual functions such as learning, memory, and cognition. Furthermore, cholinergic abnormalities are specifically associated with the cognitive dysfunction in patients with Alzheimer's disease (AD) *(76–78)*. However, in the case of vascular dementia (VD) and cerebral ischemia, the relationship between learning impairments and cholinergic dysfunctions has remained obscure in humans and experimental animals, although several studies have been reported in the experimental animal model *(79,80)*. Therefore, we have designed a new animal model of VD with chronic cerebral hypoperfusion produced by permanent ligation of bilateral common carotid arteries in Wistar rats *(81)*. We have reported previously that chronic cerebral hypoperfusion in Wistar rats induces an impairment of discrimination learning, primarily due to central muscarinic cholinergic dysfunction as well as striatal neuronal damage and rarefaction of the white matter based on chronic hypoperfusion of cerebral blood flow *(81–83)*. In particular, we have provided, for the first time direct evidence of a close relationship between learning impairment and mACh-Rs disability *(81,82)*. Thus, it seems that the abnormalities seen in our chronic cerebral hypoperfusion model are produced by a variety of mechanisms such as VD in humans. As a consequence, we propose that chronic cerebral hypoperfusion in Wistar rats is a useful animal model for studying the pathophysiology of VD *(84)*.

Cholinergic Dysfunction Induced by Chronic Cerebral Hypoperfusion

Chronic cerebral hypoperfusion influences pre- and postsynaptic cholinergic indices, that is, ACh content and choline acetyltransferase (ChAT) activity, and mACh-Rs binding ability *(81,85)*. In particular, we have noted that these changes consist of two distinct phases, before "acute" and after "chronic" 6 wk after the operation *(81)*. At 3 wk, paradoxical changes in pre- and postsynaptic cholinergic indices are noted in the frontal cortex and thalamus + midbrain, although there is no statistically significant ChAT activity in the frontal cortex. By contrast, after 6 wk, ChAT activity in the frontal cortex and thalamus + midbrain return to the levels seen in sham-operated rats. Therefore, ChAT activity is only changed at 3 wk after the operation. The B_{max} value of mACh-Rs binding is reduced in the frontal cortex, hippocampus, and striatum, but not in the thalamus + midbrain at 6 wk, and thereafter remains at this level, at least, until 12 wk. These findings suggest that hypoperfusion-induced acute changes at 3 wk in mACh-Rs binding may only be supplemented by changes in ChAT activity in the frontal cortex and thalamus + midbrain. Thus, the chronic reduction at 6 wk and thereafter in the B_{max} values of mACh-Rs bindings may play an especially important role in brain injury induced by both chronic cerebral hypoperfusion and LORMAR by transient ischemia *(81,82)*.

Effects of Immunophilin Ligands on Chronic Cerebral Hypoperfusion

In the case of chronic cerebral hypoperfusion in rats, CsA or FK506 causes a dose-dependent improvement in the histological changes induced by chronic cerebral hypoperfusion as well as transient ischemia *(86,87)*. In our study, the preventive effects of FK506 in learning impairment appears to result from the observed concomitant protection against the rarefaction of white matter and striatal neuronal cell damage *(88)*. In addition, Bennett and colleagues *(89)* have reported that the degree of apoptotic cell loss correlates with behavioral impairment in Sprague-Dawley rats following chronic cerebral hypoperfusion. Therefore, FK506 attenuates the learning impairment induced by chronic cerebral hypoperfusion, primarily by preventing the rarefaction of white matter and striatal neuronal cell damage. Moreover, CsA also partially ameliorates the learning impairment that occurs following chronic cerebral hypoperfusion in rats *(88)*.

Considering this evidence, CsA and/or FK506 may improve chronic reductions in mACh-Rs binding as well as histrogical abnormalities by chronic cerebral hypoperfusion in several regions of rat brains. Furthermore, immunophilin ligands show a therapeutic effect not only against acute cerebral ischemia, but also against brain injury due to chronic reductions in cerebral blood flow such as that occurring with chronic cerebral hypoperfusion in rats.

CONCLUSION

Both CsA and FK506 prevent the LORMAR induced by 5 min transient ischemia in gerbils and inhibit astroglial and microglial activation, although they do not have any protective effects on delayed neuronal death *(6,25)*. Furthermore, long-term continuous treatment with CsA or FK506 is not always necessary for neuroprotective action in transient-ischemic gerbils *(25,90)*. Therefore, immunosuppressive effects mediated by CaN inhibition of immunophilin ligands may not be essential to protect against transient ischemic brain injury such as LORMAR. On the other hand, we have persisted in applying LORMAR to a model of VD, and it may be applied as a screening test for therapeutic drugs for AD. Moreover, immunophilin ligands show a therapeutic effect not only against acute cerebral ischemia, but also against brain injury due to chronic reductions in cerebral blood flow such as that occurring with chronic cerebral hypoperfusion in rats. Thus, immunophilin ligands, especially CsA and FK506, may possibly function as not only neuroprotective drugs for the treatment of neurological disease but also antidementia drugs for VD and/or AD.

REFERENCES

1. Kirino T. Delayed neuronal death in the gerbil hippocampus following ischemia. Brain Res 1982;239:57–69.
2. Kogure K, Scheinberg P, Matsumoto A, et al. Catecholamines in experimental brain ischemia. Arch Neurol 1975;32:21–24.
3. Dalkara T, Endres M, Moskowitz AM. Mechanism of NO neurotoxicity. Prog Brain Res 1998;118:231–239.
4. Love S. Oxidative stress in brain ischemia. Brain Pathol 1999;9:119–131.

5. Taylor DL, Edwards AD, Mehmet H. Oxidative metabolism, apoptosis and perinatal brain injury. Brain Pathol 1999;9:93–117.

6. Ogawa N, Tanaka K, Kondo Y, et al. The preventive effect of cyclosporin A, an immunosuppressant, on the late onset reduction of muscarinic acetylcholine receptors in gerbil hippocampus after transient forebrain ischemia. Neurosci Lett 1993;152:173–176.

7. Sharkey J, Butcher SP. Immunophilins mediate the neuroprotective effects of FK506 in focal cerebral ischaemia. Nature 1994;371:336–339.

8. DeGraba TJ. The role of inflammation after acute stroke: utility of pursuing anti-adhesion molecule therapy. Neurology 1998;51:S62–S68.

9. Stol G, Jander S, Schroeter M. Inflammation and glial responses in ischemic brain lesions. Prog. Neurobiol. 1998;56:149–171.

10. Kato H, Kogure K. Biochemical and molecular characteristics of the brain with developing cerebral infarction. Cell Mol Neurobiol 1999;19:93–108.

11. Martin LJ, Al-Abdulla NA, Brambrink AM, et al. Neurodegeneration in excitotoxicity, global cerebral ischemia, and target deprivation: A perspective on the contributions of apoptosis and necrosis. Brain Res Bull 1998;46: 281–309.

12. Schulz JB, Weller M, Moskowitz MA. Caspases as treatment targets in stroke and neurodegenerative disease. Ann. Neurol. 1999;45:421–429.

13. Olney JW, Ikonomidou C, Mosinger JL, Friedrich G. MK-801 prevents hypobaric neuronal degeneration in infant rat brain. J Neurosci 1989;9: 1701–1704.

14. Kirino T, Tamura A, Sano K. Chronic maintenance of presynaptic terminals in gliotic hippocampus following ischemia. Brain Res 1990;510:17–25.

15. Johansen FF, Johansen MB, Diemer NH. Resistance of hippocampal CA-1 interneurons to 20 min of transient cerebral ischemia in the rat. Acta Neuropathol (Berl) 1983;61:135–140.

16. Haba K, Ogawa N, Mizukawa K, Mori A. Time course of changes in lipid peroxidation, pre and postsynaptic cholinergic indicies, NMDA receptor binding and neuronal death in the gerbil hippocampus following transient ischemia. Brain Res 1991;540:116–122.

17. Ishimaru H, Takahashi A, Ikarashi Y, Maruyama Y. Effect of transient cerebral ischemia on acetylcholine release in the gerbil hippocampus. NeuroReport 1994;5:601–604.

18. Araki T, Kato H, Kogure K, Kanai Y. Long-term changes in gerbil brain neurotransmitter receptors following transient cerebral ischemia. Br J Pharmacol 1992;107:437–442.

19. Kato H, Araki T, Kogure K. Preserved neurotransmitter receptor binding following ischemia in preconditioned gerbil brain. Brain Res Bull 1992; 29:395–400.

20. Nagasawa H, Araki T, Kogure K. Alternation of muscarinic acetylcholine binding sites in the postischemic brain areas of the rat using in vitro autoradiography. J Neurol Sci 1994;121:27–31.

21. Nagasawa H, Araki T, Kogure K. Autoradiographic analysis of second-messenger and neurotransmitter receptor systems in the exo-focal remote areas of postischemic rat brain. Brain Res Bull 1994;35:347–352.

22. Ogawa N, Haba K, Asanuma M, et al. Loss of *N*-methyl-D-aspartate (NMDA) receptor binding in rat hippocampal areas at the chronic stage after forebrain ischemia: Histological and NMDA receptor binding studies. Neurochem Res 1991;16:519–524.

23. Kondo Y, Asanuma M, Iwata E, et al. Early treatment with cyclosporin A ameliorates the reduction of muscarinic acetylcholine receptors in gerbil hippocampus after transient forebrain ischemia. Neurochem Res 1999;24:9–13.

24. Nishibayashi S, Kondo Y, Asanuma M, et al. Protective effects of FK506 on the late-onset reduction of muscarinic acetylcholine receptors in gerbil hippocampus after transient forebrain ischemia. J Brain Sci 1997;23:33–40.

25. Kondo Y, Ogawa N, Asanuma M, et al. Cyclosporin A prevents ischemia-induced reduction of muscarinic acetylcholine receptors with suppression of microglial activation in gerbil hippocampus. Neurosci Res 1995;22:123–127.

26. Bartfai T, Schultzberg M. Cytokines in neuronal cell types. Neurochem Int 1993;22:435–444.

27. Hopkins SJ, Rothwell NJ. Cytokines and the nervous system I: expression and recognition. TINS 1995;18:83–88.

28. Araujo DM, Lapchak PA, Collier B, Quirion R. Localization of interleukin-2 immunoreactivity and interleukin-2 receptors in the rat brain: interaction with the cholinergic system. Brain Res 1989;498:257–266.

29. Bianchi M, Panerai AE. Interleukin-2 enhances scopolamine-induced amnesia and hyperactivity in the mouse. NeuroReport 1993;4:1046–1048.

30. McGeer PL, Itagaki S, McGeer EG. Expression of the histocompatibility glycoprotein HLA-DR in neurological disease. Acta Neuropathol 1988;76:550–557.

31. Yoshimine T, Morioka K, Brengman JM, et al. Immunohistochemical investigation of cerebral ischemia during recirculation. J Neurosurg 1985;63:922–928.

32. Petito CK, Morgello S, Felix JC, Lesser ML. The two patterns of reactive astrocytosis in postischemic rat brain. J Cereb Blood Flow Metab 1990;10:850–859.

33. Schmit-Kastner R, Szymas J, Hossmann KA. Immunohistochemical study of glial reaction and serum protein extravasation in relation to neuronal damage in rat hippocampus after ischemia. Neuroscience 1990;38:527–540.

34. Rischke R, Krieglstein J. Postischemic neuronal damage causes astroglial activation and increase in local cerebral glucose utilization of rat hippocampus. J Cereb Blood Flow Metab 1991;11:106–113.

35. Morioka T, Kalehua AN, Streit WJ. The microglial reaction in the rat dorsal hippocampus following transient forebrain ischemia. J Cereb Blood Flow Metab 1991;11:966–973.

36. Korematsu K, Goto S, Nagahiro S, Ushio Y. Microglial response to transient focal cerebral ischemia: an immunocytochemical study on the rat cerebral cortex using anti-phosphotyrosine antibody. J Cereb Blood Flow Metab 1994;14:825–830.

37. Kondo Y. Activated and phagocytic microglia. In: Walz W, ed. Cerebral Ischemia: Molecular and Cellular Pathophysiology. Humana Press, Totowa, NJ, pp. 251–269.

38. Gehrmann J, Bonnekoh P, Miyazawa T, et al. Immunocytochemical study of an early microglial activation in ischemia. J Cereb Blood Flow Metab 1992;12:257–269.
39. Rossler K, Neuchrist C, Kitz K, et al. Expression of leukocyte adhesion molecules at the human blood brain barrier (BBB). J Neurosci Res 1992; 31:365–374.
40. Di Padova FE. Pharmacology of cyclosporine (Sandimune) V. Pharmacological effects on immune function: in vitro studies. Pharmacol Rev 1989;41: 373–405.
41. Lui J, Farmer JD, Lane WS, et al. Calcineurin is a common target of cyclophilin-cyclosporin A and FKBP-FK506 complexes. Cell. 1991;66: 807–815.
42. Yamasaki Y, Onodera H, Adachi K, et al. Alteration in the immunoreactivity of the calcineurin subunits after ischemic hippocampal damage. Neuroscience 1992;49:545–556.
43. Latinis KM, Norian LA, Eliason SL, Koretzky GA. Two NFAT transcription factor binding sites participate in the regulation of CD95 (Fas) ligand expression in activated human T cells. J Biol Chem 1997;272:31,427–31,434.
44. Shi YF, Sahai BM, Green DR. Cyclosporin A inhibits activation-induced cell death in T-cell hybridomas and thymocytes. Nature 1989;339:625–626.
45. Brunner T, Mogil RJ, LaFace D, et al. Cell-autonomous Fas (CD95)/Fas-ligand interaction mediates activation-induced apoptosis in T-cell hybridomas. Nature 373:441-444.
46. Dhein J, Walczak H, Baumler C, et al. Autocrine T-cell suicide mediated by APO-1/. Nature 1995;l373:438–441.
47. Dawson TM, Steiner JP, Dawson VL, et al. Immunosuppressant FK506 enhances phosphorylation of nitric oxide synthase and protects against glutamate neurotoxicity. Proc Natl Acad Sci USA 1993;90:9808–9812.
48. Wang HG, Pathan N, Ethell IM, et al. Ca^{2+}-induced apoptosis through calcineurin dephosphorylation of BAD. Science 1999;284:339–343.
49. Nakatsuka H, Ohta S, Tanaka J, et al. Release of cytochrome c from mitochondria to cytosol in gerbil hippocampal CA1 neurons after transient forebrain ischemia. Brain Res 1999;849:216–219.
50. Asai A, Qin J-H, Narita Y, et al. High level calcineurin activity predisposes neuronal cells to apoptosis. J Biol Chem 1999;274:34,450–34,458.
51. Broekemeier KM, Dempsey ME, Pfeiffer DR. Cyclosporin A is a potent inhibitor of the inner membrane permeability transition in liver mitochondria. J Biol Chem 1989;264:7826–7830.
52. Crompton M, Ellinger H, Costi A. Inhibition by cyclosporin A of a Ca^{2+}-dependent pore in heart mitochondria activated by inorganic phosphate and oxidative stress. Biochem J 1988;255:357–360.
53. Pastorino JG, Snyder JW, Serroni A, et al. Cyclosporin and carnitine prevent the anoxic death of cultured hepatocytes by inhibiting the mitochondrial permeability transition. J Biol Chem 1993;268:13,791–13,798.
54. Pastorino JG, Chen, ST, Tafani M, Snyder J. The overexpression of Bax produces cell death upon induction of the mitochondrial permeability transition. J Biol Chem 1998;273:7770–7775.

55. Pastorino JG, Tafani M, Rothman RJ, et al. Functional consequences of the sustained or transient activation by Bax of the mitochondrial permeability transition pore. J Biol Chem 274:31,734–31,739.

56. Oltvai ZN, Milliman CL, Korsmeyer SJ. Bcl-2 heterodimerizes in vivo with a conserved homolog, Bax, that accelerates programmed cell death. Cell 1993;74:609–619.

57. Siesjo BK, Elmer E, Janelidze S, et al. Role and mechanisms of secondary mitochondrial failure. Acta Neurochir Suppl (Wien) 1999;73:7–13.

58. He L, Poblenz AT, Medrano CJ, Fox DA. Lead and calcium produce rod photoreceptor cell apoptosis by opening the mitochondrial permeability transition pore. J Biol Chem 2000;275:12,175–12,184.

59. Kingham PJ, Pocock JM. Microglial apoptosis induced by chromogranin A is mediated by mitochondrial depolarisation and the permeability transition but not by cytochrome c release. J Neurochem 2000;74:1452–1462.

60. Nakai A, Kuroda S, Kristian T, Siesjo BK. The immunosuppressant drug FK506 ameliorates secondary mitochondrial dysfunction following transient focal cerebral ischemia in the rat. Neurobiol Dis 1997;4:288–300.

61. Kroemer G, Zamzami N, Susin SA. Mitochondrial control of apoptosis. Immunol Today 1997;18:44–51.

62. Shozuhara H, Onodera H, Katoh-Semba R, et al. Temporal profiles of nerve growth factor β-subunit level in rat brain regions after transient ischemia. J Neurochem 1992;59:175–180.

63. Snyder SH, Sabatini DM, Lai MM, et al. Neural actions of immunophilin ligands. Trends Pharmacol Sci 1998;19:21–26.

64. Lyons WE, George EB, Dawson TM, et al. Immunosuppressant FK506 promotes neurite outgrowth in cultutres of PC12 cells and sensory ganglia. Proc Natl Acad Sci USA 1994;91:3191–3195.

65. Gold BG. FK506 and the role of immunophilins in nerve regeneration. Mol Neurobiol 1997;15:285–306.

66. Gold BG, Zeleny-Pooley M, Wang M-S, et al. A nonimmunosuppressant FKBP-12 ligand increases nerve regeneration. Exp Neurol 1997;147:269–278.

67. Steiner JP, Connolly MA, Valentine HL, et al. Neurotrophic actions of nonimmunosuppressive analogues of immunosuppressive drugs FK506, rapamycin and cyclosporin A. Nature Med 1997;3:421–428.

68. Steiner JP, Hamilton GS, Ross DT, et al. Neurotrophic immunophilin ligands stimulate stracural and functional recovery in neurodegenerative animal models. Proc Natl Acad Sci USA 1997;94:2019–2024.

69. Gold BG, Zeleny-Pooley M, Chaturvedi P, Wang M-S. Oral administration of a nonimmunosuppressant FKBP-12 ligand speeds nerve regeneration. NeuroReport 1998;9:553–558.

70. Costantini LC, Chaturvedi P, Armistead DM, et al. A novel immunophilin ligands: distinct branching effects on dopaminergic neurons in culture and neurotrophic actions after oral administration in an animal model of Parkinson's disease. Neurobiol Dis 1998;5:97–108.

71. Sauer H, Francis JM, Jiang H, et al. Systemic treatment with GPI 1046 improves spatial memory and reverses cholinergic neuron atrophy in the medial septal nucleus of aged mice. Brain Res 1999;842:109–118.

72. Herdegen T, Fischer G, Gold BG. Immunophilin ligands as a novel treatment for neurological disorders. Trends Pharmacol Sci 2000;21:3–5.
73. Ogawa N. Immunophilin ligands: possible neuroprotective agents. NeuroSci News 1999;2:28–34.
74. Edwards MJ. Apoptosis, the heat shock response, hyperthermia, birth defects, disease and cancer: where are the common links? Cell Stress Chaperones 1998;3:213–220.
75. Dumont FJ, Staruch MJ, Koprak SL, et al. The immunosuppressive and toxic effects of FK-506 are mechanistically related: pharmacology of a novel antagonist of FK-506 and rapamycin. J Exp Med 1992;176:751–760.
76. Davies P, Maloney AJR. Selective loss of central cholinergic neurons in Alzheimer's disease. Lancet. 1976;ii:1403.
77. Reisine TD, Yamamura HI, Bird ED, et al. Pre- and postsynaptic neurochemical alterations in Alzheimer's disease. Brain Res 1978;159:477–481.
78. Whitehouse PJ, Price DL, Clark AW, et al. Alzheimer disease: evidence for selective loss of cholinergic neurons in the nucleus basalis. Ann Neurol 1981;10:122–126.
79. Okada M, Nakanishi H, Tamura A. et al. Long-term spatial cognitive impairment after middle cerebral artery occlusion in rats: no involvement of the hippocampus. J Cereb Blood Flow Metab 1995;15:1012–1021.
80. Takagi N, Miyake K, Taguchi T, et al. Changes in cholinergic neurons and failure in learning function after microsphere embolism-induced cerebral ischemia. Brain Res Bull 1997;43:87–92.
81. Tanaka K, Ogawa N, Asanuma M, et al. Relationship between cholinergic dysfunction and discrimination learning disabilities in Wistar rats following chronic cerebral hypoperfusion. Brain Res 1966;729:55–65.
82. Tanaka K, Wada N, Hori K, et al. Chronic cerebral hypoperfusion disrupts discriminative behavior in acquired-learning rats. J Neurosci Methods 1998;84:63–68.
83. Tanaka K, Wada N, Ogawa N. Chronic cerebral hypoperfusion induces transient reversible monoaminegic changes in the rat brain. Neurochem Res 2000;25:313–320.
84. Tanaka K, Ogawa N. Chronic cerebral hypoperfusion in Wistar rats as a new animal model of cerebrovascular-type dementia. J Brain Sci 1999;25:85–95.
85. Ni J-W, Ohta H, Matsumoto K, Watanabe H. Progressive cognitive impairment following chronic cerebral hypoperfusion induced by permanent occlusion of bilateral carotid arteries in rats. Brain Res 1994;653:231–236.
86. Wakita H, Tomimoto H, Akiguchi I, Kimura J. Protective effect of cyclosporin A on white matter changes in the rat brain after chronic cerebral hyoperfusion. Stroke 1995;26:1415–1422.
87. Wakita H, Tomomoto H, Akiguchi I, Kimura J. Dose-dependent, protective effect of FK506 against white matter changes in the rat brain after chronic cerebral ischemia. Brain Res 1998;792:105–113.
88. Tanaka K, Wada N, Hori K, et al. Preventive effects of low dose immunosuppressants on learning impairment induced by chronic cerebral hypoperfusion in rats. Jpn J Pharmacol 79(Suppl I):101P.

89. Bennett SAL, Tenniswood M, Chen J-H, et al. Chronic cerebral hypoperfusion elicits neuronal apoptosis and behavioral impairment. NeuroReport 9:161–166.
90. Yagita Y, Kitagawa K, Matsushita K, et al. Effect of immunosuppressant FK506 on ischemia-induced degeneration of hippocampal neurons in gerbils. Life Sci 1996;59:1643–1650.

12

The Role of Immunophilins in Focal Cerebral Ischemia

Evidence of Neuroprotection by FK506

A. L. McGregor, P. A. Jones, J. F. McCarter, T. E. Allsopp, and J. Sharkey

INTRODUCTION

The development of therapies designed to ameliorate CNS tissue damage associated with stroke, traumatic brain injury, and spinal cord injury has been described as a "chronicle of failed projects and unmet expectations" *(1)*. More than 100 agents have been examined in clinical trials, but few have shown convincing clinical benefit. Consequently, there is essentially no effective treatment targeting acute or chronic neurodegeneration in the nervous system. A measured degree of success has been achieved with tissue plasminogen activator (tPA). However, since administration must be within 3 h of stroke onset, thrombolysis is only beneficial in around 5% of stroke patients *(2)*.

The macrolide immunosupressant FK506 (tacrolimus) was originally developed to prevent allograft rejection, but has been shown to display a striking potential to prevent neurodegeneration following both ischemia (Table 1) and chemotoxicity *(3–5)*, and to improve the regeneration of axotomized nerve fibers in animal models *(3,5–9)*. FK506 is one of the few agents to consistently protect in a variety of stroke models, including transient and permanent models of focal ischemia and in both forebrain and global ischemia and in a variety of species *(10)*. Studies in our laboratory were the first to demonstrate that administration of low doses of FK506 (0.1–1 mg/kg) reduced cortical damage by approx 60% in a rat model of middle cerebral artery (MCA) occlusion *(11)*. FK506 also significantly reduced cortical damage following transient focal ischemia in both the mouse *(12)* and in the monkey (Table 1) *(13)*. The efficacy of FK506 in reducing brain damage in rat models of focal cerebral ischemia was compa-

From: *Immunosuppressant Analogs in Neuroprotection*
Edited by: C. V. Borlongan, O. Isacson, and P. R. Sanberg © Humana Press Inc., Totowa, NJ

Table 1
Evidence of FK506 and Cyclosporin A-Mediated Neuroprotection in Focal Cerebral Ischemia

Species	Model	FK506	Cyclosporin A
Rat	Endothelin-1 induced MCA occlusion	Butcher et al., 1997 (17)	Sharkey and Butcher, 1995 (11)
		Sharkey and Butcher, 1994 (11)	
		Sharkey et al., 1996 (26)	
	Temporary monofilament	Aoyama et al., 1997 (231)	Shiga et al., 1992 (16)
		Bochelen et al., 1999 (55)	Yoshimoto et al., 1999 (21)
		Kuroda and Siesjo, 1996 (25)	
		Nakai et al., 1997 (109)	
		Toung et al., 1997 (186)	
		Yoshimoto et al., 1999 (21)	
		McCarter et al., 2000 (12)	
	Permanent monofilament	Bochelen et al., 1999 (55)[a]	
		McCarter et al., 2000 (12)	
	Permanent elecrocoagulation	Sharkey and Butcher, 1994 (11)	
		Bochelen et al., 1999 (55)[a]	
		Takamatsu et al., 1998 (13)	
	Photothrombotic MCA occlusion	Takamatsu et al., 1989 (232)	
Mouse	Temporary monofilament	McCarter et al., 2000 (12)	
	Temporary MCA–CCA occlusion	Aronowski et al., 2000 (80)[a]	
Monkey	Temporary surgical MCA occlusion	Takamatsu et al., 1999 (13)	

[a]No observed protection.
MCA, middle cerebral artery; CCA, common carotid artery.

rable to that of the noncompetitive NMDA receptor antagonist, MK801 *(14)*; however, FK506 produced none of the adverse effects on physiological parameters attributed to MK801 administration *(15)*.

The literature is less emphatic regarding the protective efficacy of the immunosupressant cyclic peptide cyclosporin A (CsA, Sandimmun®) *(11,16,17)*. Convincing evidence exists that CsA is neuroprotective in forebrain ischemia *(18,19)*, however, the poor blood–brain barrier permeability of CsA *(20)* has precluded demonstration of such a decisive effect in focal models and necessitates the use of high doses (100–200 times the minimum effective dose of FK506) *(16,17)* or disruption of the blood–brain barrier using osmotic or surgical trauma *(19,20,22)*. Administration in conjunction with a intracerebral needle lesion or direct carotid artery infusion demonstrated that both pre- and post-ischemic administration of CsA was effective in a transient focal ischemia model in the rat *(21)*.

The temporal window of neuroprotective efficacy for FK506 has also been examined. FK506 is protective when administered up to 3 d prior to ischemic insult in the rat *(17)*. The long duration of neuroprotection afforded by FK506 may be attributed to its rapid accumulation and preferential sequestration in the central nervous system (CNS) *(17)*, suggesting use as a potential prophylactic treatment for patients at risk. FK506 is also protective when administered post-ictus and displayed efficacy when administered up to 2 h postocclusion in the rat *(17)*. It is generally held that the maximum window of therapeutic intervention in this species is of the order of 2–3 h. However, it has been argued that the therapeutic window for neuroprotection may be extended in gyrencephalic species such as the cat, nonhuman primate, and humans (for review, *see* refs. *23* and *24*). This time window appears to be further prolonged in situations where reperfusion occurs. Indeed, FK506 was protective when administered after 3 h of MCA occlusion in the monkey *(13)*, and it has been reported that FK506 reduces cortical infarction following ischemia–reperfusion in the rat (by 63%) when administered 5 h postinsult *(25)*.

Clinical reviewers have highlighted the lack of functional data in the preclinical assessment of putative neuroprotectants that have proven to be ineffective in humans. FK506 improves skilled motor deficits following occlusion of the middle cerebral artery in the rat *(23,26)*, and ameliorates the cognitive deficits associated with anterior cerebral artery occlusion *(27)*. These data demonstrate that the salvage of ischemic tissue by FK506 translates to an improvement in functional outcome.

The precise mechanism underlying the neuroprotective action of FK506 has yet to be elucidated (Fig. 1). This review examines the potential mechanisms of FK506 neuroprotection with respect to the immunophilins.

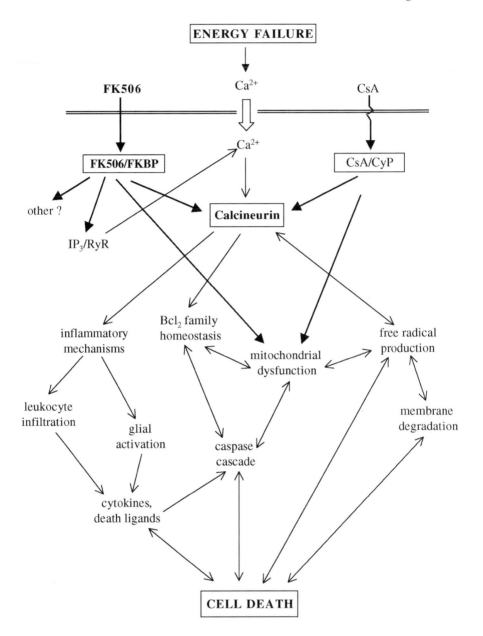

Fig. 1. Possible neuroprotective actions of FK506 and cyclosporin A. By inhibiting the activity of calcineurin, FK506 may influence a variety of ischemia-induced cytotoxic events. Cyclosporin A, in addition to its actions on calcineurin, may prevent the formation of the mitochondrial transition pore; however, its usefulness as a neuroprotectant is limited by poor blood–brain barrier penetration.

IMMUNOPHILINS

The ubiquitously expressed and highly conserved immunophilin family of proteins have received much attention owing to their ability to act as receptors for immunosupressant compounds (for review, *see* refs. *23,28,* and *29*). FK506 binding proteins (FKBPs) are the intracellular binding proteins for FK506 and the structurally related rapamycin (Sirolimus), while cyclophilins (CyPs) bind cyclosporin A (CsA). These two subfamilies possess little sequence homology but display rotamase activity, which catalyzes the *cis–trans* isomerization of peptidylprolyl bonds *(30)*. A more recently discovered peptidylprolyl isomerase, parvulin, displays no sequence homology with the other classes of immunophilins and does not bind CsA or FK506 *(31)*. In addition to a proposed primary role as chaperone molecules, immunophilins are thought to influence protein conformation, stabilization, and docking (for review, *see* ref. *29*).

To date around 15 mammalian FKBPs have been described and, although the actual cellular roles of many are unknown, they have been implicated in such diverse processes as gene transcription (FKBP25, FKBP38) *(32–34)*, protein secretion from the endoplasmic reticulum (FKBP65) *(35)*, intracellular calcium release (FKBP12, FKBP12.6) *(36–38)*, and steroid–hormone complex formation (FKBP52) *(39)*. The majority of these FKBPs are expressed at high concentrations within the brain, where they account for approx 1% of the total protein content and 10% of the total PPIase activity *(40)*. FKBP12 was the first of this family to be discovered and appears the most abundant within the brain, at concentrations some 10-fold that observed within the immune system *(40,41)*.

Around 30 mammalian cyclophilins have currently been identified; the most widely studied are CyPA, -B, -C, and -D, Cyp40, and CyPNK. Cyclophilins A–D possess conserved rotamase domains and display comparable enzymatic activity and CsA binding *(29)*. CyP40 is a component of the glucocorticoid receptor and appears to have a lower affinity for CsA than the other members *(42)*. CyPNK95 is specific to natural killer cells and is thought to be involved in cytotoxicity *(43)*.

It was initially proposed that inhibition of the rotamase activity underpinned the immunosupressant action of these ligand–immunophilin complexes. However, the FK506 derivative 506BD and related compounds *(43,44)* potently inhibited FKBP12 rotamase activity, but are not immunosupressant. Therefore, inhibition of PPIase activity alone is not sufficient to confer immunosupression.

CsA and FK506 prevent allograft rejection through suppression of the Ca^{2+}-dependent signal transduction pathway promoting IL-2-mediated proliferation of T cells *(45,46)*. The transduction pathway requires the phosphorylation state-dependent translocation of the transcription factor NF-AT, to the nucleus and the rate-limiting enzyme in this reaction is calcineurin (CaN). Thus, inhibition of the phosphatase CaN by the FK506–FKBP12 or CsA–CyPA complex mitigates the immune response *(44,47–49)*. In contrast, a third immunosupressant rapamycin, while binding to FKBP12 does not inhibit CaN. Rather, its immunosuppressant activities are mediated through inhibition of a serine–threonine kinase, RAFT (Rapamycin and FKBP12 target) *(50)*. The observation of colocalization of FKBPs and CyPs with CaN in most brain regions *(40,41)* suggests that regulation of CaN by immunophilins also occurs within the brain and that presently undiscovered endogenous effector molecules may exist.

REGULATION OF CALCINEURIN BY IMMUNOPHILINS

Calcineurin, a type 2B calcium–calmodulin dependent serine–threonine protein phosphatase is a heterodimer consisting of a 59-kDa A subunit with calmodulin and catalytic sites and, a 19-kDa B subunit, which has four calcium binding sites *(51,52)*. Immunophilins are able to interact with the CaN A subunit in the absence of endogenous immunosupressants; however, the immunophilin–CaN interaction is potentiated by the presence of the appropriate immunophilin *(53)*. In contrast to the widely held view that immunophilins are in excess, it has been suggested that the incomplete CaN inhibition observed at immunosupressant doses of FK506 and CsA may reflect limiting amounts of active immunophilins *(54)*.

THE CALCINEURIN HYPOTHESIS OF NEUROPROTECTION

The evidence supporting the hypothesis that the neuroprotective effects of FK506 and CsA are mediated through inhibition of CaN is as follows:

1. Drugs that bind to FKBPs or cyclophilins and inhibit calcineurin, such as FK506, the ascomycin derivative SDZ ASM 981, and CsA, reduce infarct volume in a dose dependent manner in rat models of cerebral ischemia *(11,16,17,55)*.
2. Compounds demonstrating a lower affinity for FKBP12 and, consequently, a lower affinity for CaN, such as SDZ ASM 981, are proportionately less potent neuroprotectants *(55)*.
3. While CsA–CyPA and FK506–FKBP12 complexes target CaN and ultimately leads to neuroprotection, the rapamycin–FKBP12 complex does not protect *(11,56)*.
4. Furthermore, concomitant administration of rapamycin and FK506 prevented the neuroprotective effect of FK506, reinforcing the suggestion that CaN inhibition is necessary for neuroprotection *(55)*.

In contrast to the prevailing view, there have been reports that suggest that inhibition of CaN may not be essential for neuroprotection. One study has reported that following a permanent focal cerebral ischemic insult, administration of low-dose rapamycin (1 mg/kg) displayed a similar degree of neuroprotection to FK506 *(57)*. Similarly, the nonimmunosupressant FKBP ligands (V-10, 367, GPI1046, and VX853) do not inhibit CaN activity but are neuroregenerative in models of peripheral neuropathy and following axotomy of central neurons *(7,58,59)*.

CALCINEURIN-INDEPENDENT MECHANISMS

Unlike other putative neuroprotectants (e.g., NMDA receptor antagonists), FK506 appears neither to exert a direct cardiovascular effect nor to influence core or brain temperature in animal models *(17,55)*. It is unlikely that the effects of FK506 are mediated through alterations in blood flow. FK506 administration in normal rats had no discernible effect on regional cerebral blood flow (CBF) as measured by iodoantipyrene autoradiography (J. Sharkey, unpublished observation) nor did it affect the observed decrease in CBF following MCA occlusion in the monkey *(13,55)*. Recent evidence suggests that FK506 results in improved cerebral blood flow after stroke. However, the concomitant preservation of metabolic activity suggests that the improved hemodynamics after stroke reflect an increase in the amount of viable tissue rather than a direct effect of FK506 on the cerebral vasculature *(13)*

PATHOPHYSIOLOGY OF CEREBRAL ISCHEMIA

Cerebral ischemia leads to a complex cascade of pathophysiological events resulting in cell death. Two types of cell death can be distinguished morphologically *(60)*. Energy failure caused by a cessation of substrate supply affects ionic gradients and leads to neuronal depolarization, neurotransmitter release, and a massive influx of ions and water into cells producing cytotoxic edema and necrotic cell death *(61)*. Alternatively, apoptosis is cell loss due to suicide or fratricide and is an energy-dependent program requiring ATP *(61)*. However, a gross perturbation of cellular ionic homeostasis, most importantly that of calcium, is a common feature of both mechanisms. Large increases in cytosolic calcium through voltage-operated ion channels coupled with a subsequent discharge from intracellular stores, certainly directs the cell toward necrosis–apoptosis *(62)*. Calcium overload may influence cell death by a vast array of widely differing mechanisms. Increased calcium activates many proteolytic enzymes, including calpains, which degrade cytoskeletal components *(63)*. Highly reactive free radicals produced by activation of phospholipase A2 *(64)* or calcineurin–nitric oxide synthase pathways have also been cited as influential in calcium-mediated cell death *(25,65)*. Perturbation of mitochondrial activity with subsequent loss of respiratory function, release of cytochrome *c*, and subsequent activation of the caspase cascade, has also gained acceptance as a significant calcium-mediated pathway in ischemic cell death *(66–68)*. The full catalog of calcium-sensitive processes that may influence ischemia is undoubtedly broader than the list above, since almost any modulation of cytosolic calcium level or function may affect cellular survival.

CALCIUM HOMEOSTASIS AND FK506 NEUROPROTECTION

FK506 and associated immunophilins could potentially divert the calcium cascade of events during ischemia via modulation of presynaptic neurotransmitter release and associated postsynaptic receptors.

Presynaptically, CaN has been shown to suppresses spontaneous cortical cell firing *(69)* via the dephosphorylation of synapsin I or dynamin I, to decrease the translocation of synaptic vesicles, vesicle recycling and/or receptor-mediated endocytosis *(70–72)*. The effect of FK506–FKBP12-mediated CaN inhibition would therefore appear to be detrimental to cell survival by increasing glutamate neurotransmission. While this augmentation of glutamate release was duly observed in potassium-depolarized synaptosomes, FK506 inhibited transmitter endocytosis in synaptosomes treated with NMDA *(71)*. To date little attention has been given to these presynaptic FK506–FKBP12-mediated events.

Postsynaptically, CaN has been shown to negatively modulate the NMDA receptor channel opening *(73)*. In the same study, FK506 duly increased the duration of time that the NMDA channel remained in the open state *(73)*. This observation appears to contradict reports that the immunosuppressant has been shown to be neuroprotective against glutamate toxicity in vitro *(74,75)*. As prolonging channel opening would serve only to increase calcium influx, it is unlikely that FK506-mediated protection is mediated in this way. In agreement with this, FK506-mediated neuroprotection of glutamate toxicity in vitro was not translated into in vivo studies *(17,75)*More recently, FK506 has been shown to inhibit calcium entry into porcine coronary artery cells via L-type calcium channels *(76)*, although similar studies on cerebral vessels have not been performed.

Protein kinase C (PKC), by virtue of its intimate relationship with calmodulin, prevents both the inhibitory feedback of NMDA receptor channels and calcium discharge through the plasma membrane calcium pump (for review, *see* ref. *77*). CaN also shares a close and complex interrelationship with PKC, modifying PKC-mediated activity in both positive and negative directions *(52)*. Owing to the complexity of this relationship, and the lack of consensus whether PKC activation or inhibition would improve recovery *(78,79)*, there is, understandably, scant information on whether modification of PKC by calcineurin would be beneficial or detrimental during ischemia. With relevance to FK506, the immunosuppressant reduced infarct size in γPKC knockout mice exposed to focal cerebral ischemia (by approx 22%), without displaying any neuroprotection in the BALB/cJ parent strain *(80)*. This is in contrast to the 59% reduction in hemispheric lesion volume observed in C57Bl/6J strain following FK506 administration (A. McGregor, unpublished observation).

Intracellularly, FKBP12 has been shown to immunoprecipitate with both the 300-kDa inositol-1,4,5-triphosphate receptor (IP$_3$R) *(36,80)* and the 565-kDa ryanodine receptor (RyR) *(81)*. Both closely homologous tetrameric receptors are located in endoplasmic reticulum membranes within cerebral tissue *(82)* and are involved in the regulation of calcium release from internal stores into the cytosol. FKBP12 appears to act as a specific physiological anchor targeting CaN to the endoplasmic reticulum membrane *(83)*. CaN is therefore able to modulate calcium homeostasis through alteration of the receptor phosphorylation state *(83)*. FKBP12 is not required for channel function, or for maximal ionic conductance, but influences receptor stability through reduction of aberrant activity. FKBP12 also increases the inertia of IP$_3$R calcium channel, making it less susceptible to opening, but once open, more difficult to close *(82)*. Conversely, the complexing of FKBP12 with the RyR may make the channel more sensitive to closure *(84)*. FK506 competes with the IP$_3$R and RyR site on FKBP12 *(83)*, dissociating the FKBP from the ER receptor complex. Under normal conditions this dissociation increases the leakage of calcium from the intracellular store *(82,84)*, although under the elevated calcium environment of the ischemic cell, the situation may differ. In the heart, the addition of FK506 caused calcium leakage and prevented the closure of the RyR channel, even in a elevated calcium environment *(84)*. Similar studies on the IP$_3$R mimicking the higher cytosolic calcium levels associated with ischemia have not been performed. Theoretically at least, destabilization of the already open IP$_3$R channel would decrease the overall release of calcium.

It is worthy of note that inhibition of calcineurin by FK506 has been demonstrated in vivo at concentrations in the nanomolar range *(85)*. In comparison, effects on calcium homeostasis were observed using micromolar concentrations of FK506 *(86)*. The contribution of these in vitro effects to the neuroprotective actions of FK506 following stroke is therefore speculative.

CHLORINE AND POTASSIUM HOMEOSTASIS

γ-Aminobutyric acid (GABA), an inhibitory neurotransmitter that modulates chlorine flux via plasma membrane-bound receptors, countering excitotoxic calcium influx *(87)*, may also be modulated by CaN (and thereby FK506–FKBP12). The dephosphorylation of L-glutamate decarboxylase (GAD) by the phosphatase *(88)* would appear to be beneficial to vulnerable neurons by increasing the biosynthesis of GABA *(87)*. GABA biosynthesis is, however, an energy-requiring process and, as such, would make further demands on already metabolically compromised tissue. It is therefore improbable that modulation of GABA biosynthesis by FK506 makes a contribution to neuroprotection under conditions of ischemia.

FK506 has also been shown to modulate potassium flux across the plasma membrane, which may importantly influence sodium-mediated cytotoxic oedema via potassium–sodium exchange. While FK506 inhibited potassium currents I_{to} and I_K increasing the duration of the action potential, these observations have been limited to cardiac tissue *(89–91)*. Within cerebral neurons, FK506 has been shown to inhibit a calcium-dependent potassium channel *(92)*. Possibly arguing against the importance of potassium channel in FK506-mediated neuroprotection is evidence from the above studies that the nonprotective immunosuppressant rapamycin exerted similar effects.

MITOCHONDRIAL HOMEOSTASIS

Mitochondria act as a calcium sink during cerebral ischemia, sequestering cytosolic calcium until a critical level is reached, whereupon the organelles undergo respiratory chain collapse, free radical production, and extrusion of contents *(93)*. Perturbation of mitochondrial homeostasis cannot be entirely attributed to accumulation of calcium, since bcl-2 increases the amount of calcium that the mitochondria can sequester without impairment *(94)*. Nevertheless, the ability to buffer changes in the intracellular environment highlights a crucial role for mitochondria in the cell death cascade *(67)*. The resurgence of interest in mitochondria has been fueled by the observation of a pore forming within the outer membrane of the organelle under certain pathological conditions in vitro *(95)*. Once open, the pore [or mitochondrial permeability transition (MPT)] releases apoptotic effectors such as cytochrome *c*, apoptosis-inducing factor (AIF), and previously sequestered calcium into the cytosol, thereby initiating the cell-death cascade *(96,97)*. While well characterized in vitro, the MPT is of dubious importance to the ischemic process in vivo. Supporting evidence for MPT involvement in the ischemic cascade is derived from the neuroprotection associated with cyclosporin A *(17,98)* and its nonimmunosuppressive analog, *N*-methyl-val-CsA *(99,100)*, both of which inhibit MPT in vitro *(100)*. These studies consistently over-look many other potential pathways for the observed in vivo neuroprotection including inhibition of neutrophil infiltration, microglial suppression, or apoptosis independent of MPT formation *(101–103)*. Aside from this, the conditions required in vitro for MPT formation may not be comparable to those occurring during cerebral ischemia in vivo, for example, *see* ref. *104*. Recent data have also suggested that brain mitochondria are highly resistant to MPT *(105)*, and that pore opening is not crucial in the release of the cyto-chrome *c (106,107)*. While MPT may not be relevant to cerebral ischemia, mitochondria still remain a linchpin in both the apoptotic and necrotic pro-cesses. FK506 does not bind to cyclophilin D, which is integral to the pore *(108)*, but has been shown to moderate mitochondria function, reducing reperfusion-associated mitochondrial dysfunction *(109–111)*. This may be explained by a partial inhibition of complexes III and V of the respiratory chain observed in the presence of the immunosuppressant *(112)*. While nei-ther the mechanism nor the immunophilin involved (if any) is known, poten-tial benefit of respiratory chain inhibition to ischemic–reperfused tissue could include a reduction in production of reactive oxygen species *(113,114)*. Few studies have examined respiratory chain inhibition as a potential neuroprotective therapy, although when compounds that are known to inhibit oxidative phosphorylation have been used in ischemic experiments (at doses which induce partial inhibition), there is often an observed benefit *(115–120)*. FK506 interaction with both anti- and proapoptotic Bcl-2 family members, modifying the caspase cascade and mitochondrial vulnerability to ischemia is discussed below.

INFLAMMATORY REACTIONS

Cytotoxic, inflammatory reactions have been implicated in the pathogen-esis of brain ischemia–reperfusion injury *(55,121)*. Ischemia induces early activation of resident glial cells *(122,123)*, expression of cytokines and other inflammatory mediators *(122,124–126)* with subsequent infiltration and accumulation of leukocytes and monocytes *(127,128)*. FK506 and CsA affect numerous components of the inflammatory cascade, and it is suggested that modification of the immune response may in part underlie the neuroprotective effects of these compounds. Beneficial effects of FK506 have been demon-strated in animal models of ischemia–reperfusion injury in peripheral organs, such as the heart, liver, intestines, and skin *(129–132)*. Pretreatment with FK506 was protective against hepatic ischemic–reperfusion injury by inhib-iting TNF-α and IL-1 release *(133,134)* and FK506-mediated inhibition of superoxide release from neutrophils is associated with cardioprotection

(110,134). An increase in molecules associated with cell death, such as cytokines *(2,135–137)*, caspases *(138)*, and free radicals *(139)*, have also been observed in the brain following the onset of ischemia, although the origin of these molecules has not been clearly established.

Microglia have been identified in ischemic regions as early as 30 min postinsult *(140)* and can be viewed as a sensitive, reliable marker of potential neuronal damage *(141)*. Like their circulating counterparts, microglia also release cytokines such as IL-1 *(142,143)*, IL-6 *(144)* , TNF-α *(145)*, free radicals *(135)*, and chemokines such as IL-8 *(146)*, cytokine-induced neutrophil chemoattractant protein (CINC) *(125,146)*, and monocyte chemoattractant protein (MCP-1) *(2,147)* in response to ischemia. The time-course of the microglial response following permanent and transient monofilament occlusion in the rat has been reported to differ, with earlier and more intense activation occurring in reperfused tissue *(12)*. Furthermore, the degree of protection afforded by FK506 in the transient model is almost twice that observed in the permanent monofilament model *(12)*. FK506 and CsA have been shown to attenuate microglial activation and tissue damage in animal models of cerebral ischemia *(98,102,148)*, therefore, the enhanced efficacy of FK506 in models with a reperfusion component may therefore reflect a preferential inhibition of microglial activation. The overall contribution of microglial activation to ischemic damage is nevertheless controversial. Release of proinflammatory cytokines is detrimental; however, microglia also release TGF-β *(149,150)* and BFGF *(151,152)*, which are known to be neuroprotective.

Cytokine-like actions have also been described for the immunophilins *per se* within the immune system. FKBP12 release from mast cells has been reported to activate Ca^{2+} signaling in neutrophils *(153)*. Formation of the FK506–FKBP12 complex would therefore attenuate the ability of the immunophilin to stimulate Ca^{2+} activation.

Similarly, astrocytes become reactive following an ischemic insult, demonstrating changes in both morphology and protein release *(122)*. The role of astrocytes in the early pathophysiology of stroke is unclear *(154,155)*, questioning the importance of recent evidence that FK506 can modulate astrocytic activity under certain ischemic conditions *(129,148)*.

In addition to the effect on resident glial cells, FK506 and CsA inhibit the infiltration of potentially deleterious circulating inflammatory cells, primarily neutrophils *(156)*. Inflammatory reactions are controlled by the expression of a number of immunological surface marker molecules on inflammatory cells *(157)*. Attenuation of neutrophil infiltration may be a consequence of altered expression of intracellular adhesion molecules

(ICAM-1) and lymphocyte function-associated antigen on cerebral vessels and neutrophils, respectively *(158,159)*. Nevertheless, it should be considered that the majority of these observations would be consistent with a direct anti-ischemic action of FK506 to reduce tissue damage and thereby reduce inflammatory signals

NITRIC OXIDE AND FREE RADICALS

Reperfusion of ischemic organs is associated with the formation of free radicals that can exacerbate ischemic damage *(160–164)*. Reduction of molecular oxygen forms superoxide anions, hydrogen peroxide, and highly reactive hydroxyl radicals *(165)*. These reactive oxygen species (ROS) damage tissue through peroxidation of lipids and oxidation of sulfydryl groups, leading to perturbations in membrane permeability and enzyme function *(165)*. The overexpression of the free radical scavenging enzyme superoxide dismutase in transgenic mice has been shown to be neuroprotective following cerebral ischemia *(166)*. By contrast, free radical scavengers have shown equivocal efficacy in preclinical studies *(167–171)* and no benefit in clinical studies *(172,173)*. FK506 both reduces superoxide production in neutrophils and inhibits ROS stimulated NF-κB activation in cultured astrocytes *(174)*. It is therefore possible that the neuroprotective effects of FK506 may be mediated, in part, by the inhibition of free-radical production. The most cited mechanism for FK506-mediated neuroprotection is by attenuation of nitric oxide (NO) production via inhibition of NO synthase (NOS) *(75,175–178)*. CaN dephosphorylates and activates NOS, and FK506–FKBP12-mediated inhibition of CaN attenuates the catalytic activity of NOS *(75)*. Prevention of glutamate-mediated cell death through selective inhibition of NOS, indicates a role for NO in neurotoxicity *(179)*. Indeed, macrolide antibiotics protect against glutamate (but not kainate or quinolinate) toxicity in both cultured neurons *(74)* and in primary cortical cultures *(75)*. A discrepancy exists, however, between in vitro and in vivo literature, as neither FK506 nor NOS inhibitors displays neuroprotection in in vivo models of excitotoxicity *(17,180,181)*. The contribution of NO to the pathology of stroke remains controversial despite enhanced production of NO following transient middle cerebral artery occlusion *(182)*. While some studies report a protective effect of NOS inhibition in ischemia, others have failed to demonstrate an effect *(183)*. Several investigators have also reported an increase in neuronal damage *(184,185)*. More recently, elegant microdialysis studies *(186)* have shown that FK506 administration does not suppress NO production following ischemia in vivo. It is therefore unlikely that FK506 neuroprotection occurs via CaN-mediated inhibition of NOS.

IMMUNOPHILINS, FK506, AND APOPTOSIS

Apoptosis, as typified by chromatin condensation, DNA fragmentation, plasma membrane blebbing, and the formation of apoptotic bodies, has been accepted by many to be a component of ischemic cell death, particularly in the ischemic penumbra *(61)*. The tightly regulated apoptotic cascade may represent a much more desirable target for therapeutic manipulation than necrosis. Considered integral to delayed neuronal death (DND) in gerbils following minutes of global ischemia, the energy-requiring apoptotic process was, until recently, considered less important in the ATP-deprived conditions of focal ischemia *(61)*. While reperfusion of ischemic tissue following tPA treatment may reinitiate mitochondrial ATP production *(187)*, there are indications of apoptosis in models of permanent occlusion *(188,189)*.

FK506 has been shown to be efficacious in preventing apoptotic-indicative DNA fragmentation following transient global ischemia in the gerbil *(176)*. There are a number of different mechanism proposed for the antiapoptotic actions of FK506, mostly involving FKBP-12 binding and calcineurin inhibition.

Calcineurin-mediated increase in the susceptibility of neuronal cells to die following serum deprivation in vitro is inhibited by FK506 *(190)*. Similar beneficial effects were observed following the administration of either an inhibitor of the proapoptotic protease, caspase-3 or Bcl-2, suggesting cell death was apoptotic *(190)*. While p38 mitogen-activated protein kinase (p38 MAPK) has been suggested as a possible downstream effector *(191)*, there are many other candidates.

TRANSCRIPTION FACTORS AND DEATH LIGANDS

By reducing both the expression of the transcription factors c-Jun and activating transcription factor-2 and the N-terminal phosphorylation of c-Jun by JNK, FK506 increased the survival of substantia nigra pars compacta cells following transection of the medial forebrain bundle *(192)*. The inhibition of the apoptotic propagator JNK was presumably mediated through the FKBP12 immunophilin with subsequent CaN inhibition, since GPI1046, which binds to FKBP12 but does not inhibit CaN, failed to replicate these effects *(193)*.

Other transcription factors known to be inhibited by FK506–FKBP12 interaction with CaN include NFAT *(194)* and NFκB *(195)*, the latter of which has been implicated in the pathophysiology of ischemia *(196)*. For example, in immature thymocytes and T-cell hybridomas, FK506 prevents CaN-dependent dephosphorylation and nuclear translocation of NFAT, the subsequent transcription of the CD95 ligand, and ultimately CD95-mediated

T-cell fratricide *(197,198)*. Death ligands such as CD95 activate caspase-8 and the subsequent caspase cascade by binding to the death domain FADD *(199)*. In addition to the CD95 ligand, recent studies have indicated that other members of the death ligand family are also regulated by CaN-dependent transcription in T cells, including TRANCE and TRAIL *(200)*. The calcium-mediated activation of transcription factors NGF1-A and NGF1-B in PC-12 cells is also suppressed by the CaN inhibitors FK506 and CsA *(201)*.

BCL-2 FAMILY PROTEINS AND CASPASES

The complex formed between bcl-2 and CaN, resulting in the inhibition of CaN, has been cited as one possible mechanism of bcl-2-mediated antiapoptotic mechanisms *(198)*. It may be postulated that in dissociating this complex, FK506–FKBP12 would not only continue the inhibition of CaN, but would also free Bcl-2 to bind to, and inhibit the actions of, the proapoptotic proteins BAD and BAX *(202)*. Hippocampal neurons transfected with BAD, have been shown to apoptose in a CaN-dependent manner in response to glutamate, an effect suppressible by FK506 *(203)*. In cells classified as slow responders to CD95-L induced killing, due to low CD95 expression, caspase-8 generates a truncated form of another proapoptotic Bcl-2 family member, BID (tBID) *(169)*. This activated form of tBID is able to translocate to mitochondria and facilitate the BAX-dependent release of cytochrome *c* from mitochondria, thereby amplifying the effector caspase cascade involving caspases 8, 9, and 3 *(204)*.

NON-CALCINEURIN-MEDIATED EFFECTS

Observations from neurons and nonneural cells lend support to the possibility that FK506 affects apoptosis either directly or indirectly by mechanisms that do not involve CaN. Ligation of the Fc eRI receptor in mast cells ultimately leads to TNF-a production and apoptosis that is FK506-sensitive and requires concomitant activation of JNK and p38 MAP kinases (205). Members of the stress-activated MAP kinase subfamily (p38/JNK/SAPK) are inactivated by the dual specificity phosphatase, MAP kinase phosphatase 1. This phosphatase has been shown to be induced in axotomized neurons of the mamillary body, an effect that is also enhanced by FK506 in these neurons, but not those of the degenerating substantia nigra pars compacta (193).

Ceramide is a key mediator of apoptosis in response to cellular stress, increasing the expression of *c-Jun*, CD95, TRAIL, TNF-α *(206)*. The apoptotic cascade is further activated by mitochondrial disruption and release of *cyt-c*, *Apaf-1*, and procaspase-9 into the cytosol. FK506-mediated inhibition of ischemia-induced ceramide generation and ceramide-activated protein kinase activity would therefore suppress apoptosis at a number of loci *(206)*. The FKBPs mediating these processes remain unknown.

MINOR IMMUNOPHILINS

Immunosupressant compounds produce their effects at nanomolar concentrations while the major immunophilins are present in micromolar concentrations in the cytosol, implying a very small proportion of the major FKBPs are complexed at a given time *(207,208)*. A small subset of minor immunophilins have been described in calf thymus and Jurkat T cells, including FKBP14, -37, -52 and the recently identified 5 to 8-kDa protein (potentially a subunit of FKBP52), which are capable of binding FK506 and rapamycin, but do not possess rotamase activity *(208)*. These minor immunophilins also inhibit CaN, and this raises the concept that these less abundant, minor FKBPs may be more compelling targets for immunosupressant compounds *(208)*, although to date there has been no evidence to implicate these immunophilins in neuroprotection.

FKBP-65

FKBP-65 is a four domain PPIase, localized to the endoplasmic reticulum *(209,210)*. To date the only accredited functions of the binding protein are the folding of tropoelastin, a 70-kDa elastic fiber protein, prior to its secretion from the ER *(35)* and complex formation with hsp-90 and the serine–threonine kinase c-Raf-1 *(211)*. What makes this FKBP worthy of further study, is that it is the only immunophilin to date (including the cyclophilins and parvulins) that is capable of binding to and being inhibited by both FK506 and CsA. With both immunosuppressants this inhibition of function is only partial, although FK506 inhibition (25%) is slightly more stringent than that of CsA (20%) *(210)*.

FKBP-52 AND HEAT SHOCK PROTEINS

The heat shock protein, hsp-90, upregulates after periods of cellular stress (including ischemia *(212)* and has been shown to complex with the 52-kDa FKBP, FKBP52 *(213)*. While heat shock protein activation is more usually associated with nerve regeneration *(214)*, hsp-70 (the expression of which is regulated by hsp-90) *(215)* is neuroprotective in some in vivo models of ischemia *(216,217)*. Hsp-70 inhibits the apoptotic cascade by preventing SAPK/JNK activation, pro-caspase cleavage and downstream caspase-mediated events *(see* ref. *218)*. Whether FK506 or even FKBP52 exerts any influence on these pathways through hsp-90 association has yet to be determined.

Both FKBP52 and hsp-90 are also integral components of steroid receptors (including those for the hormones progesterone and oestrogen; *(219,220)*. It is worth noting that hsp-90 can also combine with the CsA binding protein, CyP40, in similar steroid receptor complexes *(221)*. Upon the binding of FK506, the steroid receptor complex does not dissociate but undergoes a gain of function *(222)*, which may have important repercussions as it is well known that steroid hormones such as progesterone and estrogen can mediate neuroprotection during ischemia *(223–227)*. Similar rapamycin interactions have yet to be studied to determine whether the nonneuroprotective immunosuppressant also enhances receptor function following FKBP52 binding.

Aside from the mechanisms discussed in this chapter, FK506 may also influence p23 and MAP kinase pathways via an interaction with the hsp-90–FKBP-52 complex, preventing p23 dissociation *(228)*. Another effect of hsp-90 which has yet to be elucidated in terms of FKBP52–FK506 mediation appears to efficiently bring this review full circle. Both Hsp-90 and hsp-70, through both a calmodulin-dependent and independent mechanism have recently been shown to increase the activation of the calcium–calmodulin-dependent serine–threonine phosphatase 2B, calcineurin *(229)*.

SUMMARY

Although the precise mechanism underlying the neuroprotective action of FK506 is not known the formation of molecular complexes with immunophilins *(230)*, allows interaction at a number of fundamental steps in the ischemic cascade. All neuroprotective agent examined to date have targeted a specific pathway of the ischemic cascade, for example, NMDA-receptor antagonists or Ca^{2+} channel blockers. While these compounds reduced infarct volume in preclinical investigations, it is not surprising that agents that target a single stage in such a complex chain of events do not produce a large clinical impact. The application of FK506 and its nonimmunosuppressive derivatives is therefore a promising strategy for the treatment of neurodegeneration.

REFERENCES

1. Mcburney RN. Development of the NMDA ion-channel blocker, aptiganel hydrochloride, as a neuroprotective agent for acute CNS injury. Int Rev Neurobiol 1997;40:173–195.
2. Feuerstein GZ, Wang X. Animal models of stroke. Mol Med Today 2000;6:133–135.
3. Costantini LC, et al. A novel immunophilin ligand: distinct branching effects on dopaminergic neurons in culture and neurotrophic actions after oral

administration in an animal model of Parkinson's disease. Neurobiol Dis 1998;5:97–106.

4. Moriwaki A, Lu, YF, Tomizawa K, Matsui H. An immunosuppressant, FK506, protects against neuronal dysfunction and death but has no effect on electrographic and behavioral activities induced by systemic kainate. Neuroscience 1998;86:855–865.

5. Steiner JP, et al. Neurotrophic immunophilin ligands stimulate structural and functional recovery in neurodegenerative animal models. Proc Natl Acad Sci USA 1997;94:2019–2024.

6. Gold BG. FK506 and the role of immunophilins in nerve regeneration. Mol. Neurobiol. 1997;15:285–306.

7. Gold BG, Zeleny-Pooley M, Chaturvedi P, Wang MS. Oral administration of a nonimmunosuppressant FKBP-12 ligand speeds nerve regeneration. Neuroreport 1998;9:553–558.

8. Madsen JR, et al. Tacrolimus (FK506) increases neuronal expression of GAP-43 and improves functional recovery after spinal cord injury in rats. Exp Neurol 1998;154:673–683.

9. Snyder SH, Lai MM, Burnett PE. Immunophilins in the nervous system. Neuron 1998;21:283–294.

10. Sharkey J, Jones PA, McCarter JF, Kelly JS. Calcineurin inhibitors as neuroprotectants: Focus of Tacrolimus and Cyclosporin. CNS Drugs 2000;13:1–13.

11. Sharkey J, Butcher SP. Immunophilins mediate the neuroprotective effects of FK506 in focal cerebral ischemia. Nature 1994;371:336–339.

12. McCarter JF, McGregor AL, Jones PA, Sharkey J. FK506 protects brain tissue in animal models of stroke. Transplant Proc 2001;33:2390–2392.

13. Takamatsu H, et al. Positron emission tomographic study of the neuroprotective effects of FK506 in a monkey model of stroke. Immunophilins in the Brain, FKBP Ligands: Novel Strategies for the Treatment of Neurodegenerative Disorders, July 9–11, 1999, Schlangenbad, Germany, O19.

14. Park CK, et al. The glutamate antagonist MK-801 reduces focal ischemic brain damage in the rat. Ann Neurol 1988;24:543–551.

15. McCulloch J. Excitatory amino acid antagonists and their potential for the treatment of ischemic brain damage in man. Brit J Clin Pharmacol 1992; 34:106–114.

16. Shiga Y, Onodera H, Matsuo Y, Kogure K. Cyclosporin A protects against ischemia-reperfusion injury in the brain. Brain Res 1992;595:145–148.

17. Butcher SP, et al. Neuroprotective actions of FK506 in experimental stroke: in vivo evidence against an antiexcitotoxic mechanism. J Neurosci 1997;17:6939–6946.

18. Li PA, Kristian T, He QP, Siesjo BK. Cyclosporin A enhances survival, ameliorates brain damage, and prevents secondary mitochondrial dysfunction after a 30-minute period of transient cerebral ischemia. Exp Neurol 2000; 165:153–163.

19. Uchino H, et al. Amelioration by cyclosporin A of brain damage in transient forebrain ischemia in the rat. Brain Res 1998;812:216–226.

20. Begley DJ, et al. Permeability of the blood-brain barrier to the immunosuppressive cyclic peptide cyclosporin A. J Neurochem 1990;55:1222–1230.

21. Yoshimoto T, Siesjo BK. Posttreatment with the immunosuppressant cyclosporin A in transient focal ischemia. Brain Res 1999;839:283–291.

22. Uchino H, et al. Cyclosporin A dramatically ameliorates CA1 hippocampal damage following transient forebrain ischemia in the rat. Acta Physiol Scand 1995:155:469–471.

23. Giroux C, Scatton B. Ischemic stroke: treatment on the horizon. Eur Neurol 1996;36:61–64.

24. Koroshetz WJ, Moskowitz MA. Emerging treatments for stroke in humans. Trends Pharmacol Sci 1996;17:227–233.

25. Kuroda S, Siesjo BK. Reperfusion damage following focal ischemia: pathophysiology and therapeutic windows. Clin Neurosci 1997;4:199–212.

26. Sharkey J, Crawford JH, Butcher SP, Marston HM. Tacrolimus (FK506) ameliorates skilled motor deficits produced by middle cerebral artery occlusion in rats. Stroke 1996;27:2282–2286.

27. Gold B, Fischer Gunter, Herdegen T. Behavioural assessment of neuroprotection by FK506, in Immunophilins in the Brain, FKBP ligands: Novel Strategies for the Treatment of Neurodegenerative Diseases. Prous Science 2000; In press.

28. Snyder SH, et al. Neural actions of immunophilin ligands. Trends Pharmacol Sci 1998;19:21–26.

29. Hamilton GS, Steiner JP. Immunophilins: beyond immunosuppression. J Med Chem 1998;41:5119–5143.

30. Harding MW, Galat A, Uehling DE, Schreiber SL. A receptor for the immunosuppressant FK506 is a cis-trans peptidyl- prolyl isomerase. Nature 1989;341:758–760.

31. Rahfeld JU, et al. Confirmation of the existence of a third family among peptidyl-prolyl cis/trans isomerases. Amino acid sequence and recombinant production of parvulin. FEBS Lett 1994;352:180–184.

32. Jin YJ, Burakoff SJ. The 25-kDa FK506-binding protein is localized in the nucleus and associates with casein kinase II and nucleolin. Proc Natl Acad Sci USA 1993;90:7769–7773.

33. Kruger M, et al. Inhibition of CREB- and cAMP response element-mediated gene transcription by the immunosuppressive drugs cyclosporin A and FK506 in T cells. Naunyn Schmiedebergs Arch Pharmacol 1997;356:433–440.

34. Pedersen KM, Finsen B, Celis JE, Jensen NA. muFKBP38: a novel murine immunophilin homolog differentially expressed in Schwannoma cells and central nervous system neurons in vivo. Electrophoresis 1999;20:249–255.

35. Davis EC, Broekelmann TJ, Ozawa Y, Mecham RP. Identification of tropoelastin as a ligand for the 65-kD FK506-binding protein, FKBP65, in the secretory pathway. J Cell Biol 1998;140:295–303.

36. Cameron AM, et al. Immunophilin FK506 binding protein associated with inositol 1,4,5-trisphosphate receptor modulates calcium flux. Proc Natl Acad Sci USA 1995;92:1784–1788.

37. Huse M, Chen YG, Massague J, Kuriyan J. Crystal structure of the cytoplasmic domain of the type I TGF beta receptor in complex with FKBP12. Cell 1999;96:425–436.
38. Lopez-Ilasaca M, et al. Effects of FK506-binding protein 12 and FK506 on autophosphorylation of epidermal growth factor receptor. J Biol Chem 1998;273:9430–9434.
39. Le Bihan S, et al. Calcium/calmodulin kinase inhibitors and immunosuppressant macrolides rapamycin and FK506 inhibit proge. Mol Endocrinol 1998;12:986–1001.
40. Steiner JP, et al. High brain densities of the immunophilin FKBP colocalized with calcineurin. Nature 1992;358:584–587.
41. Dawson TM, et al. The immunophilins, FK506 binding protein and cyclophilin, are discretely localized in the brain: relationship to calcineurin. Neuroscience 1994;62:569–580.
42. Kieffer LJ, Thalhammer T, Handschumacher RE. Isolation and characterization of a 40-kDa cyclophilin-related protein. J Biol Chem 1992;67:5503–5507.
43. Anderson SK, et al. A cyclophilin-related protein involved in the function of natural killer cells. Proc Natl Acad Sci USA 1993;90:542–546.
44. Bierer BE, et al. Probing immunosuppressant action with a nonnatural immunophilin ligand. Science 1990;250:556–559.
45. Matsuda S, Koyasu S. Mechanisms of action of cyclosporine. Immunopharmacology 2000;47:119–125.
46. Schreiber SL, Crabtree GR. The mechanism of action of cyclosporin A and FK506. Immunol. Today 1992;13:136–142.
47. Kunz J, Hall MN. Cyclosporin A, FK506 and rapamycin: more than just immunosuppression. Trends Biochem Sci 1993;18:334–338.
48. Liu J. FK506 and ciclosporin: molecular probes for studying intracellular signal transduction. Trends Pharmacol Sci 1993;14:182–188.
49. Nishiyama M, Izumi S, Okuhara M. Discovery and development of FK506 (Tacrolimus), a potent immunosupressant of microbial origin. In: Merluzzi VJ, Adams J, eds. The Search for Anti-infmammatory Drugs Birkhauser, Boston, 1995, pp 65–104.
50. Sabatini DM, et al. RAFT1: a mammalian protein that binds to FKBP12 in a rapamycin-dependent fashion and is homologous to yeast TORs. Cell 1994;78:35–43.
51. Price NE, Mumby MC. Brain protein serine/threonine phosphatases. Curr Opin Neurobiol 1999;9:336–342.
52. Morioka M, Hamada J, Ushio Y, Miyamoto E. Potential role of calcineurin for brain ischemia and traumatic injury. Prog Neurobiol 1999;58:1–30.
53. Cardenas ME, et al. Immunophilins interact with calcineurin in the absence of exogenous immunosuppressive ligands. EMBO J 1994;13:5944–5957.
54. Kung L, Halloran PF. Immunophilins may limit calcineurin inhibition by cyclosporine and tacrolimus at high drug concentrations. Transplantation 2000;70:327–335.

55. Bochelen D, Rudin M, Sauter A. Calcineurin inhibitors FK506 and SDZ ASM 981 alleviate the outcome of focal cerebral ischemic/reperfusion injury. J Pharmacol Exp Ther 1999;288:653–659.

56. Brown EJ, et al. A mammalian protein targeted by G1-arresting rapamycin-receptor complex. Nature 1994;369:756–758.

57. Parker EM, et al. Rapamycin, but not FK506 and GPI-1046, increases neurite outgrowth in PC12 cells by inhibiting cell cycle progression Neuropharmacology 2000;39:1913–1919.

58. Gold BG. et al. A nonimmunosuppressant FKBP-12 ligand increases nerve regeneration. Exp Neurol 1997;147:269–278.

59. Herdegan T, Fischer G, Bold BG. Immunophilin ligands as a novel treatment of neurological disorders. Trends Pharmacol. Sci 2000;21:3–5.

60. Kermer P, Klocker N, Bahr M. Neuronal death after brain injury: models, mechanisms, and therapeutic strategies in vivo. Cell Tissue Res 1999;298: 383–395.

61. Lipton P. Ischemic cell death in brain neurons. Physiol Rev 1999;79: 1431–1568.

62. Lee JM, Grabb MC, Zipfel GJ, Choi DW. Brain tissue responses to ischemia. J Clin Invest 2000;106:723–731.

63. Saatman KE, et al. Prolonged calpain-mediated spectrin breakdown occurs regionally following experimental brain injury in the rat. J Neuropathol Exp Neurol 1996;55:850–860.

64. Farooqui AA, Horrocks LA. Excitatory amino acid receptors, neural membrane phospholipid metabolism and neurological disorders. Brain Res Brain Res Rev 1991;16:171–191.

65. Kristian T, Siesjo BK. Calcium in ischemic cell death. Stroke 1998;29:705–718.

66. Fiskum G, Murphy AN, Beal MF. Mitochondria in neurodegeneration: acute ischemia and chronic neurodegenerative diseases. J Cereb Blood Flow Metab 1999;19:351–369.

67. Kroemer G, Dallaporta B, Resche-Rigon M. The mitochondrial death/life regulator in apoptosis and necrosis. Annu Rev Physiol 1998;60:619–642.

68. Kroemer G. The mitochondrion as an integrator/coordinator of cell death pathways. Cell Death Differ 1998;5:547.

69. Victor RG, Thomas GD, Marban E, O'Rourke B. Presynaptic modulation of cortical synaptic activity by calcineurin. Proc Natl Acad Sci USA 1995; 92:6269–6273.

70. King MM, et al. Mammalian brain phosphoproteins as substrates for calcineurin. J Biol Chem 1984;259:8080–8083.

71. Steiner JP, Dawson TM, Fotuhi M, Snyder SH. Immunophilin regulation of neurotransmitter release. Mol Med 1996;2:325–333.

72. Nichols RA, Suplick GR, Brown JM. Calcineurin-mediated protein dephosphorylation in brain nerve terminals regulates the release of glutamate. J Biol Chem 1994;269:23,817–23,823.

73. Lieberman DN, Mody I. Regulation of NMDA channel function by endogenous Ca(2+)-dependent phosphatase. Nature 1994;369:235–239.

74. Manev H, et al. Macrolide antibiotics protect neurons in culture against the N-methyl-D- aspartate (NMDA) receptor-mediated toxicity of glutamate. Brain Res 1993;624:331–335.

75. Dawson TM, et al. Immunosuppressant FK506 enhances phosphorylation of nitric oxide synthase and protects against glutamate neurotoxicity. Proc Natl Acad Sci USA 1993;90:9808–9812.

76. Yasutsune T, et al. Vasorelaxation and inhibition of the voltage-operated Ca^{2+} channels by FK506 in the porcine coronary artery. Brit J Pharmacol 1999;126:717–729.

77. Chakravarthy B, Morley P, Whitfield J. Ca^{2+}-calmodulin and protein kinase Cs: a hypothetical synthesis of their conflicting convergences on shared substrate domains. Trends Neurosci 1999;22:12–16.

78. Madden KP, Clark WM, Kochhar A, Zivin JA. Effect of protein kinase C modulation on outcome of experimental CNS ischemia. Brain Res 1991;47:193–198.

79. Hara H, et al. Staurosporine, a novel protein kinase C inhibitor, prevents postischemic neuronal damage in the gerbil and rat. J Cereb Blood Flow Metab 1990;10:646–653.

80. Aronowski J, Grotta JC, Strong R, Waxham MN. Interplay between the gamma isoform of PKC and calcineurin in regulation of vulnerability to focal cerebral ischemia. J Cereb Blood Flow Metab 2000;20:343–349.

81. Jayaraman T, et al. FK506 binding protein associated with the calcium release channel (ryanodine receptor). J Biol Chem 1992;267:9474–9477.

82. Brillantes AB, et al. Stabilization of calcium release channel (ryanodine receptor) function by FK506-binding protein. Cell 1994;77:513–523.

83. Cameron AM, et al. FKBP12 binds the inositol 1,4,5-trisphosphate receptor at leucine-proline (1400–1401) and anchors calcineurin to this FK506-like domain. J Biol Chem 1997;272:27,582–27,588.

84. Valdivia HH. Modulation of intracellular Ca^{2+} levels in the heart by sorcin and FKBP12, two accessory proteins of ryanodine receptors. Trends Pharmacol Sci 1998;19:479–482.

85. Venkataramanan R, et al. Biopharmaceutical aspects of FK-506. Transplant Proc 1987;19:30–35.

86. Bultynck G, et al. Effects of the immunosuppressant FK506 on intracellular Ca^{2+} release and Ca^{2+} accumulation mechanisms. J Physiol 2000;525:681–693.

87. Green AR, Hainsworth AH, Jackson DM. GABA potentiation: a logical pharmacological approach for the treatment of acute ischemic stroke. Neuropharmacology 2000;39:1483–1494.

88. Bao J, Cheung WY, Wu JY. Brain L-glutamate decarboxylase. Inhibition by phosphorylation and activation by dephosphorylation. J Biol Chem 1995;270:6464–6467.

89. DuBell WH, Lederer WJ, Rogers TB. K(+) currents responsible for repolarization in mouse ventricle and their modulation by FK-506 and rapamycin. Am J Physiol Heart Circ Physiol 2000;278:H886–H897.

90. DuBell WH, Gaa ST, Lederer WJ, Rogers TB. Independent inhibition of calcineurin and K^{+} currents by the immunosuppressant FK-506 in rat ventricle. Am J Physiol 1998;275:H2041–H2052.

91. DuBell WH, Wright PA, Lederer WJ, Rogers TB. Effect of the immuno-supressant FK506 on excitation-contraction coupling and outward K^+ currents in rat ventricular myocytes. J Physiol (Lond) 1997;501(Pt 3):509–516.

92. Terashima A, et al. Single-channel activity of the Ca^{2+}-dependent K^+ channel is modulated by FK506 and rapamycin. Brain Res 1998;786:255–258.

93. Fiskum G. Mitochondrial damage during cerebral ischemia. Ann Emerg Med 1985;14:810–815.

94. Murphy AN, et al. Bcl-2 potentiates the maximal calcium uptake capacity of neural cell mitochondria. Proc Natl Acad Sci USA 1996;93:9893–9898.

95. Crompton M. The mitochondrial permeability transition pore and its role in cell death. Biochem J 341(Pt 2):233–249.

96. Cassarino DS, et al. Elevated reactive oxygen species and antioxidant enzyme activities in animal and cellular models of Parkinson's disease. Biochim Biophys Acta 1997;1362:77–86.

97. Susin SA, et al. Molecular characterization of mitochondrial apoptosis-inducing factor. Nature 1999;397:441–446.

98. Kondo Y, et al. Cyclosporin A prevents ischemia-induced reduction of muscarinic acetylcholine receptors with suppression of microglial activation in gerbil hippocampus. Neurosci Res 1995;22:123–127.

99. Friberg H, Connern C, Halestrap AP, Wieloch T. Differences in the activation of the mitochondrial permeability transition among brain regions in the rat correlate with selective vulnerability. J Neurochem 1999;72:2488–2497.

100. Halestrap AP, Connern CP, Griffiths EJ, Kerr PM. Cyclosporin A binding to mitochondrial cyclophilin inhibits the permeability transition pore and protects hearts from ischemia/reperfusion injury. Mol Cell Biochem 1997; 174:167–172.

101. Kubes P, Hunter J, Granger DN. Effects of cyclosporin A and FK506 on ischemia/reperfusion-induced neutrophil infiltration in the cat. Dig Dis Sci 1991;6:1469–1472.

102. Wakita H, Tomimoto H, Akiguchi I, Kimura J. Protective effect of cyclosporin A on white matter changes in the rat brain after chronic cerebral hypoperfusion. Stroke 1995;26:1415–1422.

103. Waring P, Beaver J. Cyclosporin A rescues thymocytes from apoptosis induced by very low concentrations of thapsigargin: effects on mitochondrial function. Exp Cell Res 1996;227:264–276.

104. Balakirev MY, Zimmer G. Gradual changes in permeability of inner mitochondrial membrane precede the mitochondrial permeability transition. Arch Biochem Biophys 1998;356:46–54.

105. Berman SB, Watkins SC, Hastings TG. Quantitative biochemical and ultrastructural comparison of mitochondrial permeability transition in isolated brain and liver mitochondria: evidence for reduced sensitivity of brain mitochondria. Exp Neurol 2000;164:415–425.

106. Ouyang YB, et al. Surv. J Cereb Blood Flow Metab 1999;19:1126–1135.

107. Perez-Pinzon MA, et al. Cytochrome C is released from mitochondria into the cytosol after cerebral anoxia or ischemia. J Cereb Blood Flow Metab 1999;19:39–43.

108. Griffiths EJ, Halestrap AP. Further evidence that cyclosporin A protects mitochondria from calcium overload by inhibiting a matrix peptidyl-prolyl cis-trans isomerase. Implications for the immunosuppressive and toxic effects of cyclosporin. Biochem J 1991;274(Pt 2):611-614.

109. Nakai A, Kuroda S, Kristian T, Siesjo BK. The immunosuppressant drug FK506 ameliorates secondary mitochondrial dysfunction following transient focal cerebral ischemia in the rat. Neurobiol Dis 1997;4:288–300.

110. Nishinaka Y, et al. Protective effect of FK506 on ischemia/reperfusion-induced myocardial damage in canine heart. J Cardiovasc Pharmacol 1993; 21:448–454.

111. Wakabayashi H, Karasawa Y, Maeba T, Tanaka S. Effect of FK 506 and cyclosporine A on hepatic energy status in the rat after warm ischemia, as monitored by 31P nuclear magnetic resonance spectroscopy in vivo. Transplant Proc 1992;24:1993–1995.

112. Zini R, et al. Tacrolimus decreases in vitro oxidative phosphorylation of mitochondria from rat forebrain. Life Sci 1998;63:357–368.

113. Haines DD, et al. Cardioprotective effects of the calcineurin inhibitor FK506 and the PAF receptor antagonist and free radical scavenger, EGb 761, in isolated ischemic/reperfused rat hearts. J Cardiovasc Pharmacol 2000; 35:37–44.

114. Garcia-Criado FJ, et al. Tacrolimus (FK506) down-regulates free radical tissue levels, serum cytokines, and neutrophil infiltration after severe liver ischemia. Transplantation 1997;64:594–598.

115. Piantadosi CA, Zhang J. Mitochondrial generation of reactive oxygen species after brain ischemia in the rat. Stroke 1996;27:327–331.

116. Abrahams SL, Hazen RJ, Ayers KM. Sodium azide protects against ischemia-induced acute renal failure in rats. Am J Physiol 1993;265:F130–F136.

117. Becker LB, et al. Generation of superoxide in cardiomyocytes during ischemia before reperfusion. Am J Physiol 1999;277:H2240–H2246.

118. Masuda Y, Ochi Y, Ochi Y, Kadokawa T. A possible role of endogenously formed cerebral prostaglandins in the development of adaptive protection against cerebral hypoxia/ischemia in mice. Methods Find Exp Clin Pharmacol 1987;9:721–727.

119. Stone D, Darley-Usmar V, Smith DR, O'Leary V. Hypoxia-reoxygenation induced increase in cellular Ca^{2+} in myocytes and perfused hearts: the role of mitochondria. J Mol Cell Cardiol 1989;21:963–973.

120. Boismare F, Lorenzo J. Study of the protection on afforded by nicergoline against the effects of cerebral ischemia in the cat. Arzneimittelforschung 1975;25:410–413.

121. Matsuo Y, et al. Role of cell adhesion molecules in brain injury after transient middle cerebral artery occlusion in the rat. Brain Res 1994;656:344–352.

122. Stoll G, Jander S, Schroeter M. Inflammation and glial responses in ischemic brain lesions. Prog Neurobiol 1998;56:149–171.

123. Wood PL. Microglia as a unique cellular target in the treatment of stroke: potential neurotoxic mediators produced by activated microglia. Neurol Res 1995;17:242–248.

124. Arvin B, Neville LF, Barone FC, Feuerstein GZ. The role of inflammation and cytokines in brain injury. Neurosci Biobehav Rev 1996;20:445–452.
125. Kim JS. Cytokines and adhesion molecules in stroke and related diseases. J Neurol Sci 1996;137:69–78.
126. Sharma BK, Kumar K. Role of proinflammatory cytokines in cerebral ischemia: a review. Metab Brain Dis 1998;13:1–8.
127. Kochanek PM, Hallenbeck JM. Polymorphonuclear leukocytes and monocytes/macrophages in the pathogenesis of cerebral ischemia and stroke. Stroke 1992;23:1367–1379.
128. Lehrmann E, et al. Microglial and macrophage reactions mark progressive changes and define the penumbra in the rat neocortex and striatum after transient middle cerebral artery occlusion. J Comp Neurol 1997;386:461–476.
129. Matsuda T, Baba A. [Response of Na^+/Ca^{2+} antiporter to ischemia and glial/neuronal death]. Nippon Yakurigaku Zasshi 1998;111:13–19.
130. Cicalese L, et al. Effect of FK506 on the mucosal perfusion of the rat intestinal allograft. Transplant Proc 1996;28:2575.
131. Kawano K, Bowers JL, Clouse ME. Protective effect of FK 506 on hepatic injury following cold ischemic preservation and transplantation: influence on hepatic microcirculation. Transplant Proc 1995;27:362–363.
132. Cetinkale O, et al. Involvement of neutrophils in ischemic injury. I. Biochemical and histopathological investigation of the effect of FK506 on dorsal skin flaps in rats. Ann Plast Surg 1997;39:505–515.
133. Sakr MF, et al. FK 506 pre-treatment is associated with reduced levels of tumor necrosis factor and interleukin 6 following hepatic ischemia/reperfusion. J Hepatol 1993;17:301–307.
134. Kawano K, et al. A protective effect of FK506 in ischemically injured rat livers. Transplantation 1991;52:143–145.
135. Buttini M, et al. Expression of tumor necrosis factor alpha after focal cerebral ischemia in the rat. Neuroscience 1996;71:1–16.
136. Fink K, et al. Prolonged therapeutic window for ischemic brain damage caused by delayed caspase activation. J Cereb Blood Flow Metab 1998;18:1071–1076.
137. Yamasaki Y, et al. Interleukin-1 as a pathogenetic mediator of ischemic brain damage in rats . Stroke 1995;26:676–680.
138. Endres M, et al. Attenuation of delayed neuronal death after mild focal ischemia in mice by inhibition of the caspase family. J Cereb Blood Flow Metab 1998;18:238–247.
139. Siesjo BK. Pathophysiology and treatment of focal cerebral ischemia. Part II: Mechanisms of damage and treatment. J Neurosurg 1992;77:337–354.
140. Rupalla K, Allegrini PR, Sauer D, Wiessner C. Time course of microglia activation and apoptosis in various brain regions after permanent focal cerebral ischemia in mice. Acta Neuropathol (Berl) 1998;96:172–178.
141. Gehrmann J, et al. Immunocytochemical study of an early microglial activation in ischemia. J Cereb Blood Flow Metab 1992;12:257–269.
142. Pearson VL, Rothwell NJ, Toulmond S. Excitotoxic brain damage in the rat induces interleukin-1 beta protein in microglia and astrocytes: correlation with the progression of cell death. Glia 1999;25:311–323.

143. Davies CA, et al. The progression and topographic distribution of interleukin-1beta expression after permanent middle cerebral artery occlusion in the rat. J. Cereb Blood Flow Metab 1999;19:87–98.

144. Suzuki S, et al. Cerebral neurons express interleukin-6 after transient forebrain ischemia in gerbils. Neurosci Lett 1999;262:117–120.

145. Gregersen R, Lambertsen K, Finsen B. Microglia and macrophages are the major source of tumor necrosis factor in permanent middle cerebral artery occlusion in mice. J Cereb Blood Flow Metab 2000;20:53–65.

146. Yamasaki Y, Itoyama Y, Kogure K. Involvement of cytokine production in pathogenesis of transient cerebral ischemic damage. Keio J Med 1996;45:225–229.

147. Galasso JM, et al. Acute Excitotoxic Injury Induces Expression of Monocyte Chemoattractant Protein-1 and Its Receptor, CCR2, in Neonatal Rat Brain. Exp Neurol 2000;165:295–305.

148. Wakita H, Tomimoto H, Akiguchi I, Kimura J. Dose-dependent, protective effect of FK506 against white matter changes in the rat brain after chronic cerebral ischemia. Brain Res 1998;792:105–113.

149. Lehrmann E, et al. Microglia and macrophages are major sources of locally produced transforming growth factor-beta1 after transient middle cerebral artery occlusion in rats. Glia 1998;24:437–448.

150. Flanders KC, Ren RF, Lippa CF. Transforming growth factor-betas in neurodegenerative disease. Prog Neurobiol 1998;54:71–85.

151. Toku K, et al. Microglial cells prevent nitric oxide-induced neuronal apoptosis in vitro. J Neurosci Res 1998;53:415–425.

152. Frautschy SA, Walicke PA, Baird A. Localization of basic fibroblast growth factor and its mRNA after CNS injury. Brain Res 1991;553:291–299.

153. Bang H, et al. Activation of Ca^{2+} signaling in neutrophils by the mast cell-released immunophilin FKBP12 [published erratum appears in Proc Natl Acad Sci USA 1999 Feb 2;96(3):1162]. Proc Natl Acad Sci USA 1995;92:3435–3438.

154. Giulian D. Reactive glia as rivals in regulating neuronal survival. Glia 1993;7:102–110.

155. Tacconi MT. Neuronal death: is there a role for astrocytes? [published erratum appears in Neurochem Res 1999 Mar;24(3):459]. Neurochem Res 1998;23:759–765.

156. Tsujikawa A, et al. Tacrolimus (FK506) attenuates leukocyte accumulation after transient retinal ischemia. Stroke 1998;29:1431–1437.

157. Kato H, et al. Progressive expression of immunomolecules on activated microglia and invading leukocytes following focal cerebral ischemia in the rat. Brain Res 1996;734:203–212.

158. Gonzalez-Amaro R, Diaz-Gonzalez F, Sanchez-Madrid F. Adhesion molecules in inflammatory diseases. Drugs 1998;56:977–988.

159. Karlsson H, Nassberger L. FK506 suppresses the mitogen-induced increase in lymphocyte adhesiveness to endothelial cells, but does not affect endothelial cell activation in response to inflammatory stimuli. Transplantation 1997;64:1217–1220.

160. Karmazyn M. The 1990 Merck Frosst Award. Ischemic and reperfusion injury in the heart. Cellular mechanisms and pharmacological interventions. Can J Physiol Pharmacol 1991;69:719–730.

161. Blennerhassett L, et al. The influence of ischemia/reperfusion injury on the jejunum. Ann Plast Surg 1998;40:617–623.

162. Grech ED, Jackson MJ, Ramsdale DR. Reperfusion injury after acute myocardial infarction [editorial] [see comments]. BMJ 1995;310:477–478.

163. Lucchesi BR. Myocardial ischemia, reperfusion and free radical injury. Am J Cardiol 1990;65:14I–23I.

164. Tredger JM. Ischemia-reperfusion injury of the liver: treatment in theory and in practice. Biofactors 1998;8:161–164.

165. Werns SW, Lucchesi BR. Free radicals and ischemic tissue injury. Trends Pharmacol Sci 1990;11:161–166.

166. Sheng H, et al. Mice overexpressing extracellular superoxide dismutase have increased resistance to focal cerebral ischemia. Neuroscience 1999;88:185–191.

167. Dawson DA, Masayasu H, Graham DI, Macrae IM. The neuroprotective efficacy of ebselen (a glutathione peroxidase mimic) on brain damage induced by transient focal cerebral ischemia in the rat. Neurosci Lett 1995;185:65–69.

168. Hellstrom HO, et al. Effect of tirilazad mesylate given after permanent middle cerebral artery occlusion in rat. Acta Neurochir (Wien) 1994;129:188–192.

169. Li H, Zhu H, Xu CJ, Yuan J. Cleavage of BID by caspase 8 mediates the mitochondrial damage in the Fas pathway of apoptosis. Cell 1998;94:491–501.

170. Takeshima R, Kirsch JR, Koehler RC, Traystman RJ. Tirilazad treatment does not decrease early brain injury after transient focal ischemia in cats. Stroke 1994;25:670–676.

171. Xue D, Slivka A, Buchan AM. Tirilazad reduces cortical infarction after transient but not permanent focal cerebral ischemia in rats. Stroke 1992; 23:894–899.

172. RANTTAS Investigators A randomized trial of tirilazad mesylate in patients with acute stroke (RANTTAS). Stroke 1996;27:1453–1458.

173. Yamaguchi T, et al. Ebselen in acute ischemic stroke: a placebo-controlled, double-blind clinical trial. Ebselen Study Group. Stroke 1998;29:12–17.

174. Takuma K, et al. Apoptosis in Ca^{2+} reperfusion injury of cultured astrocytes: roles of reactive oxygen species and NF-kappaB activation. Eur J Neurosci 1999;11:4204–4212.

175. Ide T, Morikawa E, Kirino T. An immunosuppressant, FK506, protects hippocampal neurons from forebrain ischemia in the mongolian gerbil. Neurosci Lett 1996;204:157–160.

176. Tokime T, Nozaki K, Kikuchi H. Neuroprotective effect of FK506, an immunosuppressant, on transient global ischemia in gerbil. Neurosci Lett 1996; 206:81–84.

177. Yagita Y, et al. Effect of immunosuppressant FK506 on ischemia-induced degeneration of hippocampal neurons in gerbils. Life Sci 1996;59:1643–1650.

178. Tanaka K, et al. Calcineurin inhibitor, FK506, prevents reduction in the binding capacity of cyclic AMP-dependent protein kinase in ischemic gerbil brain. J Cereb Blood Flow Metab 1997;17:412–420.

179. Culmsee C, et al. Lubeluzole protects hippocampal neurons from excitotoxicity in vitro and reduces brain damage caused by ischemia. Eur J Pharmacol 1998;342:193–201.
180. Globus MY, et al. A dual role for nitric oxide in NMDA-mediated toxicity in vivo. J Cereb Blood Flow Metab 1995;15:904–913.
181. MacKenzie GM, Jenner P, Marsden CD. The effect of nitric oxide synthase inhibition on quinolinic acid toxicity in the rat striatum. Neuroscience 1995;67:357–371.
182. Zhang ZG, Chopp M, Bailey F, Malinski T. Nitric oxide changes in the rat brain after transient middle cerebral artery occlusion. J Neurol Sci 1995;128:22–27.
183. Dawson DA. Nitric oxide and focal cerebral ischemia: multiplicity of actions and diverse outcome. Cerebrovasc Brain Metab Rev 6, 299-324.
184. Kamii H, et al. Effects of nitric oxide synthase inhibition on brain infarction in SOD- 1-transgenic mice following transient focal cerebral ischemia. J Cereb Blood Flow Metab 1996;16:1153–1157.
185. Huang, Z. et al. Effects of cerebral ischemia in mice deficient in neuronal nitric oxide synthase. Science 1994;265:1883–1885.
186. Toung TJ, et al. Neuroprotective FK506 does not alter in vivo nitric oxide production during ischemia and early reperfusion in rats. Stroke 1999;30:1279–1285.
187. Almeida A, Allen KL, Bates TE, Clark JB. Effect of reperfusion following cerebral ischemia on the activity of the mitochondrial respiratory chain in the gerbil brain. J Neurochem 1995;65:1698–1703.
188. Wiessner C, et al. Neuron-specific transgene expression of Bcl-XL but not Bcl-2 genes reduced lesion size after permanent middle cerebral artery occlusion in mice. Neurosci Lett 1999;268:119–122.
189. Martinou JC, et al. Overexpression of BCL-2 in transgenic mice protects neurons from naturally occurring cell death and experimental ischemia. Neuron 1994;13:1017–1030.
190. Asai A, et al. High level calcineurin activity predisposes neuronal cells to apoptosis. J Biol Chem 1999;274:34,450–34,458.
191. Lotem J, Kama R, Sachs L. Suppression or induction of apoptosis by opposing pathways downstream from calcium-activated calcineurin. Proc Natl Acad Sci USA 1999;96:12,016–12,020.
192. Winter C, et al. The immunophilin ligand FK506, but not GPI-1046, protects against neuronal death and inhibits c-Jun expression in the substantia nigra pars compacta following transection of the rat medial forebrain bundle. Neuroscience 2000;95:753–762.
193. Winter C, Schenkel J, Zimmermann M, Herdegen T. MAP kinase phosphatase 1 is expressed and enhanced by FK506 in surviving mamillary, but not degenerating nigral neurons following axotomy. Brain Res 1998;801:198–205.
194. Kiani A, Rao A, Aramburu J. Manipulating immune responses with immunosuppressive agents that target NFAT. Immunity 2000;12:359–372.
195. Zhang Y, et al. Immunosuppressant FK506 activates NF-kappaB through the proteasome- mediated degradation of IkappaBalpha. Requirement for

Ikappabalpha n- terminal phosphorylation but not ubiquitination sites. J Biol Chem 1999;274;34,657–34,662.

196. Clemens JA. Cerebral ischemia: gene activation, neuronal injury, and the protective role of antioxidants. Free Radic. Biol. Med. 2000;28:1526–1531.

197. Brunner T, et al. Activation-induced cell death in murine T cell hybridomas. Differential regulation of Fas (CD95) versus Fas ligand expression by cyclosporin A and FK506. Int Immunol 1996;8:1017–1026.

198. Shibasaki F, Price ER, Milan D, McKeon F. Role of kinases and the phosphatase calcineurin in the nuclear shuttling of transcription factor NF-AT4. Nature 1996;382:370–373.

199. Berglund H, et al. The three-dimensional solution structure and dynamic properties of the human FADD death domain. J Mol Biol 2000;302: 171–188.

200. Wong BR, et al. TRANCE is a novel ligand of the tumor necrosis factor receptor family that activates c-Jun N-terminal kinase in T cells. J Biol Chem 1997;272:25,190–25,194.

201. Enslen H, Soderling TR. Roles of calmodulin-dependent protein kinases and phosphatase in calcium-dependent transcription of immediate early genes. J. Biol. Chem. 1994;269:20,872–20,877.

202. Yang E, et al. Bad, a heterodimeric partner for Bcl-XL and Bcl-2, displaces Bax and promotes cell death. Cell 1995;80:285–291.

203. Wang HG, et al. Ca^{2+}-induced apoptosis through calcineurin dephosphorylation of BAD. Science 1999;284:339–343.

204. Yin XM. Signal transduction mediated by Bid, a pro-death Bcl-2 family proteins, connects the death receptor and mitochondria apoptosis pathways Cell Res 2000;10:161–167.

205. Ishizuka T, et al. Stem cell factor augments Fc epsilon RI-mediated TNF-alpha production and stimulates MAP kinases via a different pathway in MC/9 mast cells. J Immunol 1998;161:3624–3630.

206. Herr I, et al. FK506 prevents stroke-induced generation of ceramide and apoptosis signaling. Brain Res 1999;826:210–219.

207. Schreiber SL. Chemistry and biology of the immunophilins and their immunosuppressive ligands. Science 1991;251:283–287.

208. Davis DL, Murthy JN, Soldin SJ. Biochemical characterization of the minor immunophilins. Clin Biochem 2000;33:81–87.

209. Coss MC, Winterstein D, Sowder RC, Simek SL. Molecular cloning, DNA sequence analysis, and biochemical characterization of a novel 65-kDa FK506-binding protein (FKBP65). J. Biol. Chem. 1995;270:29,336–29,341.

210. Zeng B, et al. Chicken FK506-binding protein, FKBP65, a member of the FKBP family of peptidylprolyl cis-trans isomerases, is only partially inhibited by FK506. Biochem J 1998;330(Pt 1):109–114.

211. Coss MC, et al. The immunophilin FKBP65 forms an association with the serine/threonine kinase c-Raf-1. Cell Growth Differ 1998;9:41–48.

212. Kawagoe J, Abe K, Aoki M, Kogure K. Induction of HSP90 alpha heat shock mRNA after transient global ischemia in gerbil hippocampus. Brain Res 1993;621:121–125.

213. Callebaut I, et al. An immunophilin that binds M(r) 90,000 heat shock protein: main structural features of a mammalian p59 protein. Proc Natl Acad Sci USA 1992;89:6270–6274.
214. Bornman L, Polla BS, Gericke GS. Heat-shock protein 90 and ubiquitin: developmental regulation during myogenesis. Muscle Nerve 1996;19:574–580.
215. Sharp FR, Massa SM, Swanson RA. Heat-shock protein protection. Trends Neurosci 1999;22:97–99.
216. Rajdev S, et al. Mice overexpressing rat heat shock protein 70 are protected against cerebral infarction. Ann Neurol 2000;47:782–791.
217. Plumier JC, et al. Transgenic mice expressing the human inducible Hsp70 have hippocampal neurons resistant to ischemic injury. Cell Stress Chaperones 1997;2:162–167.
218. Yenari MA, Giffard RG, Sapolsky RM, Steinberg GK. The neuroprotective potential of heat shock protein 70 (HSP70). Mol Med Today 1999;5:525–531.
219. Smith DF, Baggenstoss BA, Marion TN, Rimerman RA. Two FKBP-related proteins are associated with progesterone receptor complexes. J Biol Chem 1993;268:18,365–18,371.
220. Ratajczak T, et al. The cyclophilin component of the unactivated estrogen receptor contains a tetratricopeptide repeat domain and shares identity with p59 (FKBP59). J Biol Chem 1993;268:13,187–13,192.
221. Ratajczak T, Carrello A, Minchin RF. Biochemical and calmodulin binding properties of estrogen receptor binding cyclophilin expressed in Escherichia coli. Biochem Biophys Res Commun 1995;209:117–125.
222. Ratajczak T, Mark PJ, Martin RL, Minchin RF. Cyclosporin A potentiates estradiol-induced expression of the cathepsin D gene in MCF7 breast cancer cells. Biochem Biophys Res Commun 1996;220:208–212.
223. Roof RL, Hall ED. Gender differences in acute CNS trauma and stroke: neuroprotective effects of estrogen and progesterone. J Neurotrauma 2000;17:367–388.
224. Chen J, Chopp M, Li Y. Neuroprotective effects of progesterone after transient middle cerebral artery occlusion in rat. J. Neurol. Sci. 1999;171:24–30.
225. Kumon Y, et al. Neuroprotective effect of postischemic administration of progesterone in spontaneously hypertensive rats with focal cerebral ischemia. J Neurosurg 2000;92:848–852.
226. Yang SH, Shi J, Day AL, Simpkins JW. Estradiol exerts neuroprotective effects when administered after ischemic insult. Stroke 2000;31:745–749.
227. Dubal DB, et al. Estradiol modulates bcl-2 in cerebral ischemia: a potential role for estrogen receptors. J Neurosci 1999;19:6385–6393.
228. Gold BG, et al. Immunophilin FK506-binding protein 52 (not FK506-binding protein 12) mediates the neurotrophic action of FK506. J Pharmacol Exp Ther 1999;289:1202–1210.
229. Someren JS, Faber LE, Klein JD, Tumlin JA. Heat shock proteins 70 and 90 increase calcineurin activity in vitro through calmodulin-dependent and independent mechanisms. Biochem Biophys Res Commun 1999;260:619–625.
230. Dumont FJ. FK506, an immunosuppressant targeting calcineurin function. Curr Med Chem 2000;7:731–748.

231. Aoyama S, Katayama Y, Terashi A. The effect of FK506, an immunosuppressant, on cerebral infarction volume in focal cerebral ischaemia in rats. Nippan Ika Daiga Ku Zasshi 1997;64(5):416–426.
232. Takamatsu H, Kondo K, Ikeda Y, Umemura K. Neuroprotective effects depend on the model of focal ischaemia following middle cerebral artery occlusion. Eur J Pharmacol 1998;362(2–3):137–142.

13
Immunosuppressants in Traumatic Brain Injury

David O. Okonkwo and John T. Povlishock

INTRODUCTION

Traumatic brain injury (TBI) remains the most common cause of death in persons under age 45 in the Western world. The societal impact is profound, with 2 million cases, 220,000 hospitalizations, and 52,000 deaths from head trauma occurring each year in the United States alone (1,2). Another 80,000 to 90,000 persons each year suffer permanent debilitation. The total cost of TBI in the United States, both direct healthcare and indirect personal and societal costs, is estimated at $44 billion per annum (3). These statistics are in lieu of the fact that mortality from TBI declined 22% between 1979 and 1992, in large measure from improvement in automobile design, use of helmets and seatbelts, prehospital management of the trauma patient, and standardization of intensive unit care (4–6). However, despite the hard-fought efforts of numerous investigators around the world, not one Phase III clinical trial investigating a pharmacological compound for the treatment of traumatic brain injury has yet been successful (7).

Despite these setbacks in past clinical trials, recent insights into the pathophysiology of traumatic brain injury have yielded new targets for therapeutic intervention. Laboratory and clinical evidence has implicated mitochondrial damage and bioenergetic failure, cysteine protease activation, and calcineurin modulation in the progression of injury in the ensuing hours and days. Immunosuppressants that target central nervous system immunophilins have been shown to alter one or more of the above secondary injury mechanisms in multiple central nervous system (CNS) disorders and, recently, in trauma. Thus, this family of compounds has emerged as one of the more promising new therapeutic modalities in traumatic brain injury. This chapter presents a survey of the current understanding of the pathological sequelae of focal and diffuse injury after head trauma, as well as a review of two immunosuppressants, cyclosporin A and FK506, as powerful pharmacological agents to limit

From: *Immunosuppressant Analogs in Neuroprotection*
Edited by: C. V. Borlongan, O. Isacson, and P. R. Sanberg © Humana Press Inc., Totowa, NJ

damage and improve recovery from traumatic brain injury, one of modern civilization's most devastating diseases.

PATHOPHYSIOLOGY OF TBI

The pathological consequences of TBI are of two principal forms: focal and diffuse injury. The distinguishing features of focal injury are intra- or extraparenchymal hematoma formation and/or cortical contusion, with resultant local necrosis of brain parenchyma. Contact and/or inertial forces from a mechanical insult to the skull cause this direct localized damage to the neuraxis, and these focal pathological consequences of morbidity and mortality are primarily based on their local, extent, and overall progression in the acute postinjury period.

By contrast, diffuse injury, and more specifically diffuse axonal injury (DAI), typically results from inertial forces, particularly involving rotational strain on the brain, and is not dependent on a direct blow to the cranium. DAI is a principal pathology typically associated with long-term morbidity after TBI *(8,9)*. When examining the postmortem brains of head-injured humans, neuropathologists in the second half of this century found injured axons diffusely scattered throughout the neuraxis, in no definable pattern *(10–12)*. These axons appeared severed, and the axonal damage was thus attributed to the tensile and shear stresses experienced at the moment of injury.

We now appreciate that direct primary axotomy describes only a small subset of the most severely injured fibers *(13,14)*. Rather, in most cases, axotomy represents the end-stage of a complex process in which the mechanical insult induces secondary injury initially involving axolemmal perturbation and followed by mitochondrial (and bioenergetic) failure, cysteine protease activation, and cytoskeletal disruption. These events culminate in the formation of a disconnected swollen axonal stub, characteristic of the classically described retraction bulb (Fig. 1). Disconnection develops over the hours following the traumatic episode and is termed delayed or secondary axotomy. These processes of diffuse axonal injury and secondary axotomy have been described over the last 20 yr in both animal models and the human clinical situation *(8,15)*. Because many of the clinical features of

---

Fig. 1. *Schema depicting delayed or secondary axotomy following traumatic insult.* The flowchart details the evolution of traumatic axonal injury from primary mechanical insult to secondary axotomy. (**A**) The primary mechanical traumatic insult seen following moderate and severe traumatic brain injury induces an overt disruption of the axolemma at one focus along the length of the injured axon. (**B**) Within this focus of axonal injury, calcium influx across the traumatically perturbed axolemma disrupts ionic homeostasis and triggers characteristic pathological

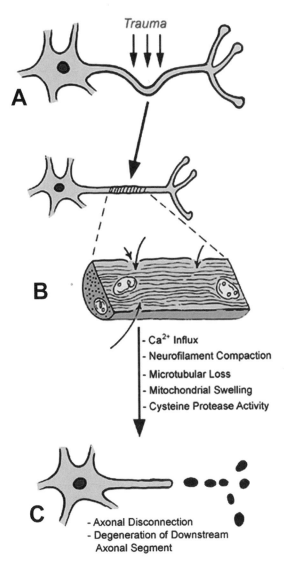

Fig. 1. (*continued from opposite page*) changes. Mitochondria actively sequester calcium ions in an attempt to buffer rising intraaxonal calcium concentrations, resulting in colloidosmotic swelling and uncoupling of oxidative phosphorylation. The increased intraaxonal calcium also triggers secondary injury mechanisms that cause neurofilament compaction and microtubular loss. (**C**) Additionally, calcium-induced activation of cysteine proteases, notably calpains and caspases, within the site of axonal injury triggers the anterograde to retrograde conversion of axoplasmic transport, preventing axonal swelling at sites of axonal damage but provoking disconnection of the axonal segment. The distal segment later undergoes wallerian degeneration.

DAI develop in the hours following the traumatic episode, elucidation of the underlying pathological mechanisms may create a therapeutic window for clinical intervention.

In addition to these focal and diffuse changes, there is now evidence of generalized changes that occur at the moment of impact or as a delayed secondary response to injury. Specifically, pathology after brain injury has also been linked to an elevation of excitatory amino acids that precipitate, through receptor-mediated neuroexcitation, the influx of sodium and calcium ions *(16,17)*. High intraneuronal calcium activates numerous secondary injury mechanisms, including, but not limited to, calpains, caspases, calcineurin, nitric oxide systems, endonucleases, and phosphatases (for a review, *see* ref. *18*). Excessive stimulation of calcium-sensitive processes leads to organelle failure and neuronal somatic cytoskeletal damage causing the neuronal death frequently observed in cortical and hippocampal tissue after TBI. One important organelle sensitive to such a neuroexcitatory surge in intracellular calcium in focal traumatic brain injury is the mitochondrion, damage to which has drastic consequences for the cell.

CALCIUM HOMEOSTASIS AND MITOCHONDRIAL DAMAGE IN TRAUMATIC BRAIN INJURY: A TARGET FOR CSA-MEDIATED NEUROPROTECTION

Recent evidence has demonstrated that a rapid rise in intracellular calcium concentrations is a key initiating mechanism in traumatic brain injury and is spatially and temporally related to the underlying mitochondrial and intracellular damage. A rapid influx of calcium across a traumatically perturbed neuronal somatic plasmalemma or its axolemma induces mitochondrial swelling and activates Ca^{2+}-dependent phosphatases and proteases, leading to the cytoskeletal collapse and mitochondrial swelling observed in injured neuronal somata and axons *(19–21)*.

Mitochondria in excitotoxic neurons and in foci of membrane failure act as calcium sinks that sequester Ca^{2+} within the matrix in an effort to preserve low cytoplasmic Ca^{2+} concentrations. This Ca^{2+} load within the mitochondrial matrix, however, leads to colloidosmotic swelling of the organelle and collapse of organelle function *(22)*. Local failure of mitochondria, in turn, could decrease production of high-energy phosphates necessary to maintain membrane pumps and prevent further ionic imbalance in injured neurons. Thus, mitochondria may be involved in a vicious cycle whereby traumatic injury leads to Ca^{2+} influx, which causes mitochondrial failure and loss of energy substrate production, which, in turn, negates the ability of the cell to restore membrane pumps thereby leading to further Ca^{2+} entry.

Previous studies have documented both morphological (swelling, membrane blebbing) and physiological (decreased oxidative phosphorylation, altered membrane potential) alterations associated with mitochondrial impairment in focal injury after TBI *(23–25)*. Furthermore, mitochondrial swelling is one of the earliest markers of diffuse axonal injury, occurring in the first minutes following injury *(21)*, and in vivo evidence has implicated mitochondrial swelling in the development of the pathobiology of axonal injury *(26)*.

It is known that mitochondrial functioning depends upon the maintenance of the membrane potential across the inner mitochondrial membrane, termed $\Delta\psi_m$. The major regulator of $\Delta\psi_m$ under adverse conditions is the permeability transition (PT) pore, a multimeric transmembrane protein on the inner mitochondrial membrane that assembles in response to specific triggers, including oxidative stress and calcium accumulation. Opening of the PT pore, loss of $\Delta\psi_m$, and the resultant mitochondrial permeability transition (MPT) results in organelle failure and can initiate death cascades in the cell *(27,28)*. MPT in response to high intraneuronal calcium is prevented by the potent immunosuppressant, cyclosporin A (CsA) *(22,29)*.

The action of CsA is dependent on binding to its partner molecule cyclophilin, a member of the immunophilin family of proteins, with formation of an immunosuppressant–immunophilin complex. Immunophilins are present in the mitochondrial matrix as well as the cytosol *(30)*. Under conditions of oxidative stress (high Ca^{2+}, low ATP, high P_i), cyclophilins can induce a conformational change in the PT pore that allows nonspecific passage of solutes less than 1.5 kDa *(29,31)*. Binding by CsA prevents cyclophilin from interacting with the PT pore complex, and thereby prevents the induction of a mitochondrial permeability transition.

Based on the above, it seemed plausible that CsA-mediated blockade of the PT pore could preserve mitochondrial functioning and interrupt the damaging cascade from Ca^{2+} accumulation during secondary injury following traumatic brain injury. This belief was also partially supported by evidence emerging from the field of brain ischemia, where there was evidence to support a role for mitochondria in mediating neuronal failure, with the suggestion of neuroprotection by CsA *(32)*.

To date, multiple studies have demonstrated the efficacy of cyclosporin A in ameliorating neurologic damage following traumatic brain injury (Table 1). In our laboratory, we examined the issue of CsA neuroprotection in a model of diffuse axonal injury and demonstrated that CsA preserves mitochondrial integrity in injured axons undergoing traumatically-induced axolemmal change (Fig. 2). We further showed that protection of mitochon-

Table 1
Evidence for Cyclosporin A Use in Traumatic Brain Injury

Ref.	Model	Dosing	Outcome variable
39	CCI	20 mg/kg ip 15 min postinjury	LTP impairment and LTD enhancement in CA1-CA3 synapses at 48 h
37	CCI	20 mg/kg ip 15 min postinjury, then 20 mg/kg ip 24 h postinjury or 4.5 or 10 mg/kg/d via osmotic pump	Cortical contusion volume at 7 d
38	CCI	20 mg/kg ip 15 min postinjury	Mitochondrial transmembrane potential, MPT, mitochondrial [Ca^{2+}], and ROS generation
35	IA	10 mg/kg it 30 min postinjury	Calcium-activated secondary injury mechanisms and diffuse axonal injury at 2 h and 24 h
34	IA	10 mg/kg it 30 min preinjury	Calpain activation and cytoskeletal collapse in DAI at 1 h
33	IA	10 mg/kg it 30 min preinjury	Mitochondrial morphology and axonal failure in diffuse axonal injury at 1 h and 24 h

Abbreviations: CCI, controlled cortical impact; IA, impact acceleration; ip, intraperitoneal; it, intrathecal; LTP, long-term potentiation; LTD, long-term depression; MPT, mitochondrial permeability transition; ROS, reactive oxygen species; DAI, diffuse axonal injury.

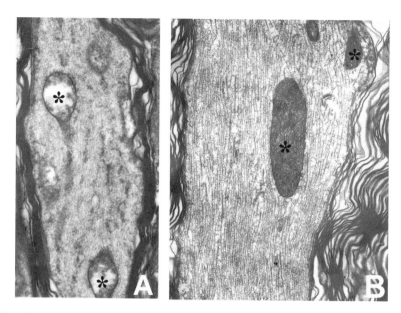

Fig. 2. *Morphological appearance of mitochondria in injured axons from untreated or CsA-treated injured animals.* (**A**) Morphology of mitochondria (asterisks) in an injured axon from an untreated animal at 1 h postinjury. No cristae are discerned within the two mitochondria and the matrix is markedly expanded, evidence of swelling from a calcium-induced mitochondrial permeability transition. (**B**) Morphological appearance of mitochondria (asterisks) in an injured axon after CsA treatment at 1 h postinjury. The myelin sheath is disrupted and the cytoskeleton is compacted, but no evidence of mitochondrial damage is seen, evidence of CsA protection of mitochondria in traumatic axonal injury.

drial integrity was associated with protection for the axon itself, reflected in a reduction in the number of damaged axons observed at 24 h postinjury *(33)*. In these experiments, a single bolus of CsA (10 mg/kg) was administered intrathecally, 30 min prior to injury.

Our initial results indicated that, in foci of axonal perturbation in CsA-treated injured animals, approx 75% of mitochondria were morphologically intact and, presumably, functioning, while 25% apparently underwent MPT and were swollen. In this scenario, we hypothesized that bioenergetic failure of mitochondria limited the axon's ability to restore ionic homeostasis. Thus, with CsA-mediated mitochondrial protection, maintenance of oxidative respiration and ATP supply from the functioning mitochondria permitted the continued functioning of ATP-dependent membrane pumps, thereby limiting enduring changes in ionic imbalance. The assumed MPT in the

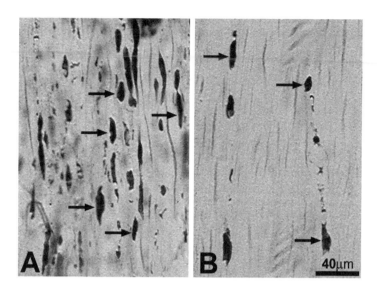

Fig. 3. *Effect of CsA treatment on calcium-induced secondary injury in traumatic axonal injury.* Traumatically injured axons displaying immunoreactivity indicating calpain-mediated spectrin proteolysis (arrows) are seen in light micrographs of medial lemniscus from a vehicle-treated injured animal **(A)** and a CsA-treated injured animal **(B)**. The number of immunoreactive damaged axons is dramatically reduced after CsA treatment compared to the vehicle-treated situation. Quantitative analysis confirms that treatment with CsA results in a 75% reduction in the number of axons displaying evidence of calcium-induced secondary injury.

remaining swollen mitochondria with consequent Ca^{2+} accumulation in the matrix would transiently protect the cytoplasm from the damaging effects of a large Ca^{2+} load. This would create a favorable environment for recovery of the injured neuron and/or axon: continued ATP supply and low intracellular calcium.

More recent studies from our laboratory confirmed this axonal protection via the demonstration that CsA also blunted the calcium-mediated cytoskeletal consequences associated with TAI *(34)*. CsA effectively reduced the number of axons displaying immunoreactivity for calpain-mediated secondary injury and for cytoskeletal damage after impact acceleration TBI (Fig. 3). These results were confirmed with postinjury administration of CsA, wherein we further demonstrated that postinjury CsA administration also limits the number of fibers that progress to axotomy *(35)*.

Scheff, Sullivan, and colleagues have investigated the use of cyclosporin A in the cortical contusion injury (CCI) model of TBI, a well-characterized experimental model of focal injury. In CCI, a parietal craniotomy is made and a pneumatically controlled pin compresses the underlying cortical tissue to a specified depth. CCI reliably reproduces the contusion, inflammatory reaction, neuroexcitation, and local necrosis of focal injury seen in human TBI. In the hands of Scheff, Sullivan, and colleagues, CsA has proven a powerful pharmacological intervention in ameliorating focal traumatic injury (*see* Table 1). Specifically, CsA was shown to produce a 50–74% reduction in the cortical lesion volume after CCI, depending on dose, route, and regimen *(36,37)*. This profound protection was later directly attributed to the amelioration of calcium-induced mitochondrial damage, as mitochondria isolated from injured animals treated with CsA had lower concentrations of matrical calcium and were resistant to the induction of a mitochondrial permeability transition *(38)*. Furthermore, the authors offered a mechanism by which CsA may improve neuropsychiatric outcome following TBI with the demonstration that CsA inhibits LTP impairment and prevented enhancement of LTP in hippocampus after injury *(39)*. These studies provide compelling evidence that CsA ameliorates secondary injury in focal injury after TBI.

Collectively, the studies from our laboratory and those from the University of Kentucky group demonstrate the utility of CsA in reducing the spectrum of secondary injury following TBI. CsA appears effective in limiting mitochondrial damage via its action on the PT pore and in lessening both neuronal death in focal injury and axonal failure in diffuse injury. The above-described results argue that CsA may represent a potent, new therapeutic strategy for the treatment of traumatic brain injury. The data thus far from animal models have been so compelling that a Phase I trial investigating the use of cyclosporin A in the treatment of severe traumatic brain injury was recently initiated at the Medical College of Virginia Hospitals.

IMMUNOSUPPRESSANTS AND CALCINEURIN IN TRAUMATIC BRAIN INJURY: A TARGET FOR FK506-MEDIATED NEUROPROTECTION

In addition to their site of action at the PT pore, CsA–cyclophilin complexes within the cytosol have other targets including calcineurin, a calcium- and calmodulin-dependent serine–threonine phosphatase *(40)*. Calcineurin inhibition is the primary mechanism of action mediating the on-label use of cyclosporin A as a potent immunosuppressant. In T lymphocytes, calcineurin dephosphorylates a transcription factor, nuclear factor of activated T cells (NFAT), thereby decreasing IL-2 secretion in antigen-reactive T cells and, thus, T-cell proliferation *(41)*.

Immunophilins, a term used to designate a class of ligands for drugs such as CsA, FK506, and rapamycin, are expressed in high concentrations in the brain *(42,43)*, a discovery that has prompted numerous investigations of the possible neural roles for immunophilins. Immunophilin–immunosuppressant complexes have been implicated in regulation of IP_3-regulated Ca^{2+} release, nitric oxide-stimulated glutamate release, neurite outgrowth, kindling, hippocampal LTP, neuronal death in Alzheimer's disease, caspase-mediated apoptosis in ischemia, and a host of other processes occurring in both normal and diseased brain *(44–46)*.

As described above, neuronal and axonal damage following TBI is the result of excessive excitatory amino acid release and membrane perturbation, respectively, producing a rapid influx of calcium with resultant activation of secondary injury mechanisms. In the preceding sections, we noted the relationship between calcium-induced mitochondrial damage to the fate of injured neurons and axons, while demonstrating the ability of the immunosuppressant cyclosporin A to inhibit these events. However, in this cascade of events, we could not exclude the possibility that this calcium influx after injury could also trigger the activation of calcineurin. Such calcineurin activity in turn could modulate the pathophysiology of both focal and diffuse traumatic injury through its effects on microtubule assembly and stability, MAP2, neurofilament spacing, and others (for a review, *see* ref. *47*).

FK506 is another member of the immunosuppressant family of compounds, which likewise exerts its effects by binding to a partner immunophilin ligand. In the case of FK506, the partner molecules are a family of proteins termed FKBPs (FK binding proteins). FK506 is distinct from CsA in that FK506 inhibits calcineurin, while having no effect on the PT pore of mitochondria *(40)*, while CsA–cyclophilin complexes inhibit both calcineurin and PT pore opening. (Only cyclophilins, the partner immunophilins of CsA, and not FKBP, the partner immunophilins of FK506, interact with the PT pore complex.)

Employing the same TBI paradigm and the same endpoints used in our previous studies, we have investigated the efficacy of FK506 in limiting the scope of diffuse axonal injury. To this end, we examined the effect of FK506 on the labeling of amyloid precursor protein (APP), a known marker of diffuse axonal injury which we also employed in our previous studies of CsA neuroprotection *(48)*. The intrathecal administration of 2 mg/kg of FK506 resulted in a dramatic 50–60% decrease in the number of damaged axons displaying APP immunoreactivity in brain stem white matter at 24 h postinjury (for a review *see* ref. *49*). Thus, FK506, as CsA, is also effective in limiting axonal transport failure after trauma.

In contrast to the protection provided to injured axons, FK506, on the other hand, did not impart similar protection to injured neurons within sites of focal injury. In their initial characterization of CsA-mediated neuroprotection following cortical contusion, Sullivan and Scheff administered FK506 to rats at 15 min and 24 h postinjury and assessed its effects on lesion volume. Postinjury administration of 0.5, 1, or 10 mg/kg was ineffective in limiting contusion volume. Thus, the authors argued that their previously described protection seen with the use of CsA should be attributed to its effects on mitochondria and not any effect that CsA may have on calcineurin and calcineurin-sensitive secondary injury mechanisms. While these arguments appear credible in the context of contusional change, questions remain whether the inhibition of calcineurin or the prevention mitochondrial damage is of greater significance in limiting diffuse axonal injury.

SO WHICH IS BETTER, FK506 OR CSA?

This argument must begin with a disclaimer: detailed, dedicated dose-response studies involving CsA have not been performed and only one dose-response study in one experimental paradigm of TBI has been conducted with FK506. Dose-response studies comparing CsA and FK506 in trauma must also be performed in order to provide a clearer understanding of these issues. Additional outcome variables involving more functional assessments of axonal integrity also need to be employed. Nonetheless, the answer to which agent is better may be found in the relative potency of these two compounds. In its initial characterization, FK506 was shown to be approx 100 times more potent than equieffective doses CsA in inhibiting the proliferation of T cells, a calcineurin-dependent event *(50)*. In our initial study of FK506, only a marker of cytoskeletal injury was employed. Thus, at the dosages used and with the end points chosen in our study, FK506 was likely more efficacious than CsA in inhibiting calcineurin and therefore may have provided greater protection against the suspected deleterious cytoskeletal consequences of calcineurin activation.

The lack of agreement in the contemporary literature regarding the neuroprotective effects of CsA and FK506 in other models of CNS disorders also illustrates the complexity of the issues at hand. For example, in ischemia, both CsA and FK506 have been shown to be neuroprotective through mechanisms involving both calcineurin and mitochondrial protection *(51–58)*. In insulin-induced hypoglycemic brain injury, however, CsA has proven protective, but FK506 has not *(59,60)*. In spinal cord injury, FK506 has been shown to enhance axonal regeneration and improve functional recovery *(61,62)*, while CsA has been shown to limit secondary injury, but its overall effects on recovery have not yet been rigorously evaluated *(63,64)*. Additionally, in recent studies from Scheff and colleagues, CsA provided no protection to the injured spinal cord. To complicate the issue further, FK506 may also possess neurotrophic properties, independent of its activity against calcineurin *(62)*. Additionally, both CsA and FK506 blunt the immune response, which may contribute to the overall neuroprotection observe with these compounds, as the immune response aggravates injury and impedes recovery *(65–69)*. The issue of the relative potency of FK506 and CsA in limiting the scope of focal and diffuse injury following CNS trauma is currently unresolved.

COMBINATION THERAPY PARADIGM IN THE TREATMENT OF TRAUMATIC BRAIN INJURY: CYCLOSPORIN A POTENTIATES HYPOTHERMIC NEUROPROTECTION

Despite the best efforts of those in the field, advances in our understanding of the pathophysiology of traumatic brain injury have not generated effective therapeutic strategies for improving the clinical outcome of patients sustaining closed head injuries. The foregoing sections presented recent data suggesting that drugs targeting the immunophilins–cyclophilins blunt the focal and diffuse changes elicited after traumatic brain injury. Now that we have a relatively complete understanding of the progressive spatial and temporal changes that occur in severe TBI, efforts have begun to focus on the use of combination therapeutic regimens to blunt the progression of these changes and thereby impact favorably upon morbidity.

Paralleling the interest in early posttraumatic hypothermia in the clinical setting, the use of hypothermia in the experimental setting has resulted in significant reductions in neuronal and axonal damage following traumatic injury *(70–75)*. With respect to DAI, it was posited that early posttraumatic hypothermia with gradual rewarming blunts the altered axolemmal permeability, thus interrupting the cascade of secondary injury mechanisms. Similarly, the use of CsA has also been shown to provide significant neuronal protection in experimental TBI, likely mediated by the effect of CsA on the mitochondrial permeability transition pore *(29,33–35,38,76,77)*. As these two therapeutic strategies appear to act on two fronts in the pathobiology of traumatically induced axonal change, and as such strategies are being touted as potential therapeutic interventions for human TBI, it also appeared rational to explore the premise that the use of posttraumatic hypothermia followed by CsA administration would result in enhanced axonal protection than that seen with either therapy alone.

In this approach, rats were subjected to impact acceleration TBI in a combined treatment paradigm wherein hypothermia (32°C) was induced immediately postinjury and maintained for 1 h, when CsA (10 mg/kg) was administered intrathecally. Through this paradigm we demonstrated that CsA, when administered 1 h following the induction of postinjury hypothermia, potentiated the neuroprotective effects of hypothermia against traumatically induced axonal change. This was evidenced by a 35% reduction in the number of immunoreactive damaged fibers exhibiting calpain activation, cytoskeletal damage, and axonal transport failure in hypothermic animals treated with CsA compared with hypothermic animals given vehicle (for review, *see* ref. *78*).

From a mechanistic sense, in relation to this distinct sequence of intraaxonal change, it appears that hypothermia most likely works at the initiating phases of axonal injury, while CsA targets the delayed opening of mitochondrial permeability transition pore. In this scenario, we hypothesize that hypothermia stabilizes the traumatized axolemma, thereby influencing axolemmal integrity and the related calcium influx that triggers the downstream secondary injury mechanism. By contrast, CsA would target the mitochondrial protection, which would prevent the release of cytochrome *c* and the activation of the caspase death cascade while maintaining the mitochondrial production of high-energy phosphates needed to maintain the membrane pumps. The success of the interventional paradigm used in the current investigation (hypothermia followed by delayed opening and CsA administration) supports this basic pathological progression and the purported sites of action of hypothermia and CsA *(33,71,72,79)*.

Mitochondrial failure may be a consequence of hypothermic treatment in and of itself. Tissue rewarming following hypothermia results in a mitochondrial permeability transition, a phenomenon first reported in studies on liver transplantation *(80)*. In those studies, an MPT was observed during the hypothermic to normothermic transition, but when CsA was added prior to rewarming, oxidative phosphorylation and mitochondrial ATP content was preserved through CsA-mediated blockade of MPT induction. Thus, CsA potentiation of hypothermic neuroprotection in TBI may also be related to CsA blocking the deleterious effects of mitochondria on rewarming following hypothermia.

From a clinical prospective, we believe combined therapeutic strategies in the treatment of TBI are of considerable interest. The enhanced protection seen with these therapies administered in a defined temporal sequence (hypothermia first, followed by CsA) supports our observations of initial axonal permeability and calcium-mediated change followed over time by local mitochondrial damage and subsequent cytoskeletal damage and disconnection. Collectively, these multiple protective effects seen with the use of CsA following posttraumatic hypothermia speak in a compelling fashion to the utility of a combined therapeutic approach in the treatment of TBI.

Further, efficacy of this combined therapeutic strategy has long-range clinical implications for the better care and management of patients with traumatically brain injury. We believe there is need for the continued examination of combined treatment paradigms in both the clinical and laboratory settings.

SUMMARY

Traumatic brain injury is the leading cause of death before middle age in Europe and North America. TBI is characterized by a phase of secondary injury that underlies long-range morbidity and morality in patients surviving the acute postinjury period. Secondary injury evolves in the hours and days following the traumatic episode, suggesting these mechanisms may be amenable to therapeutic intervention. Mitochondrial damage and calcineurin activation after trauma are two important secondary injury mechanisms in both focal and diffuse traumatic injury. The immunosuppressants cyclosporin A and FK506 are known inhibitors of calcineurin, and CsA has an additional target in protecting mitochondria from otherwise damaging levels of intracellular calcium. These compounds have proved powerful tools in the laboratory in evaluating the pathophysiological sequelae responsible for damage following TBI. More importantly, several recent reports, discussed in this chapter, have unearthed the exciting revelation that immunosuppressants represent a potentially successful therapeutic intervention for the treatment of traumatic brain injury.

REFERENCES

1. Sosin D, Sniezek J, Waxweiler DT. Trends in death associated with traumatic brain injury, 1979 thorugh 1992: success and failure. JAMA 1995;273: 1778–1780.
2. Waxweiler DT, Thurman D, Sniezek J, et al. Monitoring the impact of traumatic brain injury: a review and update. J Neurotrauma 1995;12:509–516.
3. Max W, Rice DP, MacKenzie DJ. The lifetime cost of injury. Inquiry 1990;27:332–343.
4. Klauber MR, Marchall LF, Toole BM, et al. Cause of decline in head-ijury mortality in San Diego, California. J Neurosurg 1985;62:528–531.
5. Baxt WG, Moody P. The impact of advanced prehospital emergency care on the mortality of severely brain-injured patients. J Trauma 1987;27(4):365–369.
6. Colohan AR, Alves WM, Gross CR, et al. Head injury and mortality in two centers with different emergency medical services and intensive care. J Neurosurg 1989;71:202–207.
7. Doppenberg EM, Choi SC, and Bullock R. Clinical trials in traumatic brain injury. What can we learn from previous trials? Ann NY Acad Sci 1997; 825:305–322.

8. Adams JH, Graham DI, Murray LS, Scott G. Diffuse axonal injury due to nonmissile injury in humans: an analysis of 45 cases. Ann Neurol 1982;12: 557–563.

9. Smith DH, Nonaka M, Miller R, et al. Immediate coma following inertial brain injury dependent on axonal damage in the brainstem. J Neurosurg 2000; 93:315–322.

10. Strich SJ. Diffuse degeneration of the cerebral white matter in severe dementia following head injury. J Neurol Neurosurg Psychiatry 1956;19:163–185.

11. Strich SJ. Shearing of nerve fibers as a cause of brain damage due to head injury: a pathological study of twenty cases. Lancet 1961;2:443–448.

12. Nevin NC. Neuropathological changes in the white matter following head injury. J Neuropathol Exp Neurol 1967;26:77–84.

13. Povlishock JT, Becker DP, Cheng CLY, Vaughan GW. Axonal change in minor head injury. J Neuropathol Exp Neurol 1983;42:225–242.

14. Erb DE, Povlishock JT. Axonal damage in severe traumatic brain injury: an experimental study in cat. Acta Neuropathol 1988;76:347–358.

15. Povlishock JT, Jenkins LW. Are the pathological changes evoked by traumatic brain injury immediate and irreversible? Brain Pathol 1995;5:415–426.

16. Faden AI, Dmediuk P, Pantor SS, Vink R. The role of excitatory amino acids and NMDA receptors in traumatic brain injury. Science 1989;244:798–800.

17. Katayama Y, Becker DP, Tamura T, Hovada DA. Massive increases in extracellular potassium and the indiscriminate release of glutamate following concussive head injury. J Neurosurg 1990;73:889–900.

18. Tymianski M, Tator CH. Normal and abnormal calcium homeostasis in neurons: a basis of the pathophysiology of traumatic and ischemic central nervous system injury. Neurosurgery 1996;38:1176–1195.

19. Maxwell WL, Povlishock JT, Graham DL. A mechanistic analysis of nondisruptive axonal injury: a review. J Neurotrauma 1997;14:419–440.

20. Xiong Y, Gu Q, Peterson PL, Muizelaar JP, Lee CP. Mitochondrial dysfunction and calcium perturbation induced by traumatic brain injury. J Neurotrauma 1997;14:23–34.

21. Pettus EH and Povlishock JT. Characterization of a distinct set of intra-axonal ultrastructural changes associated with traumatically induced alteration in axolemmal permeability. Brain Res 1996;722:1–11.

22. Gunter TE, Pfeiffer DR. Mechanisms by which mitochondria transport calcium. Am J Physiol 1990;258:C755–C786.

23. Colicos MA, Dixon CE, Dash PK. Delayed, selective neuronal death following experimental cortical impact injury in rats: possible role in memory deficits. Brain Res 1996;739:111–119.

24. Colicos MA, Dash PK. Apoptotic morphology of dentate gyrus granule cells following experimental cortical impact injury in rats: possible role in spatial memory deficits. Brain Res 1996;739:120–131.

25. Xiong Y, Peterson PL, Muizelaar JP, Lee CP. Amelioration of mitochondrial function by a novel antioxidant U-101033E following traumatic brain injury in rats. J Neurotrauma 1997;14:907–917.

26. George EB, Glass JD, Griffin JW. Axotomy-induced axonal degeneration is mediated by calcium influx through ion-specific channels. J Neurosci 1995;15:6445–6452.

27. Petit PX, Zamzami N, Vayssiere JL, et al. Implication of mitochondria in apoptosis. Mol Cell Biochem 1997;174:185–188.

28. Ankarcrona M, Dypbukt JM, Bonfoco E, et al. Glutamate-induced neuronal death: a succession of necrosis or apoptosis depending on mitochondrial function. Neuron 1995;15:961–973.

29. Halestrap AP, Davidson AM. Inhibition of Ca2(+)-induced large-amplitude swelling of liver and heart mitochondria by cyclosporin is probably caused by the inhibitor binding to mitochondrial-matrix peptidylprolyl cis-trans isomerase and preventing it interacting with the adenine nucleotide translocase. Biochem J 1990;268:153–160.

30. Chadhuri B, Stephan C. Only in the presence of immunophilins can cyclosporin and FK506 disrupt *in vivo* binding of calcineurin A to its autoinhibitory domain yet strengthen interaction between calcineurin A and B subunits. Biochem Biophys Res Comm 1995;215:781–790.

31. Halestrap AP, Conner CP, Griffiths EJ, Kerr PM. Cyclosporin A binding to mitochondrial cyclophilin inhibits the permeability transition pore and protects hearts form ischemia/reperfusion injury. Mol Cell Biochem 1997; 174:167–172.

32. Siesjo BK and Siesjo P Mechanisms of secondary brain injury. Eur J Anaesthesiol 1996;13:247–268.

33. Okonkwo DO, Povlishock JT. A single intrathecal bolus of cyclosporin A before injury preserves mitochondrial integrity and attenuates axonal disruption following traumatic brain injury. J Cereb Blood Flow Metab, 1999;19: 443–451.

34. Okonkwo DO, Büki A, Siman R, Povlishock JT. Cyclosporin A limits calcium-induced axonal damage following traumatic brain injury. Neuroreport 1999;10:353–358.

35. Büki A, Okonkwo DO, Povlishock, JT. Postinjury cyclosporin A administration limits axonal damage and disconnection in traumatic brain injury. J Neurotrauma 1999;16:511–521.

36. Scheff SW, Sullivan PG. Cyclosporin A significantly ameliorates cortical damage following experimental traumatic brain injury in rodents. J Neurotrauma 1999;16:783–792.

37. Sullivan PG, Thompson M, Scheff SW. Continuous infusion of cyclosporin A significantly ameliorates cortical damage following traumatic brain injury. Exp Neurol 2000;161:631–637.

38. Sullivan PG, Thompson MB, Scheff SW. Cyclosporin A attenuates acute mitochondrial dysfunction following traumatic brain injury. Exp Neurol 1999;160:226–234.

39. Albensi BC, Sullivan PG, Thompson MB, et al. Cyclosporin ameliorates traumatic brain injury-induced alterations of hippocampal plasticity. Exp Neurol 2000;162:385–389

40. Liu J, Farmer JD Jr, Lane WS, et al. Calcineurin is a common target of cyclophilin-cyclosporin A and FKBP-FK506 complexes. Cell 1991;66: 807–815.

41. Schreiber SL, Crabtree GR. The mechanism of action of cyclosporin A and FK506. Immunol Today 1992;13:136–142.

42. Steiner JP, Dawson TM, Fotuhi M, et al. High brain densities of the immunophilin FKBP colocalized with calcineurin. Nature 1992;358: 584–587.

43. Dawson TM, Steiner JP, Lyons WE, et al. The immunophilins, FK506 binding protein and cyclophilin, are discretely localized in the brain: relationship to calcineurin. Neuroscience 1994;62:569–580.

44. Sabatini DM, Lai MM, Snyder SH. The neural roles of immunophilins and their ligands. Mol Neurobiol 1997;15:223.

45. Gold BG. FK506 and the role of immunophilins in nerve regeneration. Mol Neurobiol 1997;15:285–306.

46. Selznick LA, Zheng TS, Flavell RA, et al. Amyloid beta-induced neuronal death is bax-dependent but caspase-independent. J Neuropathol Exp Neurol 1999;59:271–279.

47. Morioka M, Hamada J, Ushio Y, Miyamoto E. Potential role of calcineurin for brain ischemia and traumatic injury. Prog Neurobiol 1999;58:1–30.

48. Gentleman SM, Nash MJ, Sweeting CJ, et al. β-Amyloid precursor protein (β-APP) as a marker of axonal injury after head injury. Neurosci Lett 1993;160:139–144.

49. Singleton RH, Stone JR, Pellicane, A, Okonkwo DO, and Povlishock JT. FK506 blunts traumatic axonal injury, J Neurotrauma 2001.

50. Ochiai T, Nakajima K, Sakamoto K, et al. Comparative studies on the immunosuppressive activity of FK506, 15-deoxyspergualin, and cyclosporine. Transplant Proc 1989;21:829–832.

51. Bochelen D, Rudin M, Sauter A. Calcineurin inhibitors FK506 and SDZ ASM 981 alleviate the outcome of focal cerebral ischemic/reperfusion injury. Pharm and Ex Ther 1999;288:653–659.

52. Drake M, Friberg H, Boris-Moller F, et al. The immunosuppressant FK506 ameliorates ischaemic damage in the rat brain. Acta Physiol Scand 1996;158:–159.

53. Khaspekov L, Friberg H, Halestrap A, et al. Cyclosporin A and its nonimmunosuppressive analogue N-Me-Val-4-cyclosporin A mitigate glucose/oxygen deprivation-induced damage to rat cultured hippocampal neurons. Eur J Neurosci 1999;11:3194–3198.

54. Kuroda S, Janelidze S, Siesjo BK. The immunosuppressants cyclosporin A and FK506 equally ameliorate brain damage due to 30-min middle cerebral artery occlusion in hyperglycemic rats. Brain Res 1999;835:148–153.

55. Nakai A, Kuroda S, Kristian T, Siesjo BK. The immunosuppressant drug FK506 ameliorates secondary mitochondrial dysfunction following transient focal cerebral ischemia in the rat. Neurobiol Dis 1997;4:288–300.

56. Sharkey J, Butcher SP. Immunophilins mediate the neuroprotective effects of FK506 in focal cerebral ischaemia. Nature 1994;371:336–339.

57. Uchino H, Elmer E, Uchino K, et al. Cyclosporin A dramatically ameliorates CA1 hippocampal damage following transient forebrain ischemia in the rat. Acta Physiol Scand 1995;155:469–471.

58. Yoshimoto T and Siesjo, BK. Posttreatment with the immunosuppressant cyclosporin A in transient focal ischemia. Brain Res 1999;839:283–291.

59. Ferrand-Drake M, Friberg H., Wieloch T. Mitochondrial permeability transition induced DNA-fragmentation in the rat hippocampus following hypoglycemia. Neuroscience 1999;90:1325–1338.

60. Friberg H, Ferrand-Drake M, Bengtsson F, et al. Cyclosporin A, but not FK506, protects mitochondria and neurons against hypoglycemic damage and implicates the mitochondrial permeability transition in cell death. J Neurosci 1998;18:5151–5159.

61. Bavetta S, Hamlyn PJ, Burnstock G, et al. The effects of FK506 on dorsal column axons following spinal cord injury in adult rats: neuroprotection and local regeneration. Exp Neurol 1999;158:382–393.

62. Madsen JR, Macdonald P, Irwin N, et al. Tacrolimus (FK506) increases neuronal expression of GAP-43 and improves functional recovery after spinal cord injury in rats. Exp Neurol 1998;154:673–683.

63. Diaz-Ruiz A, Rios C, Duarte I, et al. Cyclosporin-A inhibits lipid peroxidation after spinal cord injury in rats. Neurosci Lett 1999;266:61–64.

64. Diaz-Ruiz A, Rios C, Duarte I, et al. Lipid peroxidation inhibition in spinal cord injury: cyclosporin-A vs methylprednisolone. Neuroreport 11:1765–1767.

65. Arvin B, Neville LF, Barone FC, and Feuerstein GZ. The role of inflammation and cytokines in brain injury. Neurosci Biobehav Rev 1996;20:445–452.

66. Feuerstein GZ, Wang X, Barone FC. Inflammatory gene expression in cerebral ischemia and trauma. Potential new therapeutic targets. Ann NY Acad Sci 825:179–193.

67. Ghirnikar RS, Lee YL, Eng LF. Inflammation in traumatic brain injury: role of cytokines and chemokines. Neurochem Res 23:329–340.

68. Holmin S, Mathiesen T. Long-term intracerebral inflammatory response after experimental focal brain injury in rat. Neuroreport 10:1889–1891.

69. Lee RK, Knapp S, Wurtman RJ. Prostaglandin E2 stimulates amyloid precursor protein gene expression: inhibition by immunosuppressants. J Neurosci 19:940–947.

70. Clifton GL, Allen S, Barrodale P, et al: A phase II study of moderate hypothermia in severe brain injury. J Neurotrauma 1993;10:263–271.

71. Koizumi H, Povlishock JT. Post-traumatic hypothermia protects against axonal damage in an animal model of traumatic axonal injury. J Neurosurg 89:303–309.

72. Buki A, Koizumi H, Povlishock JT. Moderate posttraumatic hypothermia decreases early calpain-mediated proteolysis and concomitant cytoskeletal compromise in traumatic axonal injury. Exp Neurol 159:319–328.

73. Chatzipanteli K, Alonso OF, Kraydieh S, et al. Importance of posttraumatic hypothermia and hyperthermia on the inflammatory response after fluid percussion brain injury: biochemical and immunocytochemical studies. J Cereb Blood Flow Metab 2000;20:531–542.

74. Yamamoto M, Marmarou CR, Stiefel MF, et al. Nueroprotective effect of hypothermia on neuronal injury in diffuse traumatic brain injury coupled with hypoxia and hypotension. J Neurotrauma 1999;16:487–500.
75. Zhao W, Alonso OF, Loor JY, et al. Influence of early posttraumatic hypothermia therapy on local cerebral blood flow and glucose metabolism after fluid-percussion brain injury. J Neurosurg 1999;90:510–519.
76. Zoratti M, Szabo I. The mitochondrial permeability transition. Biochim Biophys Acta 1995;1241:139–176.
77. Nakatsuka H, Ohta S, Tanaka J, et al. Release of cytochrome c from mitochondria to cytosol in gerbil hippocampal CA1 neurons after transient forebrain ischemia. Brain Res 1999;849:216–219.
78. Okonkwo DO, Büki A, Stone JR, Koizumi H, Povlishock JT. Cyclosporin A potentiates hypothermic neuroprotection in traumatic brain injury in rat. J Neurosurg 2001.
79. Büki A, Siman R, Trojanowsky JQ, et al. The role of calpain-mediated spectrin proteolysis in traumatically induced axonal injury. J Neuropathol Exp Neurol 1999;58:365–375.
80. Leducq N, Delmas-Beauvieux MC, Bourdel-Marchasson I. Mitochondrial permeability transition during hypothermic to normothermic reperfusion in rat liver demonstrated by the protective effect of cyclosporin A. Biochem J 1998;336(Pt 2):501–506.

V

IMMUNOSUPPRESSANTS AND SPINAL CORD INJURY

14

Inhibition of Lipid Peroxidation by Cyclosporin After Spinal Cord Injury in Rats

Antonio Ibarra and Araceli Diaz-Ruiz

INTRODUCTION

In the last 20 yr, the use of transplants as a therapy for different degenerative diseases has increased the use of immunosuppressant drugs to avoid or diminish the possible immune reaction against the transplanted tissues. In this field, therapy using tissue (1–3) or cell (4–6) transplants for neurodegenerative diseases, also promises great advantages. In this case, an immunosuppressive therapy has also been useful (7). One of the more common agents used to avoid tissue rejection is the immunosuppressant cyclosporin A (CsA), which is a cyclic undecapeptide that inhibits helper T-lymphocyte proliferation and, hence, depresses the cellular and humoral immune responses (8). In addition to its ability to suppress T-cell activity, CsA may have a number of non-immune effects including antiparasite activity (9), liver regeneration (10,11), neural regeneration (12,13) and neuroprotection (14–16). Evidence about the neuroprotective effect of CsA may be the result of several mechanisms, and among them, lipid peroxidation (LP) inhibition may play an important role (17–19). Recently, we reported on the inhibitory effect of CsA upon LP in a spinal cord (SC) injury model (20).

The purpose of this chapter is to review some of the evidence concerning the effect of CsA on LP as well as on some of the morphological and clinical aspects related to the neuroprotective effect of CsA. Likewise, some data related to the comparison of the effectiveness of CsA with methylprednisolone (MP) will be presented. This information has been obtained from studies demonstrating the protective effectiveness of CsA in experimental models of SC injury.

From: *Immunosuppressant Analogs in Neuroprotection*
Edited by: C. V. Borlongan, O. Isacson, and P. R. Sanberg © Humana Press Inc., Totowa, NJ

THE LIPID PEROXIDATION PROCESS

Lipid peroxidation is a geometrically progressing process that spreads over the surface of the cell membrane altering polyunsaturated fatty acids, causing impairment of phospholipid-dependent enzymes, disruption of ionic gradients, and even membrane lysis *(21)*. Polyunsaturated fatty acids are present in many membranes and are easy targets of free radicals. The process initiates with the attack of any reactive species, which is able to abstract a hydrogen atom from a methylene group of a polyunsaturated fatty acid, leaving an unpaired electron on the carbon. The carbon radical undergoes a molecular rearrangement to react with an oxygen molecule and to produce finally a *peroxy radical*. Peroxy radicals are able to extract a hydrogen atom from another lipid molecule giving rise to the propagation of lipid peroxidation (i.e., a chain reaction) *(22)*. Lipid peroxidation results in the ultimate destruction not only of unsaturated fatty acids but also of several other membrane molecules (i.e., proteins). The damage, among other things, alters the normal function of biological membranes by reducing membrane fluidity and inhibiting enzyme functioning. These alterations reduce the generation and transmission of the electrical stimulus and finally membrane destruction *(23)*. To prevent the attack of free radicals, cells are endowed with defense systems, including some specific enzymes such as glutathione peroxidase (GSHPx), superoxide dismutase (SOD), and catalase. All of these enzymes protect against LP by preventing the formation of reactive oxygen species.

FREE RADICALS IN CENTRAL NERVOUS SYSTEM

One of the major autodestructive mechanisms observed after a central nervous system (CNS) injury is the attack of cellular membrane by free radicals *(24)*. Nowadays, there is extensive experimental support for the pathophysiological role of oxygen radical formation and cell-membrane damage by the process of LP after injury. Some criteria to establish the pathophysiological significance of LP after CNS injury include demonstration of increased levels of oxygen radicals and lipid peroxides after CNS injury, correlation between oxygen radical formation and pathophysiological alterations, similarity between posttraumatic CNS pathology and that caused by chemical peroxidative insult, and the protective efficacy of antioxidant agents *(21)*.

Once injury occurs, free iron released from hemoglobin initiates the peroxidation damage to CNS cells and myelin sheaths, likewise oxygen radicals derived from prostaglandin synthetase and 5-lipoxygenase activity, catecholamine oxidation, mitochondrial leak, oxidation of extravasated hemoglobin, and the infiltrating inflammatory cells continue the destruction phenomenon soon thereafter *(21)*.

The CNS is especially sensitive to free radical damage because of its high metabolic rate, high levels of polyunsaturated lipids, and its relatively low level of protective systems *(25)*. Moreover, the activity of antioxidant enzymes in the CNS is low compared with other tissues *(26)*. Thus, these features provide the environment that allows active oxygen radicals produced after CNS injury to extensively damage the tissue.

SPINAL CORD INJURY AND LIPID PEROXIDATION

As part of the CNS, SC provides an especially favorable environment for the generation of LP reactions *(21)*. Thus, as early as 15 min after injury, a significant increase in LP products, especially malondialdehyde (MDA), occurs within the contused SC. Afterward, LP gradually increases during the first 2 h, reaching its maximum peak at 5 h, and then decreases *(27)*. It is important to consider that both the extent and the course of LP after injury may vary depending on the type and severity of the injury *(28)*.

Lipid peroxidation is one of the most important factors producing tissue damage after SC injury, not only as a result of the direct cytotoxic effect of free radicals, but also because the important role of these reactive species in the development of ischemia, edema, and metabolic dysfunction, which participate strongly in SC degeneration after trauma. In addition to these posttraumatic deleterious events, LP may also be directly involved in the failure and degeneration of surviving spinal axons after injury *(29)*.

Lipid peroxidation after SC lesion may be caused by several mechanisms, comparable to those for the CNS, among which the inflammatory reaction observed in the injured area plays an important role *(24)*. Inflammatory cells like neutrophils and macrophages can produce reactive oxygen species when activated and thus may contribute to LP after SC injury. Neutrophils usually reach the injured area very early, about 1 h after lesion *(30)*, then they increase until they attain their maximum peak at 24 h after injury *(31)*. On the other hand, macrophages infiltrate SC tissue soon thereafter. Peripheral macrophages are visualized starting 24 h after lesion and then increase until they reach a peak between days 4 and 7 *(31,32)*. In this case macrophages may persist in the lesioned area even in chronic stages of the lesion *(33)*. Microglia–macrophage cells (the resident macrophages), are activated within the lesion epicenter between 3 and 7 d postinjury, preceding even the peak of peripheral macrophage influx and activation *(34)*.

All these infiltrating inflammatory cells have been significantly correlated with the amount of tissue damage after injury *(31)*. Thus treatments to decrease this reaction, and secondarily LP, are likely to be beneficial to protect SC tissue and for function recovery after traumatic SC injury. The most important support to the pathophysiological role of LP upon SC damage has been provided by studies demonstrating that the pharmacological inhibition of LP attenuates the development of several deleterious events (e.g., ischemia and edema) *(21)* and significantly diminishes SC tissue damage after injury *(20,35,36)*.

STRATEGIES FOR PROTECTING AGAINST LIPID PEROXIDATION AFTER SPINAL CORD INJURY

Oxygen free radical–induced LP plays a significant role in SC tissue damage after injury. Therefore, the early inhibition of this reaction may represent a useful strategy to diminish tissue damage and thus to preserve the anatomical substrate for neurological recovery *(21)*. Several compounds have been shown to be protective in experimental SC injury. In this field, methylprednisolone (MP), a synthetic glucocorticoid steroid with anti-inflammatory properties, inhibits LP directly *(21)*, attenuates neuronal degeneration *(37,38)*, and apparently promotes neurological recovery *(39,40)*. Currently MP is the drug of choice after SC injury in humans. Lazaroids (21-aminosteriods) are MP analogs that lack glucocorticoid activity but have greater antioxidant efficacy than MP. These analogs have also been investigated for their ability to promote neurological recovery following a SC injury *(41)*. Vitamin E, a well-known membrane-targeted scavenger of lipid peroxyl radicals, attenuates the development of progressive posttraumatic ischemia *(38)* and enhances chronic recovery after SC injury *(42)*. Other compounds that combine the amino functionality of the 21-aminosteroids with the peroxyl radical scavenging portion of vitamin E (i.e., 2-methylaminochromans) have also shown promise as neuroprotective agents *(21)*.

In the last decade, numerous studies have evaluated the neuroprotective efficacy of other agents with potential lipid antioxidant activity in models of SC injury. These studies evaluate compounds like Ginkgo biloba and the thyroid releasing hormone *(43)*, magnesium *(44)*, melatonin *(36,45)*, and EPC-K1 (a phosphate diester linkage of vitamins E and C) *(35)*. In each case, attenuation of SC-tissue damage and even neurological improvement it have been reported.

Recently, we reported on the beneficial effect of CsA, a potent and selective immunosuppressive agent, upon inhibition of LP and improvement of motor recovery after SC injury. The mechanism of action of CsA supports the feasibility of its use after SC injury. Besides, there are several studies, that provide evidence about its neuroprotective effect *(14–16)*.

MECHANISM OF ACTION OF CYCLOSPORIN A
AND RATIONALE FOR ITS USE TO INHIBIT LIPID
PEROXIDATION AFTER SPINAL CORD INJURY

After injury, the inflammatory cells infiltrating the injured area are perhaps the main source of free radicals like nitric oxide (NO) and superoxide anion (O_2^-). Under conditions of excessive synthesis, NO is a well-known neurotoxic agent, either by inducing glutamate neurotoxicity or by interaction with O_2^- to form peroxynitrite ($ONOO^-$), a highly neurotoxic molecule *(46)*. CsA, may inhibit both the inflammatory reactions and NO overproduction. CsA, a cyclic undecapeptide, inhibits helper T-lymphocyte proliferation and, depresses the cellular and humoral responses *(47)*. To achieve this effect, CsA inhibits calcineurin (*see* Fig. 1), a calcium-dependent phosphoserine–phosphothreonine protein phosphatase, which participates in some immunological mechanisms like transduction of signals for cytokine production *(48)* and neutrophil cytoskeleton motility *(49)*. Calcineurin also has other nonimmunological actions, among them, the activation of nitric oxide synthase (NOS), promoting by this way the production of NO. Thus, by this means CsA inhibits both the immune response (in part the inflammatory reaction) and NO overproduction. Nevertheless, CsA may exert other actions to inhibit these detrimental phenomena.

After injury, the activation of some enzymes such as phospholipase A2 increases the inflammatory reaction through the production of arachidonic acid, a source of proinflammatory molecules. CsA is able to inhibit this enzyme *(50)* and others like cyclooxygenase that are also related with this proinflammatory pathway *(51)*. Likewise, some studies have demonstrated that by a calcineurin-independent mechanism CsA is able to inhibit the expression *(51,52)* and activation *(53)* of the inducible NOS (iNOS), an enzyme related with NO overproduction and proinflammatory effects. Thus by several mechanisms, CsA may diminish free radical overproduction and secondarily LP after SC injury.

The effect of CsA upon LP has been studied previously in organs outside the central nervous system. Different effects of CsA treatment upon oxidative stress have been reported in diverse tissues. Chronic administration of CsA increases kidney LP and secondarily nephrotoxicity *(54,55)*. By contrast, acute administration of CsA is able to significantly diminish LP in liver *(56,57)*. Thus, the effect of this immunosuppressant on LP after SC injury has emerged as an interesting research topic. In fact, the inhibitory actions of CsA upon the inflammatory response and NO overproduction supported its use to inhibit LP after SC injury. Therefore, in order to evaluate this effect some studies using a reliable experimental model of

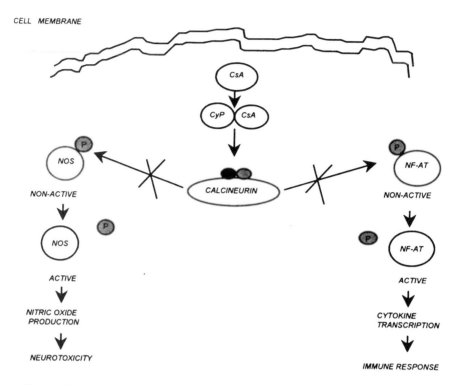

Fig. 1. Mechanism of action of cyclosporin A (CsA) to inhibit immune response and nitric oxide (NO) production. Once CsA crosses the cell membrane, it forms a complex with cyclophilin (an intracellular molecule, CyP). The CsA–CyP complex inhibits calcineurin, a calcium-dependent phosphoserine–phosphothreonine protein phosphatase that dephosphorylates and activates the nitric oxide synthase (NOS), which, in turn, produces nitric oxide, as well as the transcription factor NFAT, which activates the immune response.

SC injury in rats, a consistent method to measure the final lipid fluorescent products of LP *(58,59)* and a specially designed CsA dosing scheme for SC injured animals were carried out *(60)*. The design of a dosing scheme of CsA in SC-injured animals was the first step of our work, since it has been reported that the pharmacokinetics of several drugs, including CsA, is altered after SC injury *(61–64)*. Therefore, it was imperative to determine which dosing regimen allowed CsA levels to be maintained within the therapeutic window. It was found that administration of 2.5 mg/kg/12 h intraperitoneally during the acute phase followed by 5 mg/kg/12 h orally thereafter yields CsA circulating levels that keep within the therapeutic window *(60)*. This dosage is lower than that used to avoid tissue

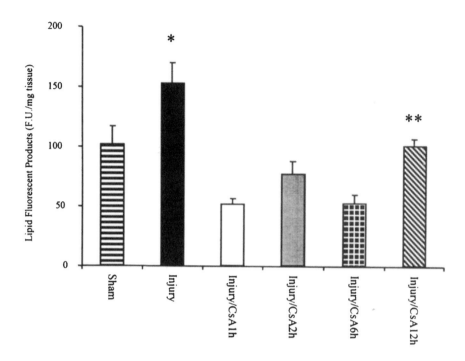

Fig. 2. Lipid peroxidation in rat spinal cord (SC) 24 h after laminectomy (sham), untreated SC injury (injury), or treated with cyclosporin A (injury/CsA) 1, 2, 6, or 12 h after lesion. The results are expressed as means ±SE of six animals per group, *different from all other groups ($p < 0.05$), ** different from sham and injury plus cyclosporin A 12 h ($p < 0.05$), ANOVA followed by Tukey's test. Reprinted from ref. *20*, with permission from Elsevier Science.

transplant rejection (10 mg/kg/12 h) *(65,66)*, and thus would not have the toxic effects of CsA. Moreover, low doses of this drug have been shown to prevent rejection of renal allografts in histoincompatible rats *(67)*. The results presented here, were obtained using this dosing regimen only in the acute phase of the injury.

After a severe SC contusion, a dose of 2.5 mg/kg every 12 h of CsA induces a 66% decrease of LP as compared to the one observed in nontreated SC injured animals *(20)* (*see* Fig. 2). The best inhibition occurs when the therapy starts during the first 6 h after injury. Furthermore, even though at 12 h LP is not inhibited to the same extent it is comparable to the nondamaged tissue. These results are very interesting because they show that even giving a dose lower than that used to inhibit transplant rejection (i.e., 5–10 mg/kg), which may be associated with toxic effects *(68)*, CsA can

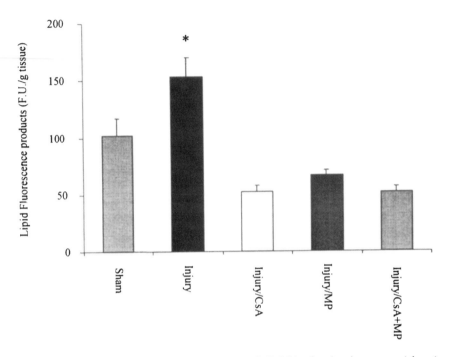

Fig. 3. Lipid peroxidation in rat spinal cord (SC) 24 h after laminectomy (sham), SC injury (injury) or SC injury plus treatment with either CsA (I/CsA), methyl-prednisolone (I/MP) or CsA plus MP (I/CsA+MP). The results are expressed as means ±SE of six animals per group. *Different from all other groups ($p < 0.05$), ANOVA followed by Tukey's tests. Reprinted ref. *69*, with permission.

inhibit LP. Furthermore, these results are of special relevance if a clinical application is considered, since there could be a wide window to start the CsA therapy after injury.

On the other hand, currently MP is the clinical standard for therapy of acute SC injury *(40)*, therefore it has been recommended that any new treatment must be as good or better than MP. Thus a comparison of the effectiveness of CsA and that of MP on LP inhibition was the next step of our work. Additionally, in order to study a possible summation effect, the effectiveness of both drugs combined was also evaluated *(69)*. Lipid peroxidation is inhibited to the same extent in CsA-, MP-, or CsA + MP-treated animals (Fig. 3). Administration of CsA (2.5 mg/kg every 12 h) or sodium succinate MP (30 mg/kg every 2 h, that is, 11 ip injections in 24 h) alone induces a significant LP decrease of 69 and 58%, respectively, compared to the injured control group ($p < 0.05$). LP is similarly inhibited when CsA and MP are administered in combination (70%). Although MP is the drug of choice to

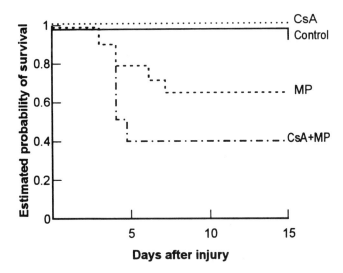

Fig. 4. Estimated probability of survival (EPS) from start of treatment to 15 d after lesion of SC cord injured rats treated with vehicle (Control, filled line), cyclosporin-A (CsA, dotted line), methylprednisolone (MP, dashed line) or CsA+ MP (doted and dashed line). Results are expressed as EPS according with the Kaplan–Meier method, where the unit represents the 100% of survival. Reprinted from ref. *69*, with permission.

diminish LP after injury, nowadays there is controversy regarding its usefulness. It has been reported that MP therapy is associated with 2.6-fold increase in the incidence of pneumonia *(70)*. Furthermore, the beneficial effect of MP on the neurological recovery of patients with injury has not been conclusively proven *(71,72)*. Therefore, other pharmacological treatments must be tested. In this field, we demonstrated that low doses of CsA inhibit LP to the same extent as MP administered at high doses several times within a 24-h period. Moreover, the combination of both drugs does not result in a synergistic effect upon LP inhibition. Therapy with CsA alone, besides its usefulness to inhibit LP, may be less aggressive because the dosing scheme useful to achieve its beneficial effect upon LP is the result of a rational scheme in experimental SC injury models *(60)*. On the contrary, MP therapy is based on a high-dose scheme *(21)* that may have a strong impact upon the immune system causing a significant susceptibility to infectious diseases and, secondarily, to death. In fact, MP-treated animals (MP alone or MP + CsA) present a lower survival than vehicle- or CsA- treated SC- injured rats *(69)*. A study of 15 d follow-up after SC injury showed that, after 3 d of therapy, none of the CsA-treated animals died *(see* Fig. 4), and all remained in good health. Conversely, the group of animals treated with MP (for 24 h only) or MP + CsA had a significant number of deaths during the first week after injury, infection being the principal cause of death. Thus, in spite of the clinical benefits of a megadose of MP, possible risks involved in its use should also be considered. Thus, CsA at a low dose seems to exert its effect upon LP similarly to MP but without the lethal effect of the latter. The negative impact of MP therapy upon survival rate makes CsA a potential compound to be used after SC injury to inhibit LP.

LIPID PEROXIDATION INHIBITION BY CYCLOSPORIN-A CORRELATES WITH NEUROPROTECTION AND MOTOR RECOVERY

Lipid peroxidation is believed to be a major cause of posttraumatic cell damage and axonal demyelination *(73)*. In patients with spinal injury, LP is believed to contribute significantly to the development of permanent neurological dysfunction *(29)*. Demyelination is a phenomenon that rebounds importantly on axonal function *(73)*. Myelin is essential for normal nervous system tasks *(74)* and loss of the axon myelin sheath has important repercussions on nerve physiology, for example, a decrease in conduction velocity or overt nerve conduction block, that may play a major role in the neurological deficits after SC injury *(75)*. Therefore, diminishing the demyelination process by inhibiting LP may give rise to an increase in the number of functional axons, which would have a significant impact on neurological recovery *(76)*.

Morphometric analysis of the myelination index (MI), a consistent parameter to evaluate the relative thickness of the myelin sheaths *(77)*, indicates a significant decrease of the demyelination process in axons located at the epicenter of the lesion of SC-injured rats treated with CsA (submitted for publication). A large percentage of fibers of treated animals present an MI between 0.6 and 0.8, which is considered a useful MI *(78,79)*, while in nontreated rats they present a significant percentage of unmyelinated axons. These results confirm the neuroprotective action of CsA that, besides inhibiting LP, also diminishes the demyelination process observed after SC injury.

On the other hand, even though the protective effect of a therapy does not necessarily correlate with a functional outcome *(80)*, CsA improves motor recovery after SC injury *(20)* (*see* Fig. 5). Evaluation of the motor outcome by a modified Tarlov's scale *(20,81)*, shows a better motor improvement in rats treated with CsA than in nontreated rats as early as 5 d after lesion, although significant difference is observed only when CsA is started 6 h

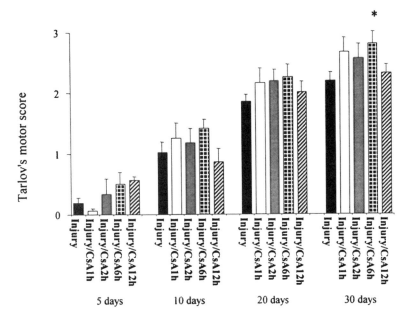

Fig. 5. Tarlov's scale score of spinal cord injured rats nontreated (Injury) or treated with cyclosporin A (Injury/CsA) administered at 1, 2, 6 or 12 h after injury. The results are expressed as means ± SE of eight animals per group. Data were analyzed by the Kruskal-Wallis ANOVA followed by by Mann–Whitney U test and considered significant when $p < 0.05$. * Different from injury without treatment. Reprinted from ref. *20*, with permission from Elsevier Science.

after injury and the motor function evaluated 30 d after lesion. The improved motor function observed after administration of CsA, could be the result of a better SC tissue preservation due to LP inhibition.

CONCLUSIONS

Besides its immunosuppressive action, cyclosporin A (CsA) may also have other nonimmunological effects. After spinal cord injury (SC), this drug inhibits lipid peroxidation (LP), given even 12 h after injury. This inhibition is equivalent to the one induced by methylprednisolone but without the deleterious effect of the latter upon the animal's survival. On the other hand, CsA is able to diminish the demyelination process, perhaps as a consequence of LP inhibition. Finally, the neuroprotective effect of CsA significantly correlates with motor improvement after injury. The benefits offered by CsA support its usefulness after SC injury, so it deserves to be studied further in experimental models.

ACKNOWLEDGMENTS

We are indebted to: Camilo Rios, Ph.D., for partial support of projects and discussion of results. Gabriel Guizar-Sahagún, Ph.D., Dolores Correa, Ph.D., and Rebecca Franco-Bourland, Ph.D., for discussion of this chapter. Araceli Diaz-Ruiz is a fellow of the National Council of Science and Technology of Mexico (CONACYT).

REFERENCES

1. Barker RA, Dunnett, SB. Functional integration of neural grafts in Parkinson's disease. Nat Neurosci 1999;2:1047–1048.
2. Nakao N, Itakura T. Fetal tissue transplants in animal models of Huntington's disease: the effects on damaged neuronal circuitry and behavioral deficits. Prog Neurobiol 2000;61:313–338.
3. Yang F, Connor J, Patel A, et al. Effects on startle responses in neonatally MSG-treated rats. Physiol Behav 2000;69:333–344.
4. Benninger Y, Marino S, Hardegger R, et al. Differentiation and histological analysis of embryonic stem cell-derived neural transplants in mice. Brain Pathol 2000;10:330–341.
5. Jacoby DB, Lindberg C, Ratliff J, et al. Fetal pig neural cells as a restorative therapy for neurodegenerative disease. Artif Organs 1997;21:1192–1198.
6. Schwartz EJ, Alexander GM, Prockop DJ, Azizi SA. Multipotential marrow stromal cells transduced to produce L-DOPA: engraftment in a rat model of Parkinson disease. Hum Gene Ther 1999;10:2539–2549.
7. Honey CR, Shen H. Immunosuppression for neural xenografts: a comparison of cyclosporin and anti-CD25 monoclonal antibody. J Neurosug 1999;91:109–113.
8. Zav'yalov VP, Denesyuc AI, Lundell J, Korpela T. Some new aspects of molecular mechanisms of cyclosporin-A effect on immune response. APMIS 1995;103:401–415.
9. Page AP, Kumar S, Carlow CKS. Parasite cyclophilins and antiparasite activity of cyclosporin-A. Parasitol Today 1995;11:385–388.
10. Kapan M, Ipek T, Sad A, et al. Effects of cyclosporin and somatostatin on liver regeneration after partial hepatectomy in rats. Eur Surg Res 1996;28:262–269.
11. Morii Y, Kawano K, Kim YI, et al. Augmentative effect of cyclosporin A on rat liver regeneration: influence on hepatocyte growth factor and transforming growth factor-beta (1). Eur Surg Res 1999;31:399–405.
12. Palladini G, Caronti B, Pozzessere G, et al. Treatment with cyclosporin-A promotes axonal regeneration in rats submitted to transverse section of the spinal cord. II. Recovery of function. J. Brain Res. 1996;37:145–153.
13. Teichner A, Morselli E, Buttarelli FR, et al. Treatment with cyclosporine-A promotes axonal regeneration in rats submitted to transverse section of the spinal cord. J Hirnforsch 1993;34:343–349.
14. Buki A, Okonkwo DO, Povlishock JT. Postinjury cyclosporin-A administration limits axonal damage and disconnection in traumatic injury. J Neurotrauma 1999;16:511–521.

15. Scheff SW, Sullivan PG. Cyclosporin-A significantly ameliorates cortical damage following experimental traumatic brain injury in rodents. J Neurotrauma 1999;16:783–792.

16. Sullivan PG, Thompson M, Scheff SW. Continuous infusion of cyclosporin-A postinjury significantly ameliorates cortical damage following traumatic brain injury. Exp Neurol 2000;161:631–637.

17. Kondo Y, Asanuma M, Iwata E, et al. Early treatment with cyclosporin A ameliorates the reduction of muscarinic acetylcholine receptors in gerbil hippocampus after transient forebrain ischemia. Neurochem Res 1999;24:9–13.

18. Okonwo DO, Povlishock JT. An intrathecal bolus of cyclosporin A before injury preserves mitochondrial integrity and attenuates axonal disruption in traumatic brain injury. J Cereb Blood Flow Metab 1999;19:443–451.

19. Seaton TA, Cooper JM, Schapira AH. Cyclosporin inhibition of apoptosis induced by mitochondrial complex I toxins. Brain Res 1998;809:12–17.

20. Diaz-Ruiz A, Rios C, Duarte I, et al. Cyclosporin-A inhibits lipid peroxidation after spinal cord injury in rats. Neurosci Lett 1999;266:61–64.

21. Hall ED, Yonkers PA, Andrus PA, Cox JW, Anderson DK. Biochemestry and pharmacology of lipid antioxidants in acute brain and spinal cord injury. J. Neurotrauma 1992;9(Suppl 2):S425–S442.

22. Yagi K. Lipid Peroxides in Biology and Medicine. Academic Press, New York, 1982.

23. Halliwell B, Gutteridge JMC. Oxigen radicals and the nervous system. Trends Neurosci 1985;8:22–26.

24. Hall DE, Braughler JM. Central nervous system trauma and stroke. II. Physiological and pharmacological evidence for involvement of oxygen radicals and lipid peroxidation. Free Radic Biol Med 1989;6:303–307.

25. Halliwell B, Gutteridge JMC. Free Radicals in Biology and Medicine. Cledon Press, Oxford.

26. Aspberg A, Tottmar O. Oxidative stress decreases antioxidant enzyme activities in reaggregation cultures of brain cells. Free Radic Biol Med 1994;17:511–516.

27. Qian H, Liu D. The time curse of malondialdehyde production following impact injury to rat spinal cord as measured by microdialysis and high pressure liquid chromatography. Neurochem Res 1997;22:1231–1236.

28. Kaynar MY, Hanci M, Kafadar A, et al. The effect of duration of compression on lipid peroxidation after experimental spinal cord injury. Neurosurg Rev 1998;21:117–120.

29. Hall ED. The role of oxygen radicals in traumatic injury: clinical implications. J Emerg Med 1993;11, Suppl. 1:31–36.

30. Dussart I, Schwab ME. Secondary cell death and the inflammation reaction after dorsal hemisection of the rat spinal cord. Eur J Neurosci 1994;6: 712–724.

31. Carlson SL, Parrish ME, Springer JE, et al. Acute inflammatory response in spinal cord following impact injury. Exp Neurol 1998;151, 77–88.

32. Blight AR. Macrophages and inflammatory damage in spinal cord injury. J. Neurotrauma 1992;9(Suppl 1):S83–S91.

33. Guizar-Sahagún G, Grijalva I, Madrazo I, et al.Development of post-traumatic cysts in the spinal cord of rats subjected to severe spinal cord contusion. Surg Neurol 1994;41:241–249.

34. Popovich PG, Wei P, Stokes BT. Cellular inflammatory response after spinal cord injury in Sprague-Dawley and Lewis rats. J Comp Neurol 1997;377: 443–464.

35. Fujimoto T, Nakamura T, Ikeda T, Taoka Y, Takagi K. Effects of EPC-K1 on lipid peroxidation in experimental spinal cord injury. Spine 2000;25:24–29.

36. Fujimoto T, Nakamura T, Ikeda T, Takagi K. Potent protective effects of melatonin on experimental spinal cord injury. Spine 2000;25:769–775.

37. Braughler JM, Hall ED. Effects of multidose methylprednisolone sodium succinate administration on injured cat spinal cord neurofilament degradation and energy metabolism. J Neurosurg 1984;61:290–295.

38. Hall ED, Wolf DL. A pharmacological analysis of the pathophysiological mechanism of post-traumatic spinal cord schemia. J Neurosurg 1986; 64:951–961.

39. Bracken MB, Shepard MJ, Collins WF, et al. A randomized control trial of methylprednisolone or naloxone in the treatment of acute spinal cord injury. Results of the Second National Acute Spinal Cord Injury Study. N Engl J Med 1990;322:1405–1411.

40. Bracken MB, Shepard MJ, Holford TR, et al.Administration of methylprednisolone for 24 or 48 hours or tirilazad mesylate for 48 hours in the treatment of spinal cord injury. Results of the Third National Acute Spinal Cord Injury Randomized Controlled Trial. National Acute Spinal Cord Injury Study. JAMA 1997;277:1597–1604.

41. Anderson DK, Braughler JM, Hall ED, et al. Effect of treatment with U-74006F on neurological recovery following experimental spinal cord injury. J Neurosurg 1988;69:562–567.

42. Anderson DK, Waters TR, Means ED. Pretreatment with alpha-tocopherol enhances neurologic recovery after spinal cord compression injury. J Neurotrauma 1988;6:61–68.

43. Koc RK, Akdemir H, Kurtsoy A, et al. Lipid peroxidation in experimental spinal cord injury. Comparison of treatment with Ginkgo biloba, TRH and methylprednisolone. Res Exp Med 1995;195:117–123.

44. Suzer T, Coskun E, Islekel H, Tahta K. Neuroprotective effect of magnesium on lipid peroxidation and axonal function after experimental spinal cord injury. Spinal Cord 1999;37:480–484.

45. Kaptanoglu E, Tuncel M, Palaoglu S, et al. Comparison of the effects of melatonin and methylprednisolone in experimental spinal cord injury. J Neurosurg 2000;93:77–84.

46. Dawson TM, Snyder SH. Gases as biological messengers: nitric oxide and carbon monoxide in the brain. J Neurosci 1994;14:5147–5159.

47. Borel J. Mechanism of action of cyclosporin-A and rationale for its use in nephritic syndrome. Clin Nephrol 1991;35:23–30.

48. Morris RE. Mechanisms of action of new immunosuppressive drugs. Ther Drug Monit 1995;17:564–569.

49. Hendey B, Maxfiel FR. Regulation of neutrophil and adhesion by intracellular calcium transients. Blood Cells 1993;19:143–161.

50. Fan TPD, Lewis GP. Effect of cyclosporin-A and inhibitors of arachidonic acid metabolism on blood flow and cyclo-oxigenase products in rat skin allografts. Brit J Pharmacol 1984;81:361–371.

51. Attur MG, Patel R, Thakker G, et al. Differential anti-inflammatory effects of immunosuppressive drugs: cyclosporin, rapamycin and FK-506 on inducible nitric oxide synthase, nitric oxide, cyclooxigenase-2 and PGE2 production. Inflamm Res 2000;49:20–26.

52. Trajkovic V, Badovinac V, Jankovic V, et al. Cyclosporin A suppresses the induction of nitric oxide synthesis in interferon-gamma-treated L929 fibroblasts. Scand J Immunol 1999;49:126–130.

53. Trajkovic V, Badovinac V, Jankovic V, Mostarica-Stojkovic M. Cyclosporin A inhibits activation of inducible nitric oxide synthase in C6 glioma cell line. Brain Res 1999;816:92–98.

54. Baligan, R, Ueda N, Walker PD, Shah SV. Oxidant mechanisms in toxic acute renal failure. Drug Metab Rev 1999;31:971–997.

55. Kasiske BL. Cyclosporine and lipid peroxidation. Am J Kidney Dis 1998;31:149–154.

56. Broekemeier KM, Carpenter-Deyo L, Reed DJ, Pfeiffer DR. Cyclosporin A protects hepatocytes subjected to high Ca^{2+} and oxidative stress. FEBS Lett 1992;304:192–194.

57. Konukoglu D, Tasci I, Cetinkale O. Effect of cyclosporin A and ibuprofen on liver ischemia-reperfusion injury in the rat. Clin Chim Acta 1998;275:1–8.

58. Santamaria A, Rios C. MK an *N*-methyl-D-aspartate receptor antagonist, blocks quinolinic acid-induced lipid peroxidation in rat corpus striatum. Neurosci Lett 1993;159:51–54.

59. Triggs, WJ, Willmore LJ. In vivo lipid peroxidation in rat brain following intracortical Fe^{2+} injection. J Neurochem 1984;42:976–978.

60. Ibarra A, Reyes J, Martinez S, et al. Use of cyclosporin-A in experimental spinal cord injury: Design of a dosing strategy to maintain therapeutic levels. J Neurotrauma 1996;13:569–572.

61. Ibarra A, Guizar-Sahagun G, Correa D, et al. Alteration of cyclosporin-A pharmacokinetics after experimental spinal cord injury. J Neurotrauma 1996;13:267–272.

62. Segal JL, Brunnemann S, Gordon S, Eltorai IM. Decreased theophylline bioavailability and impaired gastric empty in spinal cord injury. Curr Ther Res 1985;38:831–846.

63. Segal JL, Brunnemann S, Gray D, et al. Impaired absorption of intramuscularly administered gentamicin in spinal cord injury. Curr Ther Res 1986; 39:961–969.

64. Segal JL, Brunnemann S, Eltorai IM, Vulpe M. Decreased systemic clearance of lorazepam in humans with spinal cord injury. J Clin Pharmacol 1991; 31: 651–656.

65. Brundin P, Widner H, Nilsson O, et al. Intracerebral xenografts of dopamine neurons: Role of immunosuppression and blood-brain barrier. Exp Brain Res 1989;75:195–207.

66. Finsen B, Poulsen PH, Zimmer J. Xenografting of fetal mouse hippocampal tissue to the brain of adult rats: effect of cyclosporin-A treatment. Exp Brain Res 1988;70:117–133.
67. Green CL. Experimental transplantation and cyclosporine. Transplantation 1988;46:3S–10S.
68. Christians U, Sewing KF. Cyclosporin metabolism in transplant patients. Pharmacol Ther 1993;57:291–345.
69. Diaz-Ruiz A, Rios C, Duarte I, et al. Lipid peroxidation inhibition in spinal cord injury: cyclosporin-A vs methylprednisolone. NeuroReport 2000;11: 1765–1767.
70. Gerndt SJ, Rodriguez JL, Pawlik JW, et al. Consequences of high-dose steroid therapy for acute spinal cord injury. J Trauma 1997;42:279–284.
71. Coleman WP, Benzel D, Cahill DW, et al. A critical appraisal of the reporting of the National Acute Spinal Cord Injury Studies (II and III) of methylprednisolone in acute spinal cord injury. J Spinal Disord 2000;13:185–199.
72. Nesathurai S. Steriods and spinal cord injury: revisiting the NASCIS 2 and NASCIS 3 trials. J Trauma 1998;45:1088–1093.
73. Hall DE. Free radicals in central nervous system injury. In: Rice-Evans CA, Burdon RH, eds. Free Radical Damage and Its Control. Elsevier Science B.V., Amsterdam, Netherlands, pp. 217–230.
74. Webster H de P. Myelin injury and repair. Adv Neurol 1993;59, 67–73.
75. Young W. Recovery mechanisms in spinal cord injury: implications for regenerative therapy. In: Seil FJ, ed. Neural Regeneration and Transplantation. Wiley-Liss, New York, pp. 157–169.
76. Young W. Secondary injury mechanisms in acute spinal cord injury. J Emerg Med 1993;11:13–22.
77. Little GJ, Heath JW. Morphometric analysis of axons myelinated during adult life in mouse superior cervical ganglion. J Anat 1994;184:387–398.
78. Goldman L, Albus JS. Computation of impulse conduction in myelinated fibers: Theoretical bases of the velocity-diameter relation. Biophys J 1968;8: 596–607.
79. Williams RW, Chalupa LM. An analysis of axon caliber within the optic nerve of the cat: evidence of size groupings and regional organization. J Neurosci 1983;3:1554–1564.
80. Amar AP, Levy ML. Phathogenesis and pharmacological strategies for mitigating secondary damage in acute spinal cord injury. Neurosurgery 1999;44, 1027–1040.
81. Stokes BT, Reier PJ. Fetal grafts alter chronic behavioral outcome after contusion damage to the adult rat spinal cord. Exp Neurol 1992;116:1–12.

15

Axonal Regeneration in Cyclosporin A-Treated Rats Submitted to Transverse Section of the Spinal Cord

Guido Palladini and Brunella Caronti

SURVEY OF THE PROBLEM OF THE CENTRAL AXONAL REGENERATION

The neurons of the central nervous system of mammals, with respect to the invertebrates, are traditionally considered extremely susceptible to oxygen deficit *(1)* and do not have the capability for spontaneous regeneration *(2)*. As a matter of fact, both these characteristics have been doubted.

A series of experimental results demonstrated the potential ability to regenerate the neurons of central nervous system in mammals. Multipotent stem cells are present in adult mammalian spinal cord and ventricular neuroaxis and *de novo* generation of neuronal cells from brain occurs in adults *(3,4)*. With particular regard to the regeneration of the axons, the researches by David and Aguayo *(5)* furnished evidence that fetal mesencephalic neurons survive and extend long axons across peripheral nerve grafts implanted into the adult rat striatum. These results represented the direct evidence that neurons of the central nervous system of mammals maintain the potentiality to regenerate during the adult age and suggested that environmental inhibitory factors block the spontaneous regenerative capacity of the adult mammalian cerebral neurons.

HYPOTHESES ON THE LACK REGENERATION OF CENTRAL AXONS IN MAMMALS

The wide spectrum of researches performed in the field of the regeneration of the central nervous system demonstrated that the problem is very complex and the phenomenon of the regeneration in adult mammals results from a complex balance of both positive and negative factors *(6)*.

The main factor is represented by the kind of neuron *(7,8)*. For instance, neurons of the cerebellar cortex never regenerate the axons in the peripheral

From: *Immunosuppressant Analogs in Neuroprotection*
Edited by: C. V. Borlongan, O. Isacson, and P. R. Sanberg © Humana Press Inc., Totowa, NJ

graft. On the contrary, precerebellar nuclei in the brainsteam regenerated our axons into the graft *(9)*. In particular, the corticospinal axons are not able to regenerate in peripheral graft *(10)*. This latter observation reevaluates the old concept of pathoclisis by C. and O. Vogt *(11)*: different kinds of neurons show different susceptibility to the same *noxa*.

The second factor that plays a key role in the problem of the regeneration of the central neurons is due to the ability of the perikaryon to resist to the axotomy and to the vascular injuries in central nervous tissue following traumatic lesion, as occurs in both experimental and clinical conditions *(12,13)*.

Following the suggestion from results obtained by David and Aguayo, a series of factors inhibiting the central axonal regeneration has subsequently been characterized and each new factor has always been considered the true agent responsible of the lack regeneration of the central neurons *(5)*.

Different groups of neuroscientists invoked the myelin-associated glycoprotein (MAG) as the major inhibitory factor, but subsequent studies refuted this hypothesis *(14)*.

Proteins of oligodendrocyte origin with inhibitory action on the central nervous system regeneration have been characterized and identified by Schwab and Caroni *(15)*. These authors obtained sprouting and strong enhancement of axonal regeneration in mammals following graft in the place of hybridomas producing antibodies against oligodendrocyte-associated proteins. These latter results have not been always confirmed. The same proteins have been identified in teleosteans, in which central axonal regeneration spontaneously occurs *(16–18)*. Other studies performed on neurons of dorsal ganglia demonstrated that the axonal regeneration was complete in myelinated white matter tracts of adult mammalian spinal cord, without any myelin inhibitor neutralization. These results were obtained in vivo, but not in vitro *(19)*.

Other authors interpreted the abortive regeneration of mammalian central nervous system as due to the lack of neurotrophic factors acting on neuronal survival and axonal elongation *(20)*, such as proteins, endogenous opioids, nerve growth factor (NGF), brain-derived neurotrophic factor (BDNF), fibroblast growth factor (FGF), and neurotrophin-3 (NT3) *(21–23)*. Mechanical and biochemical actions of the glial barrier have been proposed to explain the regeneration failure of central axons *(19,24,25)*. Other authors underlined the importance of the contact guidance exerted by connective fibers and/or neurilemmal sheaths *(25–28)*.

Puzzling results have been obtained from molecular investigations performed on regenerating and nonregenerating neurons *(7,29)*. The possibility that the principal molecular basis for posttraumatic neuronal degeneration is the oxygen free radical–induced lipid peroxidation *(30)* and the upregulation of nitric oxyde synthase (NOS) *(31)* opened new researches and clinical perspectives.

A further possibility, to which our laboratory has given strong experimental support, is that the inflammation and the immune reaction occurs following traumatic central nervous system lesion *(19,32)*. Thus, inflammation and immune reaction, in particular, autoimmune response, may contribute to inhibit the axonal regeneration.

The autoimmune hypothesis was originally suggested by Berry and Riches *(33)* and several authors consistently demonstrated that in mammals traumatic lesions of central nervous system elicits an autoimmune reaction in serum and in *in situ* lesion *(2)*. The autoimmune hypothesis was indirectly supported from a variety of treatments potentially acting on the immune system, such as puromicine, cyclophosphamide, corticosteroids, colchicine and cloroquine, other antimitotic drugs (Sanamicyn, TEM) *(27)*, transglutaminase, neonatal desensitization *(2)*, X-ray irradiation *(34)*, and autoimmune T cells against central nervous system myelin-associated peptide *(35)*.

Moreover, the regenerative enhancement was observed in central nervous system–lesioned animals in putative conditions of natural immunodeficiency, such as in rat fetus, in newborn opossum and hamster, and in hibernating animals *(2)*.

OUR EXPERIMENTAL MODELS CONCERNING THE "IMMUNOLOGICAL BEAM" OF THE BALANCE OF CENTRAL AXONAL REGENERATION

The autoimmune hypothesis proposed by Berry and Riches in 1974 *(33)* supported our previous observations concerning the spinal cord regeneration in adult rat during treatment with antiblastic substances *(27)* and encouraged our laboratory to study the immunological approach to regeneration of the central nervous system in mammals. Thus, we designed different experimental models aimed at investigating the immunological aspects affecting the regeneration of the central nervous system. Experimental protocols with different treatments acting on the immune system were performed to investigate whether the immune reaction may significantly contribute to the abortive regeneration of the central nervous system in mammals.

Autoimmune Response in Spinal Cord–Lesioned Mammals
Autoantibodies Production After Spinal Cord Lesion

Serum autoantibodies of the IgG family directed against protein fraction (45 and 65 kDa) of spinal cord homogenate (prepared according to Willard and Simon) *(36)* have been demonstrated in spinal cord–injured rabbits and rats *(37)*.

In the rabbit, serum antibodies appeared 2–3 d after lesion and persisted at least the maximal survival time (21 d). In the rat, a faint positivity was present before the lesion that disappeared 1 h after lesion and reappeared 3 d later, suggesting that this autoimmune reaction is anamnestic in nature. The immunohistochemical method revealed IgG uniformly deposited on the axon, on the third day after the lesion.

Intact spinal cord sections incubated with sera from lesioned rats 3 d after surgery showed a similar pattern; control methods demonstrated the specificity of the immunohistochemical reaction. This specificity was also confirmed by the absence of autoimmune response following lesions of the peripheral nervous system and by the absence of crossreactivity between the central and peripheral nervous systems *(2,38)*.

Anatomocomparative Researches

A diffuse pattern of anatomocomparative researches by our group produced clear evidence of a relationship between abortive axonal regeneration in the central nervous system and autoimmune response and vice versa.

Complete morphological and functional regeneration of the spinal cord is possible in urodele amphibians *(Triturus) (39)*; in this species, we did not observe the immune response in serum, using an antitriturus Ig serum obtained in our laboratory, although urodeles are capable of the humoral and cellular immune responses *(40)*. If after remotion of a 2- to 3-mm segment of spinal cord, a homologous or heterologous graft of spinal cord covered with a powerful mineral adjuvant (venetian talcum) was inserted into a subcutaneous pouch, the spinal cord regeneration was inhibited and immunocomplexes in *in situ* lesion were observed. On the contrary, insertion of spinal cord graft alone or the adjuvant alone, respectively, did not influence the spontaneous spinal cord regeneration and the presence of immunocomplexes in lesion *in situ*.

In reptiles (*Lacerta*), in which spinal tracts regeneration is functionally complete *(41)*, an immune reaction was not present in serum or *in situ* lesion.

In adult birds, a marked morphological regeneration of spinal descending axons (*fasciculus longitudinalis medianus*) (although not permanent and without functional recovery) was present in the absence of IgG both *in situ* lesion and in serum *(42)*.

Specific Immunosuppression: Neonatal Desensitization in Mammals

Specific immunosuppression against the central nervous system extract was achieved according to Hockfields *(43)* in newborn Wistar rats. The animals underwent complete transverse section of the spinal cord at T7/T8 3 mo after treatment. Serum IgG levels were unchanged in desensitized-transected animals, whereas significant increases were measured in control-transected animals 7 d after surgery; also in desensitized-transected rats, immunocomplexes precipitation in the lesion *in situ* was markedly lower than in control-transected animals.

Thin, dark irregular fibers were observed in longitudinal sections of the spinal cord, organized in thick bundles that transversed the lesion and penetrated in the distal stump. Quantitative evaluation of regenerated fibers in desensitized-transected rats demonstrated a higher number of fibers in the pyramidal field reached the length of 5–6 mm in the distal stump. On the contrary, in the control animal only a few fibers were found at 1 mm caudal to the lesion. However, no clinical improvement was observed *(2)*.

Treatment with Cyclosporin A as Immunosuppressant Agent in Mammals

To further investigate whether the blocking of autoimmune response is able to facilitate central axonal regeneration in mammals, we studied the effect of cyclosporin A in adult rats submitted to transverse section of the spinal cord. Cyclosporin A was selected from the wide spectrum of immunosuppressant drugs because of its peculiar properties. Cyclosporin A acts specifically on T lymphocytes, thus blocking the T cell-mediated antibody production *(44)*. For its properties, cyclosporin A differs from other drugs previously used as immunosuppressants that inhibit protein synthesis and produce numerous collateral effects.

Female Wistar rats were used and submitted to transverse sections of the spinal cord at midthoracic level *(38,45)*. Treated-transected animals received cyclosporin A (2.5–5 mg/kg/d, sc), and the control group was composed of saline-treated-transected rats.

In the first series of experiments, treatment began immediately after lesion and carried out for 14 d, in the second series, treatment was continued for 35 d after surgery. Blood samples were systematically collected in all animals; at 3, 7, 14, 21, and 30 d after surgery, two animals were sacrificed for the detection of the antibodies in the *in situ* lesion; morphofunctional recovery of lesioned axons was analyzed by Fast Blue retrograde tracing procedure; the stain was injected 4 mm below the original transection. Clinical recovery was observed following different approaches and tests.

Morphofunctional, Behavioral, and Electrophysiological Studies

Spinal cord of vehicle-treated-transected rats showed a typical pattern of alterations *(19,37)*. As shown in Fig. 1, wide areas of necrosis are present in two stumps of spinal cord, with numerous foamy cells and reactive astrocytes; descending fibers show for 2–3 mm cranially to the lesion a clear

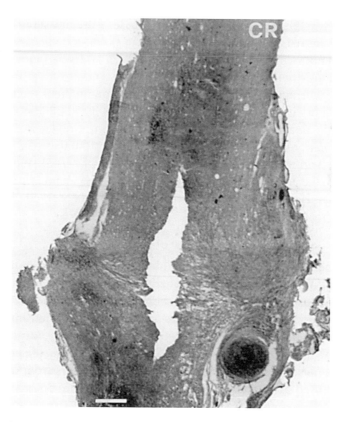

Fig. 1. Cryostatic longitudinal section of spinal cord from a saline-treated rat, 35 d after surgery (silver impregnation according to Bodian's method, mosaic of 2 frames). Wide areas of necrosis are present in the two stumps of the spinal cord. Lack of bridging fibers at the level of the lesion. CR = cranial stump. Calibration bar = 100 μm.

pattern of degeneration. The scar appeared strongly incomplete with numerous arachnoidal cystis; nerve fibers bridging the scar were not observed.

A similar pattern of alterations was present at 35 d after lesion, with numerous microgliallike cells and macrophages, positive for MHC class II antigens; immunostaining for neurofilaments decreased and eventually disappeared 14 d after lesion. Retrograde tracing procedure was completely negative for pyramidal fibers cranially or rostrally to the lesion. Positivity for IgG in the *in situ* lesion was strongly present at the level of axoplasm and axonal membranes.

Bilateral paralysis of the hind limbs occurred immediately at surgery and lasted though the sacrifice. Spinal walking was never observed, according to the observations in rat by Kaijhara and colleagues *(46)* and De La Torre and colleagues *(47)*. Pain stimulation produced weak reflex activity in a few animals (15%). Somatosensory-evoked potentials recorded by sciatic nerve stimulation *(48)* at 25 d after lesion never showed appearance of the triphasic wave at the dorsal level.

In cyclosporin A-treated transected rats histological picture was completely different (Fig. 2). The cut ends of the spinal cord were bridged by a strong glial-connectival scar and thin, argirophilic and convoluted fibers (Fig. 3B). These latter fibers were similar to those observed in the spontaneous axonal regeneration in the spinal cord of adult lampreys *(49)* and *Lacerta (41)*. No necrosis or aracnoidal cystis were observed. Positivity for neurofilaments was present in almost all rostral fibers observed at 30 d after lesion. In all cyclosporin A-treated rats after retrograde tracing procedure was performed, a large number of positive fluorescent fibers were observed in corticospinal tracts bridging the scar and extending in the cranial stump (Fig. 3A). Many fluorescent fibers were observed at the level of the pyramidal cervical field and finally (35 d after lesion) numerous traced perikaryons were observed at the brainstem reticular formation and sensorimotor cortex (Fig. 3C).

It is very interesting that the interneurons around the lesion captured the fluorescent dye, giving evidence of the integrity of these cells in cyclosporin A-treated rats.

The survival of the spinal cord intrinsic neurons is a powerful factor of the functional spinal recovery, as it is well known that in rat all corticospinal innervation to motor neurons in the ventral horn is through interneurons *(50)*.

Following cyclosporin A treatment, the level of serum antibodies against protein components weighing between 45 and 65 kDa were much lower than the level measured in vehicle-treated rats.

Animals were monitored for sensorimotor recovery twice weekly after surgery. Locomotion and sensibility were evaluated according to the criteria of Kunkel-Bagden and associates *(51)*:

1. *Climb*. Climbing is the ability of the animals suspended by its tail to climb onto a platform. A normal animal lifts both hind limbs together with his hips and rapidly places his hind limbs onto the platform. This normal behavior was observed in 32% of cyclosporin A-treated rats and never in vehicle-treated animals.

2. *Runway*. This parameter concerns the ability of the animal to deambulate over a plane or inclined surface. Hind limb movement, the coordination of movement (left hind limb⇒ left fore limb⇒ right hind limb⇒ right forelimb *(52)* and the animal's individual limb movement were videotaped. In 27% of cyclosporin A-treated animals recovery of normal hind limb motor activity

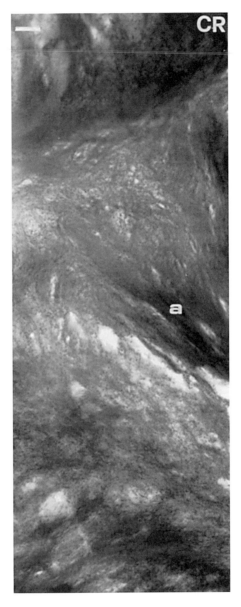

Fig. 2. Cryostatic longitudinal section around the lesion area (mosaic of two frames) of a rat spinal cord, cyclosporin A-treated, 35 d after surgery. Placing contact reaction and incomplete spontaneous motor activity are observed in this rat. The spinal cord was injected with Fast Blue, 4000 μm caudally to the scar 30 d after surgery. The slide was observed and photographed in fluorescence and subsequently refixed and impregnated according to Bodian's method. CR = cranial stump. a = Gauge point in Fig. 3 A,B. Calibration bar = 100 μm.

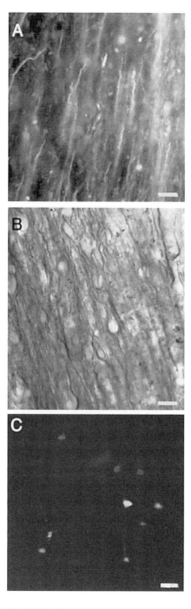

Fig. 3. Enlarged details of Fig. 2. Calibration bar = 100 μm. (**A**) Fast Blue tracing. Regenerating fibers that extend at least as far the injection site, 4 mm further down, bridge the transected area and give a fluorescent signal for retrograde tracing procedure from the injection site (Gauge point **a** in Fig. 2). (**B**) Silver impregnation according to Bodian's method of the same section after refixation. (**C**) Fast Blue tracing. Corticomotor area of the same rat with fluorescent perikaryons for retrograde tracing procedure from the injection site.

was observed starting approx 20 d after surgery, according to data in the literature concerning the growth rate of adult spinal cord axons following NGF or
NT$_3$ treatment *(53,54)*. Recovery of function was not complete in the coordi-
nated movements. The coordination of movements was maintained only for a
few steps (but the position of hind limb was very similar to that an intact rat),
then interrupted by spastic hind limb movement before being restored for
another short series of steps. Vehicle-treated rats were absolutely unable to
walk at any time after lesion.

3. *Placing*. Placing is the ability of an animal to place the hind limb onto a surface for support in response to proprioceptive (joint bending) and to contact
(light touch) stimuli. After spinal cord section in the adult rat, the contact placing response, which is considered as strictly indicative of supraspinal motor
control *(51,55,56)*, was never recovered. The 77% of cyclosporin A-treated
animals displayed proprioceptive reflexes and positive contact placing reaction, as the intact animals; contact placing reaction was never observed in
vehicle-treated animals (Fig. 4A–C).

4. *Sensibility*. In 91% of cyclosporin A -treated animals strong reflex activity
was observed after pain stimulation; in vehicle-treated animals only 13%
showed a weak pain reflex reaction.

5. *Somato-sensory evoked potentials (SSEP)*. SSEP were used to measure the
capacity of different sensory pathways to transmit impulses from L6 (caudally
to the lesion) to T5 (rostrally to the lesion) along the spinal cord; then they
furnish a proof of the functional recovery of long tracts of spinal cord. Triphasic wave rostral to the lesion was recorded in all cyclosporin A-treated tested
animals, 30 d after surgery, but never in saline-treated rats.

CONCLUSION ABOUT THE RESULTS OBTAINED
FROM THE AUTOIMMUNE APPROACH
TO CENTRAL AXONAL REGENERATION

The results of the studies reviewed herein definitively demonstrate that
autoimmune phenomena contribute to the abortive central nervous system
in mammals. The autoimmune hypothesis proposed by Berry and Riches in
1974 has been supported by numerous experimental reports on mammals.
Moreover, anatomocomparative data demonstrated a relationship between
autoimmunity and abortive central axonal regeneration. However, it is worth
noting that experimental protocols based on the autoimmune approach to
the central axonal regeneration produced a morphologically and functionally incomplete regeneration. The only immunosuppressant treatment able
to exert a positive action on functional recovery on lesioned spinal cord,
according to the criteria proposed by Guth and coworkers *(57)* and De La
Torre *(58)*, is the cyclosporin A administration. Therefore, it is conceivable
that Cyclosporine A may exert a positive action on functional recovery on
spinal cord by some other effects, besides the immunosuppression.

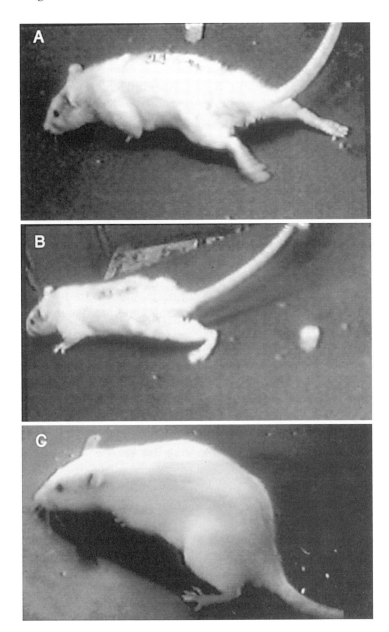

Fig. 4. Frames taken from videotape of (**A**) a transected, vehicle treated rat, 24 d after surgery; (**B**) a transected, cyclosporin A-treated rat, 24 d after surgery. Treatment with cyclosporin A promotes reappearance of contact placing reaction. Similar results were obtained in 77% of the rats treated with cyclosporin A; 27% of the treated rats also presented incomplete spontaneous locomotion (*see* text for details). (**C**) Normal rat.

NONIMMUNOSUPPRESSIVE
PROPERTIES OF CYCLOSPORIN A

Besides its immunosuppressive properties, depending on a specific domain of the molecule, cyclosporin A has other different properties. Some cyclosporin A derivatives deprived of the immunosuppressive property are able to bind immunophilins. By means of the binding to the immunophilins, these cyclosporin A derivatives exert evident neuroprotective action *(59)* and stimulate neuritogenesis *(60)*. The neuroprotective effects of cyclosporin A are associated with different activities and different mechanisms of action.

Cyclosporin A inhibits the opening of voltage-gated megachannels allowing molecules and ions weighing 1500 Da to pass in the inner mithocondrial membrane with the relative induction of the mitochondrial permeability transition, which causes swelling of isolated mitochondria *(61,62)*.

Despite its immunosuppressive activity, cyclosporin A may protect damaged tissues from lipid peroxidation by free radicals *(63,64)*. A very important neuronal protective activity of cyclosporin A results from the binding to the immunophilins. Immunophilins are proteins interfaced with a wide range of signal transduction system inside cells, especially those relating to calcium and phosphorilation. Some authors *(65,66)* showed that following binding to immunophilins, cyclosporin A exerts a significantly inhibitory action on NOS. This latter enzyme strongly contributes to neuronal damage in traumatic lesions of the central nervous system *(31)*.

Another protein with phosphorilation activity that is increased by immunophilins is a growth-associated protein (p43), involved in neuronal process extension *(67)*. It is worth noting that regeneration of peripheral nervous system is strongly associated to the increased expression of a particular immunophilin.

Further nonimmune system-related activities of cyclosporin A have been reported in literature. Treatment with cyclosporin A in the rat increases motor activity *(68,69)* and improves memory retention *(70)*. The positive effects of these latter activities of cyclosporin A on central axonal regeneration cannot be excluded.

FINAL CONCLUSIONS

Taken together, all results by the different groups of neuroscientists provide evidence that the immune reaction play an important role in the abortive regeneration of central nervous system in mammals, but it is not the only responsible factor.

The results obtained following treatments with the different specific immunosuppressant agents demonstrate that the treatment with cyclosporin A is the most effective to improve the central axonal regeneration. As this drug also exerts a variety of nonimmunosuppressive activities, it is conceivable that the immunosuppressive and nonimmunosuppressive effects act in synergy in favor of the axonal regenerative phenomena. Therefore, the possibility of therapeutic use of cyclosporin A focused the attention of clinicians. In fact, recent study reported that the treatment with cyclosporin A of human spinal cord lesion significantly reduce the lesion's volume *(71)* and exerts a protective activity in subarachnoid hemorrhage *(72,73)*.

REFERENCES

1. Palladini G, Conforti A, Medolago-Albani L. Ultrastructural hypoxic changes in Ammon's horn and Purkinje cells. Brain Res 1976;103:45–56.
2. Palladini G, Caronti B. Regeneration in axotomized cord: influence of Cyclosporine A and neonatal immune desensitization in mammals. In: Stalberg E, Sharma HS, Olsson Y, eds. Spinal cord Monitoring. Springer, Vienna, 2998, pp. 157–180.
3. Weiss S, Dunne C, Hewson J, et al. Multipotent CNS stem cells are present in the adult mammalian spinal cord and ventricular Neuroaxis J Neurosci 1996;16:7599–7609.
4. Richard LJ, Kilpatrick TJ, Bartlett PF. De novo generation of neuronal cells from the adult mouse brain. Proc Natl Acad Sci USA 1992;89:8591–8595.
5. David S, Aguayo AJ. Axonal elongation into peripheral nervous system bridges after central nervous system injury in adult rat. Science 1981;214:931–933.
6. Olson L. Regeneration in the adult central nervous system: experimental repair strategies. Nature Med 1997;3:1329–1335.
7. Anderson PM, Lieberman AR. Intrinsic determinants of differential axonal regeneration by adult mammalian central nervous system axons. In: Saunders NR, Dziegielewska KM, eds. Degeneration and Regeneration in the nervous system. Harwood Ac. Pu, Amsterdam, 2000, pp. 53–76.
8. Tetzlaff W, Steeves JD. Intrinsic neuronal and extrinsic glial determinants of axonal regeneration in the injured spinal cord. In: Saunders NR, Dziegielewska KM, eds. Degeneration and regeneration in the nervous system. Harwood Ac. Pu., Amsterdam, 2000, pp. 93–118,
9. Vaudano E, Campbell G, Hunt SP, Lieberman AR. Axonal ijury and peripheral nerve grafting in the thalamus and cerebellum of the adult rat. Eur J Neurosci 1998;10:2644–2656.
10. Ye JH, Hule JD. Treatment of the chronically injured spinal cord with neurotrophic factors can promote axonal regeneration from supraspinal neurons Exp Neurol 1997;143:70–81.
11. Vogt C, Vogt O. Erkrankungen der Grosshirnrinde im Lichte der Topistik, Pathoklise und Pathoarchitektonik. J Psychol Neurol (Leipz) 1922;28:1–171.
12. Zhang Z, Guth L. Experimental spinal cord injury: Wallerian degeneration in the dorsal column is followed by revascularisation, glial proliferation and nerve regeneration. Exp Neurol 1997;147:159–171.

13. Marsala M. Spinal cord blood flow and metabolism in transient spinal ischemia. In: Stalberg E, Sharma HS, Olsson Y, eds. Spinal cord Monitoring. Springer, Vienna, 1998, pp. 3–25.
14. Bartsch U, Bandtlow CE, Schnell L, et al. Lack of evidence that myelin-associated glycoprotein is a major inhibitor of axonal regeneration in the CNS. Neuron 1995;15:1375–1381.
15. Caroni P, Schwab ME. Oligodendrocytes and myelin-associated inhibitors of neurite growth in the adult nervous system. Adv Neurol 1993;61:175–179.
16. Nona SN. Regenerative failure in the mammalian CNS. Trends Neurosci 1995;18:128–129.
17. Sivron T, Schwartz M. Glial cell types lineages and response to injury in rat and fish: implication for regeneration. Glia 1995;13:157–165.
18. Stichel CC, Muller HW. Regenerative failure in the mammalian CNS. Trends Neurosci 1995;18:128.
19. Fitch MT, Silver J. Inflammation and the glia scar: factors at the site of injury that influence regeneration in central nervous system. In: Saunders NR, Dziegielewska KM, eds. Degeneration and regeneration in the nervous system. Harwood Ac. Pu, Amsterdam, 2000, pp. 77–91.
20. Kiernan JA. Hypothesis concerned with axonal regeneration in the mammalian nervous system. Biol Rev 1979;54:155–197.
21. Ferguson JA, Lu JJ, Zhou XF, Rush RA. The low affinity neurotrophin receptor, p75: a multifunction molecule with a role in nerve regeneration? In: Saunders NR, Dziegielewska KM, eds. Degeneration and regeneration in the nervous system Harwood Ac. Pu, Amsterdam, 2000, pp. 221–238.
22. Hagg T, Oudega M. Neurotrophic factors and CNS reparation. In: Stalberg E, Sharma HS, Olsson Y, eds. Spinal cord Monitoring Springer, Vienna, 1998, pp.129–156.
23. Lauro GM, Margotta V, Venturini C, et al. Correlations between immune response and CNS regeneration in vertebrate phylogenesis. Boll Zool 1992;59:215–220.
24. Reier DJ, Holle JD. The glial scar: its bearing axonal elongation and transplantation approaches to CNS. In: Watzan SG, ed. Advances in Neurology: functional recovery in neurological diseases Raven Press, NY, 1988, vol. 7, pp. 87–138.
25. Aubert I, Ridet JL, Gage FH. Regeneration in the adult mammalian CNS: guided by development. Curr. Opinion Neurobiol. 1995;5:625–635.
26. Conti A, Selzer ME. The role of cytoskeleton in regeneration of central nervous system axons. In: Saunders NR, Dziegielewska KM, eds. Degeneration and regeneration in the nervous system. Harwood Ac. Pu, Amsterdam, 2000, pp. 153–170.
27. Palladini, G. and Alfei, L. (1965) Observations concerning the regeneration of the spinal cord of the adult rat during treatment with antiblastic substances. In: Kiortsis V, Trampush HAL, eds. Regeneration in Animals and Related Problems. North-Holland, Amsterdam, 1965, pp. 515–520.
28. Stefanelli A. Il problema dell'orientamento delle fibre nervose in vitro studiato in colture disgregate di midollo spinale embrionale di Gallus e Coturnix. Acta Embrio Morph Experim 1960;3:159–179.

29. Aigner L, Caroni P. Absence of persistent spreading, branching and adhesion in GAP-43-depleted growth cones. J Cell Biol 1995;128:647–660.
30. Brown DJ. Repair after spinal cord injury: a clinical perspective. In Saunders NR, Dziegielewska KM, eds. Degeneration and Regeneration in the Nervous System. Harwood Ac. Pu, Amsterdam, 2000, pp. 1–16.
31. Sharma HS, Nyberg F, Gordh T, et al. Neurotrophic factors attenuate neuronal oxide synthase upregulation, microvascular permeability disturbances, edema formation and cell injury in the spinal cord following trauma. In: Stalberg E, Sharma HS, Olsson Y, eds. Spinal cord monitoring Springer, Vienna, 1998, pp. 181–210.
32. Borlongan CV, Stahl CE, Cameron DF, et al. CNS immunological modulation of neural graft rejection and survival. Neurol Res 1996;18:297–304.
33. Berry M, Riches AC. (1974) An immunological approach to regeneration in central nervous system. Brit. Med. Bull. 1974;30:135–140.
34. Kalderon N, Fuks Z. Severed corticospinal axons recover electrophysiologic control of muscle activity after x-ray therapy in lesioned adult spinal cord. Proc Natl Acad Sci USA 1996;93:11,185–11,190.
35. Hauben E, Nevo U, Yoles E, et al. Autoimmune T cells as potential neuroprotective therapy for spinal cord injury. Lancet 2000;354:286–287.
36. Willard M, Simon C. Antibodies decoration of neurofilaments. J Cell Biol 1981;89:198–205.
37. Palladini G, Grossi M, Maleci A, et al. Immunocomplexes in rat and rabbit spinal cord after injury. Exp Neurol 1987;95:639–651.
38. Palladini G, Caronti B, Pozzessere G, et al. Treatment with Cyclosporine A promotes axonal regeneration in rat submitted to transverse section of the spinal cord. II. Recoverry of function. J Hirnforsch 1996;37:145–153.
39. Margotta V, Filoni S, Venturini G, et al. Autoimmunity and central nervous system regeneration in Urodele Amphibians. J Hirnforsch 1989;30:99–106.
40. Marchalonis JJ. Immunity in evolution. Arnold, London, 1977.
41. Raffaelli E, Palladini G. Rigenerazione delle cellule e degli assoni del midollo spinale dorsale di Lacerta sicula. Boll. Zool 1969;36:105–110.
42. Margotta V, Lauro GM, Di Lorenzo N, et al. Central axonal regeneration and autoimmunity in adult birds. . J Hirnforsch 1989;30:595–602.
43. Hockfield S. A mab to unique cerebellar neuron generated by immunosuppression and rapid immunisation. Science 1987;237:67–70.
44. Borel JM, Feurewr C, Guble HU, Stahelin H. Biological effects of cyclosporine A: a new anti-lymphocytic agent. Agent Actions 1976;6:468–475.
45. Teichner A, Morselli E, Buttarelli FR, et al. Treatment with cyclosporine A promotes axonal regeneration in rat submitted to transverse section of the spinal cord J Hirnforsch 1993;34:343–349.
46. Kaijhara K, Kawanaga HM, De La Torre JC, Mullan S. Dimethylsulfoxide in the treatment of the experimental acute spinal cord injury. Surg Neurol 1973;1:16–22.
47. De La Torre JC, Johnson CM, Goode DJ, Mullan S. Pharmacological treatment and evaluation of permanent experimental spinal trauma. Neurology 1975;25:508–511.

48. Pozzessere G, Valle E, Santoro A, et al. Prognostic value of early somatosensory evoked potentials during carotid surgery: relationship with electroencephalogram, stump pressure and clinical outcome. Acta Neurochir (Wien) 1987;89:28–33.
49. Cohen AH, Baker MT, Dobrov TA. Functional regeneration demonstrated in the adult spinal cord of lampreys. Soc Neurosci Abstr 1988;14:482–485.
50. Bernstein JJ, Goldberg WJ. Experimental spinal cord transplantation as a mechanism of spinal cord regeneration. Paraplegia 1995;33:250–253.
51. Kunkel-Bagden E, Dai HN, Bregmann BS. Method to asses the development and recovery of locomotor function after spinal cord injury in rats. Exp Neurol 1993;119:153–164.
52. Iwashita Y, Kawaguchi S, Murata M. Restoration of function by replacement of spinal cord segments in the rat. Nature 1994;367:167–169.
53. Fernandez E, Pallini R, Lauretti L, et al. Spinal cord transection in adult rat:effects of local infusion of NGF on the corticospinal tract axons. Neurosurgery 1993;33:889–893.
54. Schnell L, Schneider R, Kolbeck R, et al. Neurotrophin-3 enhances sprouting of corticosdpinal tract during development and after adult spinal cord lesion. Nature 1994;367:170–173.
55. Bregman BS, Kunkel-Badgen E, Reier PJ, et al. Recovery of the function after spinal cord injury: mechanism underlying transplant-mediated recovery of function differ after spinal cord injury in newborn and adult rat. Exp Neurol 1993;123:3–16.
56. Donatelle JM, Growth of the corticospinal tracts and the development of placing reaction in the postural life. J Comp Neurol 1977;175:207–232.
57. Guth L, Albuquerque EX, Deshpande SS, et al. Ineffectiveness of enzyme therapy on the regeneration in the transected spinal cord of the rat. J Neurosurg 1980;52:73–86.
58. De La Torre JC. Spinal cord injury models. Progr Neurobiol 1984;4: 289–344.
59. Steiner JP, Connolly MA, Valentine HL, et al. Neurotrophic actions of non immunosuppressive analogues of immunosuppressive drugs FK506, rapamycin and cyclosporin A. Nat Med 1997;3:421–428.
60. Steiner JP, Hamilton GS, Ross DT, et al. Neurotrophic immunophilin ligands stimulate structural and functional recovery in neurodegenerative animal models. Proc Natl Acad Sci USA 1997;94:2019–2024.
61. Friberg H, Ferrand-Drake M, Bengtsson F, et al. Cyclosporin A, but not FK506, protects mithocondria and neuron against hypoglycemic damage and implicates the mitochondrial permeability transition in cell death. J Neurosci 1998;18:5151–5159.
62. Siesjo BK, Elmer E, Janelidze S, et al. Role and mechanism of secondary mithocondrial failure. Acta Neurochir Suppl 1999;73:7–13.
63. Diaz-Ruiz A, Rios C, Duarte I, et al. Cyclosporine A inhibits lipid peroxidation after spinal cord injury in rats. Neurosci Lett 1999;266:1–64.
64. Kasiske BL. Cyclosporine and lipid peroxidation. Am J Kidney Dis 1998;31:149–154.

65. Fast DJ, Lynch R, Lau RW. Cyclosporine A inhibit nitric oxide production by L529 cells in response to tumor necrosis factor and interferon. J Interferon Res 1993;13:235–240.
66. Muhl H, Kunz D, Rob P, Pfeischiter J. Cyclosporin derivative inhibits interleukin 1 induction of nitric oxyde synthase in renal mesangial cells. Eur J Pharmacol 1993;249:95–100.
67. Snyder SH, Sabatini DM. Immunophilins and the nervous system. Nat Med 1995;1:32–37.
68. Borlongan CW, Freeman TB, Scorcia TA, et al. Cyclosporine A increases spontaneous and dopamine-agonist-induced locomotor behaviour in normal rats. Cell Transplant 1995;4:65–73.
69. Borlongan CV, Stahl CE, Fuijsaki T, et al. Cyclosporine A induced hyperactivity in rats: it is mediated by immunosuppressionn, neurotrphism or both? Cell Transplant 1999;8:153–159.
70. Borlongan CV, Fujisaki T, Watanabe S. Chronic administration of cyclosporine A does not impair memory retention in rat. Neuroreport 1997;8:673–676.
71. Davies S, Illis LS, Raisman G. Regeneration in the central nervous system and related factors. Summary of the Bermuda Paraplegia Conference. Paraplegia 1995;33:10–17.
72. Manno EM, Gress DR, Ogilvy CS, et al. The safety and the efficacy of cyclosporine A in the prevention of vasospasm in patients with Fisher grade three subarachnoid hemorrages: a pilot study. Neurosurgery 1997;40:289–293.
73. Ryba M, Grieb P, Bidzinski J. et al. Cyclosporine A for the prevention of neurological deficits following subarachnoidal hemorrage. Stroke 1991;22:531.

VI

IMMUNOSUPPRESSANTS AND SCIATIC NERVE INJURY

16

Neuroimmunophilin Ligands Accelerate and Promote Nerve Regeneration in the Rat Peripheral Nerve and Spinal Cord

Role of the Steroid Receptor–FKBP52 Complex

Bruce G. Gold

INTRODUCTION

Neuroimmunophilins refer to the binding targets for immunosuppressant drugs (FK506, rapamycin, and cyclosporin A) present in the nervous system. Neuroimmunophilin ligand, the compounds that bind to them, have great potential for significantly advancing the practice of clinical neurology. The ability to separate the nerve regenerative and immunosuppressant properties of FK506 (tacrolimus) was a fundamental step in the development of clinically useful neuroimmunophilin ligands for nerve regeneration. This discovery was made independently by the Snyder/Guilford and Gold laboratories *(1–3)* who demonstrated that nonimmunosuppressant (noncalcineurin inhibitor) FK506 derivatives (e.g., GPI-1046 and V-10,367, respectively) retain the nerve regenerative property of FK506 and are orally active *(4,5)*, the latter finding being unprecedented.

It is now well established that FK506 and the related nonimmuno-suppressant neuroimmunophilin ligands increase nerve regeneration in a variety of experimental models of nerve injury and neurodegenerative disease including nerve crush, nerve transection, spinal cord injury, and neurotoxic chemical models of Parkinson's disease. In fact, clinical application of neuroimmunophilin ligands for increasing nerve regeneration has already begun with two separate reports *(6,7)* that FK506 speeds functional recovery in the first two successful human hand transplantations performed to date. Clearly, with the anticipated increase in hand and limb transplantations in several centers around the world, both the clinical need and use of neuroimmunophilin ligands for nerve regeneration will continue to grow.

From: *Immunosuppressant Analogs in Neuroprotection*
Edited by: C. V. Borlongan, O. Isacson, and P. R. Sanberg © Humana Press Inc., Totowa, NJ

Furthermore, two clinical trials using nonimmunosuppressant derivatives of FK506 are in progress: Timcodar (Vertex Pharmaceuticals, Inc.) is in Phase II clinical trials for diabetic neuropathy; NIL-A (Amgen/Guilford Pharmaceuticals, Inc.) is in Phase II clinical trials for Parkinson's disease.[1] Many companies (e.g., Pfizer, Inc. and Fujisawa Pharmaceuticals, Inc.) are presently developing similar nonimmunosuppressant ligands for clinical trials. An understanding of the underlying mechanism is essential for development of second-generation neuroimmunophilin ligands designed to be more selective for the appropriate target. An appreciation of this novel mechanism also provides new insight into how these compounds effect a change in the rate of nerve regeneration. This is the subject of this chapter. (For a more detailed review, *see* ref. *8*). Before addressing this issue, however, it is first important to assess the utility of in vitro models for approximating rate effects in vivo.

ASSESSMENT OF NEURITE OUTGROWTH IN VITRO

My laboratory's 1992 discovery, first reported in 1993 *(9)*, that the immunosuppressant drug FK506 speeds functional recovery and nerve regeneration in the rat sciatic nerve crush model *(10)* helped to launch a new branch of neuroscience research: the neuroimmunophilin ligands. While numerous other classes of compounds [e.g., the neurotrophins, such as nerve growth factor (NGF)] have been shown to increase neurite outgrowth in vitro, these often do not demonstrate activity in subsequent animal models *(11)* and, to date, have been disappointing in human clinical trials. Thus, it is not possible to conclude, solely on the basis of in vitro studies, that a given compound possesses nerve regenerative activity. It is, therefore, essential to consider what exactly is being assessed in these cell-based assay systems.

Beginning with the initial in vitro study by Snyder and co-workers *(12)*, many investigators have examined neurotrophic activity by determining the percentages of cells with processes. However, such determination is really a measure of cell differentiation, which is not the same process as elongation. Thus, my laboratory has relied on measurement of length and maintains that this is the best in vitro correlate of rate. In this context, it should be noted that one recent report *(13)* claimed not to find a neurotrophic effect for FK506. While this study at first appears to be in marked contradiction to our findings, these investigators examined a very different issue: the ability to induce process outgrowth (i.e., differentiation) at suboptimal

---

[1]Guilford Pharmacuetical Inc.: Guilford Pharmacueticals announces completion of NIL-A phase II clinical trial for Parkinson's disease. Press release from 26 July 2001 at http://www.corporate-ir.net/ireye/ir_site.zhtml?ticker=GLFD&script=410&layout=6&item_id=195083.

concentrations of NGF. In that study, FK506 and a nonimmunosuppressant derivative (GPI-1046) were found not to induce neurite outgrowth. This apparent paradox is readily resolved by an appreciation of the fact that the mechanism underlying differentiation is very different from that resulting in accelerated process elongation *(13)*; in fact, in agreement with these in vitro studies, my laboratory has also never observed an ability of any neuroimmunophilin ligand to induce differentiation in the absence of added growth (differentiation) factors (e.g., NGF). Support for such a mechanistic distinction is provided by these investigators' *(13)* additional finding that another immunosuppressant (rapamycin), while also increasing elongation, is able to induce differentiation, presumably via its ability to inhibit progression of the cell cycle. This observation appears to be consistent with the original report by Snyder and coworkers *(12)* that rapamycin increases the number of cells with processes in PC12 cells (not to be confused with an increase in process length). This, however, is not meant to undermine the importance of such in vitro studies, since Snyder and coworkers *(12)* also made the important mechanistic finding that FK506 increases NGF responsiveness in PC12 cells (*see* the section entitled Mechanism of Nerve Regeneration by Neuroimmunophilin Ligands).

FK506 ACCELERATES THE RATE OF AXONAL REGENERATION IN THE SCIATIC NERVE CRUSH MODEL VIA A CALCINEURIN-INDEPENDENT MECHANISM

The most definitive way to establish an effect on the rate of nerve regeneration in animals is the use of radiolabeling techniques. This enables the most accurate measurement of the elongation distances from the crush site. When conducted at multiple time-points, it is possible to estimate the rate of axonal regeneration using regression line analysis. The data are most powerful and convincing when the effect is shown to be dose-dependent. While indices of functional recovery are important for assessing nerve regeneration, such determinations do not reveal the underlying mechanism leading to the improved performance; faster recovery of function does not necessarily indicate a faster regrowth of individual nerve fibers and, furthermore, does not always correlate with the morphological appearance of the nerve (e.g., *see* ref. *14*). The only other acceptable method for determining an effect on rate is the pinch test *(15)*. However, this is far less sensitive (relying on electrophysiological thresholds for activation of nerve conduction) and only measures the fastest growing fibers, in contrast to radiolabeling techniques that reveal the growth of the entire population of regenerating axons (*see* Fig. 6 in ref. *16*).

One consideration is that by the above criterion (*see* the section entitled Assessment of Neurite Outgrowth In Vitro), to date, only FK506 has been shown to definitively increase the rate of regeneration *(16,17)*. However, all neuroimmunophilin compounds tested in vitro so far demonstrate an increase process length over time, consistent with a rate alteration. Nevertheless, without the availability of definitive rate determination in vivo, the possibility exists that not all the nonimmunosuppressant derivatives act via the same mechanism.

In this context, Constantini and Isacson *(18)* recently suggested that an increase in elongation is a calcineurin-dependent process, while increased branching is calcineurin-independent; however, these in vitro data, obtained from dopaminergic neurons in culture, are difficult to compare with previous studies, since the results are presented as a percentage of control instead of absolute lengths. Studies from my laboratory on the nonimmunosuppressant (non-calcineurin-inhibiting) FK506 derivative V-10,367 *(3,4)* reveal that functional recovery is accelerated by an increase in elongation (reflected by increased axonal calibers and earlier myelination in the distal portions of the nerve) and not by branching (total numbers of nonmyelinated and myelinated axons are not increased). These results are not consistent with the proposal *(18)* that elongation is calcineurin-dependent in vivo. Differences in cell type (i.e., central versus peripheral neurons) are a possible explanation, but this seems unlikely. In this regard, it is important to note that calcineurin inhibition may also not be the entire reason for the ability of FK506 to provide neuroprotection (in the brain) against ischemia–hypoxia *(19)*, since a recent study shows that rapamycin (an immunosuppressant that exhibits neurotrophic activity but does not inhibit calcineurin) also reduces infarct size after cerebral ischemia *(13)*. Taken together, these studies implicate calcineurin-independent mechanisms in both nerve regeneration and, at least to some extent, neuroprotection.

The most likely explanation for these apparent contradictory results is that, given the very high concentrations (1 μM) of the compounds employed by Constantini and Isacson *(18)*, the finding that the combination of FK506 with a non-calcineurin-inhibiting neuroimmunophilin ligand leads to a block in elongation by FK506 may simply reflect the fact that the total concentration of neuroimmunophilin ligands exceeds the optimal range for increasing neurite outgrowth; neuroimmunophilin ligands exhibit a bell-shaped dose-response curve with FK506, even by itself, showing inhibition of outgrowth at concentrations exceeding 1 μM *(17,20)*. An alternative interpretation to the involvement of separate calcineurin-dependent and calcineurin-independent mechanisms underlying the processes of elongation and branching *(18)*, respectively, is the involvement of separate FK506-binding proteins (FKBPs); i.e., distinct FKBPs, with different affinities for neuroimmuno-philin ligands, may mediate branching and elongation, the latter involving FKBP52 *(21)* (*see* the section entitled Mechanism of Nerve Regeneration by Neuroimmunophilin Ligands). One mechanistic distinction between these processes is that while both elongation and branching would be expected to speed functional recovery and increase the morphological appearance of nerve regeneration, only the former would lead to an increase in actual rate of growth for individual axons.

NERVE TRANSECTION MODELS

Nerve transection models offer that advantage over the simple nerve crush model by better approximating the clinical situation, that is, reconnecting severed nerves. In this context, FK506 has also been shown to increase axonal regeneration in several nerve transection models. In these models, the proximal and distal stumps of the severed peripheral (sciatic) nerve are reconnected by reconnection with a nerve graft *(22)*, or by using either a polyethylene tube or collagen-based nerve guide to bridge the gap *(23)*. Obviously, these initial studies should be extended by employing other types of artificial guides, such as collagen-based *(24–26)* and silicone-based *(27)* nerve guides. By contrast, cyclosporin A does not significantly increase nerve regeneration in peripheral nerve transection models *(22)*, in agreement with results obtained in the nerve crush model *(14,16)*. While cyclosporin A has been shown to increase the number of cells with processes in vitro *(2,12)*, this is clearly not the same as an effect on rate. This is supported by our finding the drug does not accelerate the rate of nerve regeneration in the sciatic nerve crush model *(16)*.

CHRONIC NERVE INJURY MODELS

Besides examining nerve transection models, it is important for clinical application to determine whether the drug is effective after chronic nerve injuries. In collaboration with Tessa Gordon's laboratory, we have recently found *(28)* that FK506 also accelerates and promotes regeneration in a model of chronic nerve injury. Chronic injury in the peripheral nervous system results in poor functional recovery due to the reduced regenerative potential of the axotomized neurons and the progressive loss of a growth supportive environment (most significantly, Schwann cells and their basal lamina) in the denervated distal stump *(29)*. In a chronic (2-mo) axotomy model (where the proximal stump was sutured to a freshly cut distal nerve), FK506 doubled the number of regenerated neurons (identified by retrograde labeling) and more than doubled the number of myelinated axons in the distal nerve stump. Thus, more axons enter the distal stump from the chronically transected nerve, indicating that FK506 also promotes elongation of neurons, as in the spinal cord (*see* the section entitled Spinal Cord Injury Models). Although the total numbers of axons (myelinated plus nonmyelinated) increased, there was a 30% reduction in the numbers of nonmyelinated axons. This indicates that a greater proportion of the regenerating axons have matured to become myelinated sooner, having grown through the distal stump faster. Taken together, FK506 not only increases the rate of nerve regeneration, but also promotes regeneration of neurons whose regenerative capacity is significantly reduced by chronic axotomy *(29)*; to reiterate, promotion of mature neurons is not equivalent to differentiation of neuronal processes in vitro (*see* the section entitled Assessment of Neurite Outgrowth In Vitro). By contrast, after chronic denervation (the reverse experiment in which a freshly cut proximal nerve is sutured to a 2-mo chronically denervated distal stump), FK506 did not overcome the reduced capacity of Schwann cells to support axonal regeneration. The ability of FK506 to increase axonal regeneration following chronic axotomy, but not chronic denervation, indicates that the drug acts directly on the neuron to accelerate and promote nerve regeneration.

SPINAL CORD INJURY MODELS

The potential for neuroimmunophilin ligands in the treatment of spinal cord injuries was first demonstrated by Benowitz and coworkers *(30,31)*, who showed that FK506 improves functional recovery (as assessed by the ability to walk on an inclined plane) following a photothrombotic lesion of the thoracic spinal cord. In addition, a preliminary report *(32)* also found increased penetration of dorsal root axons into the spinal cord, reportedly reaching motor neurons. However, a recent study by Lieberman and coworkers *(33)*, may indicate that this is due, at least in part, to enhanced sprouting and/or sparing of dorsal column fibers; by contrast, GPI-1046 lacks such activity *(33)*.

My laboratory recently reported *(34)* that FK506 increases the regeneration of spinal cord axons into a peripheral nerve autograft placed in the lumbar spinal cord. Most strikingly, FK506 was found to also promote the regeneration of rubrospinal neurons into the peripheral nerve grafted into the lumbar spinal cord *(34)* (*see* the section entitled Chronic Nerve Injury Models). This finding is unique because rubrospinal neurons injured at such a long distance from their cell bodies do not respond to a distal (lumbar) graft even in the presence of exogenous neurotrophins (i.e., BDNF and NT4)

(35). It remains to be determined whether FK506 (and its nonimmuno-suppressant derivatives) can promote long-distance axonal elongation directly in the injured spinal cord. Since it is unlikely that any single treatment will be effective in repairing spinal cord injuries, it will also be important to study the neuroimmunophilin ligands in conjuncture with nonneuronal growth-promoting cells for example, Schwann cells *(36)* or olfactory endothelial cells *(37–40).*

MECHANISM OF NERVE REGENERATION BY NEUROIMMUNOPHILIN LIGANDS

How do the neuroimmunophilins alter nerve regeneration? The calcineurin hypothesis originally proposed by Snyder and coworkers *(12)* and by Gold and coworkers *(10),* whereby inhibition of calcineurin leads to an increased level of GAP43 phosphorylation and consequent increased neurite elongation, albeit discredited *(1–3),* was a rationale hypothesis at the time and is, surprisingly, still being evoked *(41).* Through a series of studies, this hypothesis nevertheless uncovered an entirely new view on how regeneration is regulated *(21);* for a more detailed review, *see* ref. 8.

As part of the calcineurin hypothesis, it was initally assumed by myself *(10)* and by Snyder and coworkers *(12)* that the immunophilin mediating immunosuppression (i.e., FKBP12) also mediates the neurotrophic activity of the neuroimmunophilin ligands. However, FKBP12 is clearly not necessary for FK506 to promote neurite outgrowth, as shown by the ability of FK506 to maintain its neurotrophic activity in vitro using primary hippocampal neurons from FKBP12 knockout mice *(21).* In contrast, the neurotrophic action of FK506 (examined in human neuroblastoma SH-SY5Y cells) is completely prevented by addition of a monoclonal antibody to the immunophilin FKBP52 (FKBP59 or hsp56) *(21),* a component of mature steroid receptor complexes. The finding that the FKBP52 antibody *(21),* which does not bind FKBP12, is also neurotrophic further showed that binding to FKBP12 is not necessary to elicit enhanced neurite elongation. Moreover, the discovery of nonimmunosuppressant FK506 derivatives that do not bind FKBP12 (e.g., V-13,670) yet demonstrate potent neurotrophic activity (B. G. Gold and D. M. Armistead, unpublished observation) *(42,43)* further demonstrates that FKBP12 does not mediate the neurotrophic activity of neuroimmunophilin ligands.

An important clue to unraveling how FKBP52 mediates this neurotrophic activity was the finding *(21)* that geldanamycin (a benzoquinone ansamycin that selectively binds to hsp90, disrupting mature steroid receptor complexes and releasing p23 from hsp90 [*see* references cited in *(8,21)*] is also neurotrophic at low (0.1–10 n*M*) concentrations. Conversely, preventing disruption of mature steroid receptor complexes by treatment with molybdate decreases the neurotrophic activity of the neuroimmunophilin ligands, as well as geldanamycin and the FKBP52 antibody *(21)*. Based upon these findings, I proposed *(21)* that the neurotrophic action of these compounds is associated with dissociation of steroid receptor complexes.

The down-stream signaling components activated by dissociation of the steroid receptor complex are unknown. However, several, albeit not mutually exclusive, possibilities exist. One involves the mitogen-associated protein (MAP) kinase pathway. This possibility is strongly implicated by the ability of the MAP kinase kinase (MEK) inhibitor PD 098059, at relatively low (0.1–10 µ*M*) concentrations, to completely inhibit the neurotrophic activity of FK506, geldanamycin, and radicicol (a macrolactone antifungal compound that acts similarly to geldanamycin). Thus, one or more of the mature steroid receptor chaperone components (i.e., FKBP52, hsp90 and p23) may elicit a "gain-of-function" to augment the MAP kinase signal transduction pathway, known to be employed by the neurotrophins *(44)*. Such a mechanism appears to support crosstalk between neuroimmunophilins and NGF, as originally suggested by Snyder and coworkers *(12)*. Additional possibilities include altered retrograde signaling to the nucleus by FKBP52, via its association with the retrograde motor dynein *(45,46)*, and an increase in GAP43 synthesis *(47)* (*see* the section entitled Mechanisms Underlying an Acceleration in Rate), this being different from an increase in GAP43 phosphorylation.

MECHANISMS UNDERLYING AN ACCELERATION IN RATE

How do these molecular alterations, dissociation of steroid receptor complex chaperone proteins (e.g., hsp90, hsp70, FKBP52, p23) leading to a "gain in function" in one or more of these components *(21)*, manifest as an increase in rate? One clue is suggested by the recent finding *(48)* that hsp70 releases membrane bound vesicles from kinesin fast transport. This could lead to an increase in membrane insertion into growth cone and, consequently, an increase in rate. The kinesin tandem repeat domains mediating cargo transport show sequence identity with tetratricopeptide (TPR) domains *(49)* present in FKBP52 (for a more complete discussion, *see* ref. *8*). Thus, FKBP52, which undergoes fast axonal transport (B. G. Gold and H. S. Gordon, unpublished observation) and is associated with retrograde signaling via its ability to bind dynein *(45)*, may function similarly to hsp70 to release transported cargo in regenerating axons following its dissociation from the steroid receptor complex *(21)*. In addition, an increase in synthesis of GAP43

(47) could also lead to such an increase in the insertion of new membrane into the growth cone *(50)*.

An additional possibility is an increase in Schwann cell proliferation *(51)*, which could lead to an increase in the local release of neurotrophic factors. However, an increase in Schwann cell proliferation was only observed at very high concentrations (0.1 m*M*) of FK506 in vitro. Furthermore, such a mechanism is not supported by the failure of FK506 to increase nerve regeneration following chronic denervation (*see* the section entitled Chronic Nerve Injury Models). Finally, although an increased removal of myelin debris *(51)* could increase regeneration, such an effect would most likely reduce the delay to onset and not lead to a real increase in rate; this is supported by the earlier appearance of growing axons into the nerve graft *(51)*. Nevertheless, it is likely that multiple mechanisms underlie the ability of neuroimmunophilin ligands to accelerate and promote nerve regeneration in the peripheral nerve and spinal cord.

CONCLUSIONS

In conclusion, it will be important to unravel the specifics of this mechanism, in particular to determine the ultimate downstream determinants. Regardless, given the present use of FK506 for hand and limb transplantations and the clinical trials underway for two neuroimmunophilin ligands (*see* the Introduction section of this chapter), advances in development of clinically useful drugs have not been hampered by this lack of knowledge. Nevertheless, for developing more selective neuroimmunophilin ligands, components of steroid receptor complexes should become valuable screening tools for the discovery of new classes of compounds with neurotrophic activity as well as targets for the design of novel immunophilin ligands for use as neuroregenerative drugs.

ACKNOWLEDGMENT

I thank Rhonda Rae for secretarial assistance.

REFERENCES

1. Steiner JP, Hamilton GS, Ross DT, et al. Neurotrophic immunophilin ligands stimulate structural and functional recovery in neurodegenerative animal models. Proc Natl Acad Sci USA 1997;94:2019–2024.
2. Steiner JP, Connolly MA, Valentine HL, et al. Neurotrophic actions of nonimmunosuppressive analogues of immunosuppressive drugs FK506, rapamycin and cyclosporin A. Nature Med 1997;3:421–428.
3. Gold BG, Zeleny-Pooley M, Wang M-S, et al. A nonimmunosuppressant FKBP-12 ligand increases nerve regeneration. Exp Neurol 1997;147:269–278.

4. Gold BG, Zeleny-Pooley M, Chaturvedi P, Wang M-S. Oral administration of a nonimmunosuppressant FKBP-12 ligand speeds nerve regeneration. NeuroReport 1998;9:553–558.

5. Hamilton GS. Immunophilin ligands for the treatment of neurological disorders. Exp Opin Ther Patents 1998;8:1109–1124.

6. Dubernard J-M, Owen E, Herzberg G, et al. Human hand allograft: report on first 6 months. Lancet 1999;353:1315–1320.

7. Jones JW, Gruber SA, Barker JH, Breidenbach WC. Successful hand transplantation: One year follow-up. N Engl J Med 2000;343:468–473.

8. Gold BG. Neuroimmunophilin ligands and the role of steroid hormone chaperone proteins in nerve regeneration. In: Gold BG, Fischer G, Herdegen T, ed. In Immunophilins the Brain. FKBP-Ligands: Novel Strategies for the Treatment of Neurodegenerative Disorders. Prous Science, Barcelona, Spain, 2000, pp. 3—22.

9. Gold BG, Storm-Dickerson T, Austin DR, Katoh K. FK506, an immunosuppressant, increases functional recovery and axonal regeneration in the rat following axotomy of the sciatic nerve. Soc Neurosci Abstr, 1993;19:1316.

10. Gold BG, Storm-Dickerson T, Austin DR. The immunosuppressant FK506 increases functional recovery and nerve regeneration following peripheral nerve injury. Restor Neurol Neurosci 1994;6:287–296.

11. Gold BG. Axonal regeneration of sensory neurons is delayed by continuous intrathecal infusion of nerve growth factor. Neuroscience 1997;76:1153–1158.

12. Lyons WE, George EB, Dawson TM, et al. Immunosuppressant FK506 promotes neurite outgrowth in cultures of PC12 cells and sensory ganglia. Proc Natl Acad Sci USA 1994;91:3191–3195.

13. Parker EM, Monopoli A, Ongini E, et al. Rapamycin, but not FK506 and GPI-1046, increases neurite outgrowth in PC12 cells by inhibiting cell cycle progression. Neuropharmacol 2000;39:1913–1919.

14. Lee M, Doolabh VB, Mackinnon SE, Jost S. FK506 promotes functional recovery in crushed rat sciatic nerve. Muscle Nerve 2000;23:633–640.

15. Kanje M, Lundborg G, Edström A. A new method for studies of the effects of locally applied drugs on peripheral nerve regeneration in vivo. Brain Res 1988;439:116–121.

16. Wang MS, Zeleny-Pooley M, Gold BG. Comparative dose-dependence study of FK506 and cyclosporin A on the rate of axonal regeneration in rat sciatic nerve. J Pharmacol Exp Ther 1997;282:1084–1093.

17. Gold BG. FK506 and the role of immunophilins in nerve regeneration. Mol Neurobiol 1997;15:285–306.

18. Costantini LC, Isacson O. Immunophilin ligands and GDNF enhance neurite branching or elongation from developing dopamine neurons in culture. Exp Neurol 2000;164:60–70.

19. Sharkey J, Butcher SP. Immunophilins mediate the neuroprotective effects of FK506 in focal cerebral ischaemia. Nature 1994;371:336–339.

20. Chang HY, Takei K, Sydor AM, et al. Asymmetric retraction of growth cone filopodia following focal inactivation of calcineurin. Nature 1995;376:686–690.

21. Gold BG, Densmore V, Shou W, et al. Immunophilin FK506-binding protein 52 (not FK506-binding protein 12) mediates the neurotrophic action of FK506. J Pharmacol Exp Therap 1999;289:1202–1210.
22. Doolabh VB, Mackinnon SE. FK506 accelerates functional recovery following nerve grafting in a rat model. Plast Reconstr Surg 1999;103:1928–1936.
23. Archibald SJ, Wang M-S, Gold BG. FK506 accelerates axonal regeneration through an artificial nerve guide in the rat sciatic nerve transection model. J Peripheral Nerv System 1999;4:202.
24. Madison RD, Archibald SJ. Point sources of Schwann cells result in growth into a nerve entubulation repair site in the absence of axons: Effects of freeze-thawing. Exp Neurol 1994;128:266–275.
25. Madison RD, Archibald SJ, Lacin R, Krarup C. Factors contributing to preferential motor reinnervation in the primate peripheral nervous system. J Neuroci 1999;19:11,007–11,016.
26. Ceballos D, Navarro X, Dubey N, et al. Magnetically aligned collagen gel filling a collagen nerve guide improves peripheral nerve regeneration. Exp Neurol 1999;158:290–300.
27. Rodríguez FJ, Gómez N, Labrador RO, et al. Improvement of regeneration with predegenerated nerve transplants in silicone chambers. Restor Neurol Neurosci 1999;14:65–79.
28. Sulaiman OAR, Voda J, Gold BG, Gordon T. FK506 Increases Peripheral Nerve Regeneration after Chronic Axotomy but not After Chronic Schwann Cell Denervation. Exp Neurol 2002;175:127–137.
29. Fu SY, Gordon T. The cellular and molecular basis of peripheral nerve regeneration. Mol Neurobiol 1997;14:67–116.
30. Madsen JR, MacDonald P, Irwin N, Benowitz LI. FK-506 improves behavioral recovery and upregulates neuronal expression of GAP-43 after spinal cord injury in rats. Soc Neurosci Abstr 1996;22:264.
31. Madsen JR, MacDonald P, Irwin N, et al. Tacrolimus (FK-506) increases neuronal expression of GAP-43 mRNA in parallel to enhanced recovery after spinal cord injury in rats. Soc Neurosci Abstr 1997;23:1129.
32. Sugawara T, Itoh Y, Mori E, et al. Immunosuppressive agents enhance regeneration of adult dorsal root axons into spinal cord. Soc Neurosci Abstr 1995;21:315.
33. Bavetta S, Hamlyn PJ, Burnstock G, et al. The effects of FK506 on dorsal column axons following spinal cord injury in adult rats: neuroprotection and local regeneration. Exp Neurol 1999;158:382–393.
34. Wang M-S, Gold BG. FK506 increases the regeneration of spinal cord axons in a predegenerated peripheral nerve autograft. J Spinal Cord Med 1999; 22:287–296.
35. Kobayashi NR, Fan D-P, Giehl KM, et al. BDNF and NT-4/5 prevent atrophy of rat rubrospinal neurons after cervical axotomy, stimulate GAP-43 and Ta1-tubulin mRNA expression, and promote axonal regeneration. J Neurosci 1997;17:9583–9595.
36. Menei P, Montero-Menei C, Whittemore SR, et al. Schwann cells genetically modified to secrete human BDNF promote enhanced axonal regrowth across transected adult rat spinal cord. Eur J Neurosci 1998;10:607–621.

37. Li Y, Feld PM, Raisman G. Repair of adult rat corticospinal tract by transplants of olfactory ensheathing cells. Science 1997;277:2000–2002.
38. Ramón-Cueto A, Plant GW, Avila J, Bunge,MB. Long-distance axonal regeneration in the trasected adult rat spinal cord is promoted by olfactory ensheathing glia transplants. J Neurosci 1998;18:3803–3815.
39. Navarro X, Valero A, Gudiño G, et al. Ensheathing glia transplants promote dorsal root regeneration and spinal reflex restitution after multiple lumbar rhizotomy. Ann Neurol 1999;45:207–215.
40. Li Y, Field PM, Raisman G. Regeneration of adult rat corticospinal axons induced by transplanted olfactory ensheathing cells. J Neurosci 1998; 18:10,514–10,524.
41. Diaz-Ruiz A, Rios C, Duarte I, et al. Lipid peroxidation inhibition in spinal cord injury: cyclosporin-A vs methylprednisolone. NeuroReport 2000;11: 1765–1767.
42. Gold BG. Compositions and methods for promoting nerve regeneration. US Patent 5,968,921.
43. Cole DG, Ogenstad S, Chaturvedi P. (2000) Pharmacological activities of neurophilin ligands. In: Gold BG, Fischer G, Herdegen T, ed. Immunophilins in the Brain. FKBP-Ligands: Novel Strategies for the Treatment of Neurodegenerative Disorders. Prous Science, Barcelona, Spain, 2000, pp. 109–116.
44. Chao MV. Growth factor signaling: Where is the specificity? Cell 1992;68: 995–997.
45. Silverstein AM, Galigniana MD, Radanyi C, et al. Different regions of the immunophilin FKBP52 determine its association with the glucocorticoid receptor, hsp90, and cytoplasmic dynein. J Biol Chem 1999;274:36,980–36,986.
46. Pratt WB, Silverstein AM, Galigniana MD. A model for the cytoplasmic trafficking of signaling proteins involving the hsp90-binding immunophilin FKBP52. In: Gold BG, Fischer G, Herdegen T, ed. Immunophilins in the Brain. FKBP-lLgands: Novel Strategies for the Treatment of Neurodegenerative Disorders Prous Science, Barcelona, Spain, 2000, pp. 37–47.
47. Gold BG, Yew JY, Zeleny-Pooley M. The immunosuppressant FK506 increases GAP-43 mRNA levels in axotomized sensory neurons. Neurosci Lett 1998;241:25–28.
48. Tsai M-Y, Morfini G, Szebenyi G, Brady ST. Release of kinesin from vesicles by hsc70 and regulation of fast axonal transport. Mol Biol Cell 2000;11: 2161–2173.
49. Gindhart Jr, JG, Goldstein LSB. Tetratrico peptide repeats are present in the kinesin light chain. Trends Biochem Sci 1996;21:52–53.
50. Benowitz LI, Routtenberg A. GAP-43: An intrinsic determinant of neuronal development and plasticity. Trends Neurosci 1997;20:84–91.
51. Fansa H, Keilhoff G, Horn T, et al. Stimulation of Schwann cell proliferation and axonal regeneration by FK 506. Restor Neurol Neurosci 2000;16:77–86.

17
Neuroimmunophilin Ligands Stimulate Recovery of Injured Sciatic Nerves

Joseph P. Steiner, Heather Valentine, Theresa Morrow, and Gregory Hamilton

INTRODUCTION

In clinical medicine the immunosuppressive drugs FK506 and cyclosporin A have been used for over 15 yr for organ transplantation *(1–4)*. Traditional immunosuppressive drugs function by inhibiting cell division. Lymphocytes proliferate more rapidly than other cell types, thus targeting them for elimination. However, this lack of specificity results in high toxicity. The development of the more selective immunosuppressive drugs FK506 and CsA has led to a decrease in toxicity and has had a great impact on the success of clinical organ transplantation.

Many studies have shown that both FK506 and CsA achieve their immunosuppressive goals by blocking early calcium-dependent events that regulate IL-2 production, ultimately preventing the activation of antigen-specific T cells *(5,6)*. FK506 binds to a small high-affinity receptor protein, FK506 binding protein 12 (FKBP12), while cyclosporin A specifically interacts with cyclophilin A *(7–9)*. FKBP12 and cyclophilin A both catalyze the isomerization of peptide proline residues between *cis* and *trans* conformations, and upon binding they inhibit this rotamase activity *(8–11)*. Also, complexes of FK506–FKBP12 and CsA–cyclophilin A bind to and inhibit a common target protein, calcineurin, which possesses calcium–calmodulin-dependent protein phosphatase activity *(12,13)*. In T cells, a key substrate of calcineurin is the phosphorylated form of the transcription factor family, nuclear factor of activated cells (NFAT), whose activation plays a key role in cytokine gene expression, including IL-2 *(14)*. NFAT enters the nucleus only after it is dephosphorylated by calcineurin, and inhibition of calcineurin phosphatase activity by drug-immunophilin complexes leads to the retention of NFAT in the cytoplasm, thereby providing the basis for immunosuppression.

From: *Immunosuppressant Analogs in Neuroprotection*
Edited by: C. V. Borlongan, O. Isacson, and P. R. Sanberg © Humana Press Inc., Totowa, NJ

Binding studies using [^{3}H]FK506 showed that binding was 50-fold greater in the central nervous system (CNS) and the peripheral nervous system (PNS) over peripheral tissues *(15,16)*, and FKBP12 colocalized with the target protein calcineurin *(16)*. Cyclophilin also colocalizes with calcineurin in the CNS *(15,17)*. While colocalization data often imply relevant associations between two proteins, immunophilins are also found in organisms that lack calcineurin, suggesting that they might associate with other proteins as well.

Functionally, addition of FK506 to brain homogenates increases the phosphorylation level of many phosphoproteins. One of these FK506-targeted proteins, GAP43 (growth associated protein of 43 kDa), has been linked to the neuronal regeneration process. GAP43 is an abundant component of growth cones expressed at high levels during development when neural connections are being formed *(18)*. Overexpression of GAP43 in neurons leads to spontaneous sprouting of axonal terminals and abnormalities in axonal pathfinding *(19,20)* and when coexpressed with another growth cone associated protein, CAP23, triggers a 60-fold increase in regeneration of DRG axons in adult mice after spinal cord injury in vivo *(21)*. GAP43 is phosphorylated at serine-41 by protein kinase C and is dephosphorylated by calcineurin and other phosphatases *(22)*. In vitro, FK506 inhibits calcineurin, leading to significant increases in the amount of phosphorylated GAP43 *(16)*. Following lesions to neurons, an early cellular response is the rapid and dramatic up-regulation of GAP43 expression. In fact, in experiments in which the facial nerve is transected, there is a significant increase in mRNA for GAP43 in the facial nucleus. Likewise, there is a concomitant up-regulation of FKBP12 mRNA in the same facial nucleus with the same spatiotemporal distribution. Yet another activity linked to GAP43 is that of synaptic targeting and neuronal process extension *(23)*. These studies link the immunophilin proteins with the neuronal regenerative process and suggest that further studies to elucidate the mechanism by which FK506 and similar drugs regulate GAP43 expression and function may be of clinical importance.

Immunohistochemical studies looking at FKBP12 expression in the nervous system has provided hints about how immunophilins might function. Because of their high levels of expression in neurons and link to the neuroregenerative process, we wished to evaluate the role of immunophilin proteins in the neurite outgrowth process. We chose to address this issue by evaluating the effects of the neuroimmunophilin ligand FK506 on neurite outgrowth in two model systems, pheochromocytoma cells (PC12) and explant cultures of dorsal root ganglia. In experiments with PC12 cells, we found that treating latent PC12 cells with FK506 did not affect neurite outgrowth. Cells treated with the maximal dose of nerve growth factor

(50 ng/mL NGF) were also unaffected by FK506 treatment. However, treatment of PC 12 cells with a suboptimal dose of NGF (0.5–1 ng/mL) and 100 nM FK506, elicited striking neurite outgrowth that was comparable to 50 ng/mL NGF *(24)*. We quantitated the number of cells bearing processes as a fraction of total PC12 cell number. The data suggested the FK506 increased the sensitivity of the PC12 cells to NGF. In the DRG explant model system, treatment of sensory neurons with FK506 elicited neurite outgrowth in the absence of any exogenously added neurotrophic factor *(24)*. Maximal neurite outgrowth was observed in cultures treated with 100 nM FK506. In summary, the neuroimmunophilin ligand FK506 stimulated significant neurite outgrowth in each of these cell culture systems.

Inhibition of calcineurin and the accompanying immunosuppressive actions of FK506 are not responsible for the neurotrophic effects of neuroimmunophilin ligands. In a series of studies *(25)*, both immunosuppressive and nonimmunosuppressive ligands of neuroimmunophilins stimulated neurite outgrowth in these two cell culture models. These ligands dose dependently and potently potentiated the actions of NGF in the PC12 cells and stimulated neuronal process formation in sensory ganglion explants. The neurotrophic actions of these compounds in cell culture models suggested that these molecules might facilitate neuronal regeneration in vivo.

The immunosuppressant drug FK506 accelerated the recovery of damaged peripheral nerves in studies published a few years ago *(26,27)*. In these studies, both morphological and functional improvement of lesioned sciatic nerves following FK506 drug treatment was monitored. The nerve was crushed at the level of the hip and behavioral recovery was assessed by determining the time until the rats to bear weight on the injured limb, the distance of toe spread between the outermost digits and time to walk properly on hindlimb and toes of the injured limb. Morphological recovery was assessed by determining axonal caliber of the tibial nerve by EM analysis, and by measuring the rate of axonal regeneration by radioisotopic labeling of the dorsal root ganglion. While rats with lesioned sciatic nerves treated with vehicle were just beginning to bear weight on the injured hindpaw, rats with crushed sciatic nerves treated with FK506 were walking normally by d 18 postlesion. Morphologically, increased axonal caliber was the result of FK506 treatment and the rate of axonal regeneration was likewise increased after treatment of the lesioned rats with FK506. The optimal dose of FK506 to produce these accelerated regenerative effects in the sciatic nerve lesions was 5 mg/kg *(26–28)*. This dose of FK506 is known to be immunosuppressive and inhibit T-cell proliferation via inhibition of calcineurin. We wished to test the hypothesis that a neurotrophic but nonimmunosuppressive neuroimmunophilin ligands could stimulate recovery of the lesioned sciatic nerves.

NEURONAL REGENERATION
FOLLOWING SCIATIC NERVE CRUSH

We treated rats whose sciatic nerve had been crushed at the level of the hip with FK506 (1 mg/kg in Gelfoam) and the nonimmunosuppressive analog of FK506, L-685,818 (1 mg/kg in Gelfoam) (*see* Fig. 1 for structures and also Table 1). Lesioned animals treated with vehicle displayed a majority of axons with very small diameter and cross-sectional area. Animals treated with either FK506 or L-685818 display an increased number of larger-sized axons compared to vehicle-treated lesioned animals. The average caliber of the axons treated with neuroimmunophilin ligands is significantly larger than those of the lesioned animals and is about 60% of sham-operated control animals. Furthermore, myelination levels are increased following neuroimmunophilin ligand treatment. Sciatic nerve crush caused a 90% decrease in myelination levels in lesioned animals compared to sham-operated controls. Treatment of lesioned animals with FK506 and L-685,818 restored 20–30% of control myelination levels in the sciatic nerve axons. Augmented myelination implies a greater rate of neuronal regeneration associated with treatment by neuroimmunophilin ligands.

We also observed a more rapid functional recovery of the injured hindlimb following neuroimmunophilin ligand treatment. We monitored the ability of the animals to bear weight and regain use of the injured hindlimb by measuring the internal toe spread distance. At 14 d postlesion, the lesioned animals treated with vehicle, FK506, or L-685,818 all showed the same toe spread distance relative to normal control animals or sham-operated rats. These data suggested that the neuroimmunophilin ligands did not protect against degeneration of the axons following nerve crush. At 18 d postlesion, FK506- and L-685818-treated animals displayed significant recovery, regaining nearly completely the ability to bear weight on the injured limb and with interdigit toe spread values at 95% of control levels. The vehicle-treated lesioned animals showed significantly less weight bearing and toe-spread distance. These data indicated that the neuroimmunophilin ligands promote and accelerate neuronal regeneration of the lesioned sciatic nerves.

Using the principles of structure-based drug design, low-molecular-weight small-molecule neuroimmunophilin ligands were synthesized *(25)*. These molecules bound to FKBP12 specifically, and inhibited the enzymatic peptidylprolyl-*cis-trans* isomerase activity of the neuroimmunophilin FKBP12 *(25)*. These two compounds elicited significant neurite outgrowth in cell cultures developed from embryonic chick dorsal root ganglion explants. Increases in process number, the length of the neurites, and den-

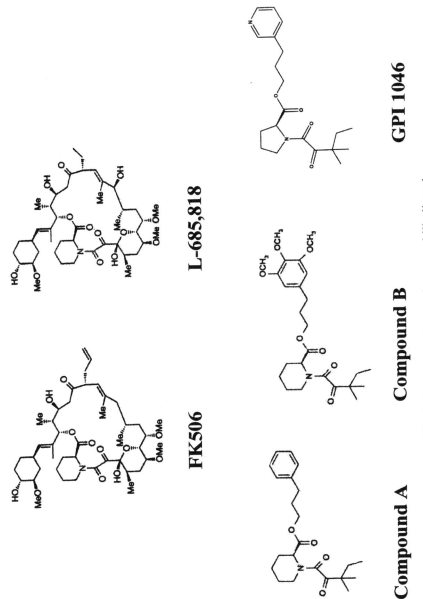

FK506 **L-685,818**

Compound A **Compound B** **GPI 1046**

Fig. 1. Structures of neuroimmunophilin ligands.

Table 1
Regeneration of Lesioned Rat Sciatic Nerves

Treatment	Axonal diameter (μm)	Cross-sectional area (μm²)	Myelination
Study I			
Sham	2.98 ± 0.221	9.14 ± 0.835	60.07
Lesion/Vehicle	1.56 ± 0.73	2.74 ± 0.357	5.30
Lesion/FK506	1.99 ± 0.192	4.16 ± 0.403	11.67
Lesion/L-685818	1.87 ± 0.141	3.43 ± 0.295	16.68
Study II			
Sham	2.62 ± 0.179	8.69 ± 0.503	55.98
Lesion/Vehicle	1.40 ± 0.204	2.54 ± 0.376	2.95
Lesion/Compound A	2.06 ± 0.360	5.04 ± 0.403	21.13
Lesion/Compound B	1.81 ± 0.123	3.84 ± 0.281	ND
Study III			
Sham	3.46 ± 0.148	12.04 ± 0.949	63.44 ± 8.50
Lesion/Vehicle	1.94 ± 0.071	4.61 ± 0.324	3.18 ± 1.59
Lesion/GPI 1046-3	2.66 ± 0.079	8.62 ± 0.452	21.66 ± 5.94
Lesion/GPI 1046-10	2.74 ± 0.042	8.87 ± 0.337	24.31 ± 7.61

Animals lesioned by sciatic nerve crush were treated as described for individual drugs and sacrificed on d 18 of gfeh experiment. Diameter and cross sectional area of axons were quantitated from antineurofilament staining. Myelin leves were quantitated from myelin basic protein-immunoreactive staining density. FK506 and L-685818 (1 mg/kg in intralipid) were administered in Gelfoam directly to the site of the lesion. Compounds A and B were administered at 30 mg/kg sc once a day for 18 d. GPI-1046 was administered at 3 or 10 mg/kg sc once a day for 18 d.

sity or branching of the dendritic arbors was observed following neuro-immunophilin ligand treatment.

Following demonstration of an in vitro neurite outgrowth promoting activity in cell culture, these neuroimmunophilin ligands (GPI-1046, compounds A and B in Fig. 1) were evaluated for efficacy in the sciatic nerve crush model *(25)*. The sciatic nerve of the rats was crushed by two 30-s applications of jeweler's forceps, and the animals were monitored for behavioral and morphological improvement over the ensuing 21 d. Behaviorally, lesioned rats treated with GPI-1046, compounds A and B were able to bear weight on the injured hindlimb sooner than vehicle-treated rats. Toe-spread distances were increased and comparable to sham-lesioned rats following neuroimmunophilin drug treatment. Morphologically, the axonal caliber and cross-sectional area of axons in the sciatic nerve were quantitated at a distance 2 mm distal to the crush site. (*See* Table 1.) Significant decreases in caliber and cross-sectional area of about 50% were observed at this area relative to the crush site. Treatment of rats with crushed sciatic nerves with the neuroimmunophilin compounds stimulated increased axonal diameter and cross-sectional area (*see* Fig. 2 and Table 1) *(25,29)*. Average increases of 40–50% in axonal diameter and area following neuro-immunophilin drug treatment compared to vehicle-treated rats was found.

Perhaps the most striking feature of neuroimmunophilin drug treatment of animals with lesioned sciatic nerves was the level of myelination achieved after the drug treatment (*see* Fig. 3 and Table 1). Lesioning of the sciatic nerve in this model resulted in a very significant level of myelin degeneration. This deficit in myelination was apparent in light micrographs of axons in cross section, which shows incomplete myelination of axons and myelin fragments and debris staining with myelin basic protein. The overall level of myelin basic protein–immunoreactive material in the sections was only 5–10% of the levels in sham-operated control animals. Lesioned animals treated with neuroimmunophilin compounds displayed highly significant increases in levels of remyelination, in some cases to 30–40% of sham-operated control animals. The axons of animals treated with neuro-immunophilin ligands are decorated with relatively uniform myelin bands surrounding the axons, and much less evidence of myelin fragmentation and degeneration, compared to lesioned animals treated with vehicle.

DISCUSSION

Both immunosuppressant and nonimmunosuppressant immunophilin ligands promote nerve regeneration, both with respect to axon number and caliber and myelination level following sciatic nerve crush. The enhanced neuronal regeneration is associated with augmented functional recovery. While FK506 also accelerated morphological and functional recovery of injured sciatic nerves, the doses required for optimal effects were 5–10 mg/kg, which would suppress immune function. Immunosuppression with FK506 has been shown to lead to toxic side effects on kidney and liver function *(30–32)*. However, accelerated functional recovery of lesioned peripheral nerves with nonimmunosuppressive neuroimmunophilin ligands is antici-pated to be free of the adverse events, which are related to calcineurin inhi-bition *(33)*. Chronic administration of a neurorestorative agent, such as a neuroimmunophilin ligand, would avoid the toxicities associated with FK506 treatment.

In addition to avoiding toxicities associated with immunosuppression, nonimmunosuppressive neuroimmunophilin ligands also do not elicit

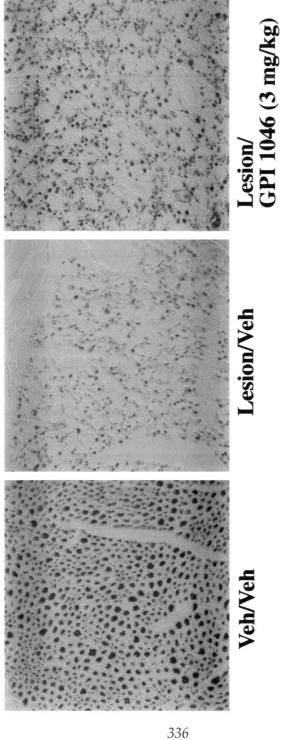

Veh/Veh   **Lesion/Veh**   **Lesion/ GPI 1046 (3 mg/kg)**

Fig. 2. Neuroimmunophilin ligands promote neuronal regeneration following sciatic nerve crush. Rats with crushed sciatic nerves were treated with vehicle or 3 mg/kg/d GPI-1046 subcutaneously daily for 18 d. Sciatic nerve sections (4–5 μm) of the injured nerves were made at a distance of 2–3 mm distal to the crush site. These sections were stained with anti-Pan axonal neurofilament Ig to stain the axons. The magnification of each micrograph is ×630.

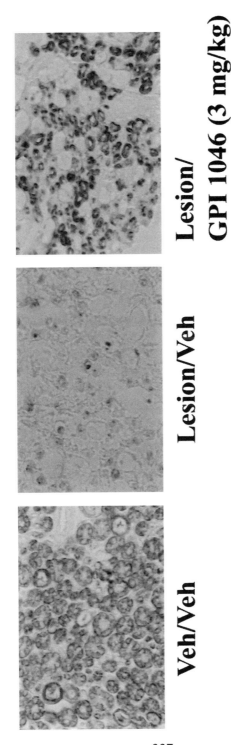

Veh/Veh　　　　　**Lesion/Veh**　　　　　**Lesion/ GPI 1046 (3 mg/kg)**

Fig. 3. Neuroimmunophilin ligands promote remyelination of injured sciatic nerves. Rats with crushed sciatic nerves were treated with vehicle or 3 mg/kg/d GPI-1046 subcutaneously daily for 18 d. Sciatic nerve sections (4–5 μm) of the injured nerves were made at a distance of 2–3 mm distal to the crush site. These sections were stained with antimyelin basic protein Ig to detect myelin levels. The magnification of each micrograph is ×630.

abnormal or aberrant sprouting of noninjured neurons. We see no evidence of sprouting or increased axonal outgrowth from healthy neurons. Likewise, axonal caliber and myelination levels in the sciatic nerves of neuroimmunophilin ligand-treated sham-operated rats are indistinguishable from normal control rats. These drugs apparently have specificity for acting on injured neurons, and thus target only the susceptible and vulnerable neurons in both the peripheral and central nervous system *(29,34)*. This selectivity for action on injured nerves may also enhance the projected safety profile for use of neuroimmunophilin ligands in the treatment of neurodegenerative disorders.

Drugs, such as the nonimmunosuppressive neuroimmunophilin ligands, which accelerate the recovery of injured peripheral nerves, may prove therapeutically useful in treating peripheral sensory neuropathy. Neuroimmunophilin ligands might be employed to treat painful sensory neuropathies induced by chemotherapeutic agents, such as paclitaxel and platinum-containing compounds. Recently, we have found that the neuroimmunophilin ligand GPI-1046 has demonstrated efficacy in ameliorating the sensitivity to painful stimuli in both paclitaxel- and cisplatin-treated rats *(35)*. The hyperalgesia observed in sensory testing of rats chronically treated with these agents is decreased by GPI-1046 treatment *(35)*. We have also found that the sensory deficits associated with hyperglycemia (streptozotocin-induced diabetic neuropathy) can be attenuated by GPI-1046 therapy *(36,37)*. GPI-1046 administered in a concurrent manner with the streptozotocin toxin blocks the onset of hypoalgesia associated with hyperglycemia. Likewise, protection of sensory nerve conduction velocity in the sciatic nerve of the GPI-1046-treated STZ-lesioned rats was observed. If the symptoms of sensory neuropathy are allowed to develop prior to GPI-1046 treatment, the neuroimmunophilin drug can reverse the hypoalgesia associated with painful sensory neuropathy *(36,37)*. GPI-1046 treatment of STZ-lesioned rats also stimulated the increase in sensory nerve conduction velocity, indicating a physiological recovery as well. Nonimmunosuppressive neuroimmunophilin ligands may represent an effective therapy for sensory neuropathic injuries.

Neuroimmunophilin ligands have elicited morphological and functional recovery in preclinical models of peripheral nerve injury. Chronic treatment with these agents has not demonstrated toxic events associated with their use. These compounds are small organic molecules that readily cross the blood–brain barrier and access their target, injured nerves and neurons in the nervous system. Small molecule agents, which are orally bioavailable, stimulate neuronal regrowth and protect injured neuronal cells, may provide a novel treatment for disorders of the peripheral nervous system.

REFERENCES

1. Bierer BE, Hollander G, Fruman D, Burakoff SJ. Cyclosporin A and FK506: molecular mechanisms of immunosuppression and probes for transplantation biology. Curr Opin Immunol 1993;5:763–773.
2. Henry ML. Cyclosporine and tacrolimus (FK506): a comparison of efficacy and safety profiles. Clin Transplant 1999;13:209–220.
3. Kahan BD. Cyclosporine: the base for immunosuppressive therapy—present and future. Transplant Proc 1993;25:508–510.
4. Spencer CM, Goa KL, Gillis JC. Tacrolimus. An update of its pharmacology and clinical efficacy in the management of organ transplantation. Drugs 1997;54:925–975.
5. Borel JF, Feurer C, Gubler HU, Stahelin H. Biological effects of cyclosporin A: a new antilymphocytic agent. 1976. Agents Actions 1994;43:179–186.
6. Kay JE, Benzie CR, Borghetti AF. Effect of cyclosporin A on lymphocyte activation by the calcium ionophore A23187. Immunology 1983;50:441–446.
7. Handschumacher RE, Harding MW, Rice J, et al. Cyclophilin: a specific cytosolic binding protein for cyclosporin A. Science 1984;226:544–547.
8. Harding MW, Galat A, Uehling DE, Schreiber SL. A receptor for the immunosuppressant FK506 is a cis-trans peptidyl- prolyl isomerase. Nature 1989;341:758–760.
9. Siekierka JJ, Hung SH, Poe M, et al. A cytosolic binding protein for the immunosuppressant FK506 has peptidyl-prolyl isomerase activity but is distinct from cyclophilin. Nature 1989;341:755–757.
10. Fischer G, Wittmann-Liebold B, Lang K, et al. Cyclophilin and peptidyl-prolyl cis-trans isomerase are probably identical proteins [see comments]. Nature 1989;337:476–478.
11. Takahashi N, Hayano T, Suzuki M. Peptidyl-prolyl cis-trans isomerase is the cyclosporin A-binding protein cyclophilin. Nature 1989;337:473–475.
12. Friedman J, Weissman I. Two cytoplasmic candidates for immunophilin action are revealed by affinity for a new cyclophilin: one in the presence and one in the absence of CsA. Cell 1991;66:799–806.
13. Liu J, Farmer JD Jr, Lane WS, et al. Calcineurin is a common target of cyclophilin-cyclosporin A and FKBP- FK506 complexes. Cell 1991;66:807–815.
14. Tocci MJ, Matkovich DA, Collier KA, et al. The immunosuppressant FK506 selectively inhibits expression of early T cell activation genes. J Immunol 1989;143:718–726.
15. Dawson TM, Steiner JP, Lyons WE, et al. The immunophilins, FK506 binding protein and cyclophilin, are discretely localized in the brain: relationship to calcineurin. Neuroscience 1994;62:569–580.
16. Steiner JP, Dawson TM, Fotuhi M, et al. High brain densities of the immunophilin FKBP colocalized with calcineurin. Nature 1992;358:584–587.
17. Goldner FM, Patrick JW. Neuronal localization of the cyclophilin A protein in the adult rat brain. J Comp Neurol 1996;372:283–293.
18. Skene JH. Axonal growth-associated proteins. Annu Rev Neurosci 1989;12: 127–156.

19. Aigner L, Arber S, Kapfhammer JP, et al. Overexpression of the neural growth-associated protein GAP43 induces nerve sprouting in the adult nervous system of transgenic mice. Cell 1995;83:269–278.

20. Widmer F, Caroni P. Phosphorylation-site mutagenesis of the growth-associated protein GAP- 43 modulates its effects on cell spreading and morphology. J Cell Biol 1993;120: 503–512

21. Bomze HM, Bulsara KR, Iskandar BJet al. Spinal axon regeneration evoked by replacing two growth cone proteins in adult neurons. Nat Neurosci 2001; 4:38–43.

22. Dokas LA, Pisano MR, Han YF. Selective phosphorylation and dephosphorylation of the protein B-50. Prog Brain Res 1991;89:27–36.

23. Meiri KF, Bickerstaff LE, Schwob JE. Monoclonal antibodies show that kinase C phosphorylation of GAP43 during axonogenesis is both spatially and temporally restricted in vivo. J Cell Biol 1991;112:991–1005.

24. Lyons WE, George EB, Dawson TM, et al. Immunosuppressant FK506 promotes neurite outgrowth in cultures of PC12 cells and sensory ganglia. Proc Natl Acad Sci USA 1994;91:3191–3195.

25. Steiner JP, Connolly MA, Valentine HL, et al. Neurotrophic actions of nonimmunosuppressive analogues of immunosuppressive drugs FK506, rapamycin and cyclosporin A. Nat Med 1997;3:421–428.

26. Gold BG, Katoh K, Storm-Dickerson T. The immunosuppressant FK506 increases the rate of axonal regeneration in rat sciatic nerve. J Neurosci 1995; 15:7509–7516.

27. Gold BG, Storm-Dickerson T, Austi, DR. The immunosuppresssant FK506 increases functional recovery and nerve regeneration following peripheral nerve injury. Restorative Neurol Neurosci 1994;6:287–296.

28. Gold BG, Zeleny-Pooley M, Wang MS, et al. A nonimmunosuppressant FKBP-12 ligand increases nerve regeneration. Exp Neurol 1997;147: 269–278.

29. Steiner JP, Hamilton GS, Ross DT, et al. Neurotrophic immunophilin ligands stimulate structural and functional recovery in neurodegenerative animal models. Proc Natl Acad Sci USA 1997;94:2019–2024.

30. Platz KP, Mueller AR, Blumhardt G, et al. Nephrotoxicity after orthotopic liver transplantation in cyclosporin A and FK 506-treated patients. Transpl Int 12984;7:S52–S57.

31. Platz KP, Mueller AR, Blumhardt G, et al. Nephrotoxicity following orthotopic liver transplantation. A comparison between cyclosporine and FK506. Transplantation 1994;58:170–178.

32. Porayko MK, Textor SC, Krom RA, et al. Nephrotoxicity of FK 506 and cyclosporine when used as primary immunosuppression in liver transplant recipients. Transplant Proc 1993;25:665–668.

33. Dumont FJ, Staruch MJ, Koprak SL, et al. The immunosuppressive and toxic effects of FK-506 are mechanistically related: pharmacology of a novel antagonist of FK-506 and rapamycin. J Exp Med 1992;176:751–760.

34. Hamilton GS, Steiner JP. Immunophilins: beyond immunosuppression. J Med Chem 1998;41:5119–5143.

35. Liang S, Valentine HL, Ramsey C, et al. Experimental Treatment of Cisplatin-induced peripheral neuropathy with a neuroimmunophilin ligand. Soc Neuroscience Abstr 1998;28.
36. Steiner J, Valentine HL, Chen Y, et al. Comparison of neuroprotective drug effects in the streptozotocin-induced rat model of diabetic neuropathy. Soc Neuroscience Abstr 2000;30.
37. Valentine HL, Spicer D, Fuller M, et al. Neuroimmunophilin ligands promote recovery from the peripheral sensory neuropathy associated with Streptozotocin-induced diabetes. Soc Neuroscience Abstr 1998;28.

VII

IMMUNOSUPPRESSANTS AND OTHER DISORDERS OF THE CENTRAL NERVOUS SYSTEM

18
Cyclosporin A Prolongs Survival of SOD1 Mutant Mice and Implicates Mitochondrial Permeability Transition in Amyotrophic Lateral Sclerosis

Marcus F. Keep, Keith S. K. Fong, Katalin Csiszar, and Eskil Elmér

INTRODUCTION

Amyotrophic Lateral Sclerosis

Amyotrophic lateral sclerosis (ALS) is a progressive upper and lower motor neuron degenerative disease characterized by loss of motor neurons in the spinal cord, brainstem, and motor cortex (1,2). It is the most common human motor neuron disease, so far without cure and with only limited treatment options. The combined loss of both upper and lower motor neurons and pyramidal tract degeneration creates a picture of progressive weakness with skeletal muscle wasting. Upper motor neuron loss is manifested histologically as corticospinal tract degeneration. Lower motor neuron loss is manifested as anterior horn and anterior nerve root atrophy. Brainstem motor nuclei cell loss usually spares the oculomotor cranial nerves. Ascending weakness leads to paralysis and death in 3–5 yr after diagnosis from loss of motor cranial nerves that coordinate swallowing and breathing (3). Sensation and cognition are generally unaffected.

Familial ALS and Mutant Copper/Zinc Sodium Dismutase

While about 90% of ALS is sporadic, 10% is familial (FALS), and characterized by additional pathological features that involve sensory fibers of the posterior columns as well as cerebellar projections in the lateral columns (4). FALS tends to manifest at an earlier age, and have a faster progression to death than the sporadic form; 20% of FALS cases are associated with a mutation in the Cu/Zn superoxide dismutase enzyme (Cu/Zn–SOD) that is inherited in an autosomal dominant fashion (5). Cu/Zn–SOD is a

From: *Immunosuppressant Analogs in Neuroprotection*
Edited by: C. V. Borlongan, O. Isacson, and P. R. Sanberg © Humana Press Inc., Totowa, NJ

cytosolic metalloenzyme that catalyzes the conversion of superoxide to hydrogen peroxide *(6)*. Working with other antioxidant enzymes such as catalase and glutathione peroxidase harmful oxygen free radicals are reduced to water and oxygen *(7)*. The SOD1–G93A missense mutation in the familial form of ALS substituting one amino acid for another has little effect on its free radical scavenging activity but may introduce adverse function (*see* below). Cu/Zn–SOD is located primarily in spinal cord motor neurons, cerebral cortex pyramidal cells, hippocampal pyramidal cells and the basal ganglia including the substantia nigra *(8)*.

The G93A Mutant SOD1 Animal Model of FALS

Several Cu/Zn–SOD transgenic mouse strains overexpressing mutant SOD genes identified in familial ALS have been generated. The mice display a phenotype similar to the human disease and in our work described below the Gly→Ala mutation at position 93 of the SOD enzyme (G93A) served as the model for human ALS. The strain was developed by Gurney et al. *(9)* and these mice develop a progressive, ascending paralysis similar to human ALS *(9–12)*. Disease usually starts with tremors and ends with hindlimb proximal atrophy *(9)* and complete paralysis of both hindlimbs at the time of euthanasia. At the onset of clinical disease (around 3 mo of age), significant death of somatic motor neurons innervating limb muscles has occurred; mice at end-stage disease show up to 50% loss of cervical and lumbar motor neurons. Dal Canto and Gurney *(13)* describe early vacuolar degeneration of neurons and processes of the anterior horn cells, with late stage Lewy body-like inclusions, cell loss, and anterior horn atrophy. Changes in mitochondria are among the earliest and begin at 1 mo of age. Mitochondria are severely affected with dilation of cristae progressing at late stages to fragmentation. Fluid accumulates within the mitochondrial membranes causing swelling. Mitochondria in adjacent interneurons are normal in appearance. Spinal white matter changes of descending corticospinal tracts in anterior and lateral columns at late stage disease showed moderate wallerian degeneration *(13)*.

PATHOGENESIS OF ALS

Selective Vulnerability of Motor Neurons

It is not known how the progression of the disease causes the selective death of specific populations of motor neurons while other neurons such as those controlling the extraocular muscles remain relatively unaffected. A number of factors that make spinal, bulbar, and cortical motor neurons more vulnerable than other neurons have been suggested.

High Level of Metabolism/Free-Radical Production

Large cell size and length (up to 1 meter in length for neurons controlling distal lower limb muscles) with special demands on intracellular transport and communication, require a high level of metabolism/ATP production. High metabolism requires a high density of mitochondria, which are the most important producers of free radicals in animal cells. In a newly developed in vitro model of chronic motor neuron toxicity, inhibition of complex II or IV in the mitochondrial electron-transport chain resulted in a dose-dependent decrease in cellular ATP levels. Motor neurons were significantly more vulnerable to mitochondrial inhibition than control neurons in the dorsal horn. Supporting a role for oxidative mechanisms in vulnerability, free radical scavengers were protective in this new model of ALS *(14)*.

Impaired Axonal Transport

There is increasing evidence implicating abnormalities of neurofilament function in the pathogenesis of ALS *(15,16)*. It has been proposed that neurofilament accumulations cause axonal degeneration by impeding the transport of components required for axonal maintenance *(17)*. In support of this notion, transgenic mice overexpressing the human NF-H gene, a model of ALS, revealed defects of intracellular transport both of cytoskeletal proteins and organelles such as mitochondria *(18–20)*.

Aberrant Glutamate–Calcium Neurotransmission

Two molecular features of motor neurons have been identified that may render them susceptible to calcium-mediated toxic events following glutamate receptor activation. a) Disturbed expression and function of the major glutamate reuptake transporter protein as well as the presence of certain calcium permeable glutamate receptors which differs from many CNS neuronal cell types *(21–24)*; b) the low expression of calcium-binding proteins *(25)*. Antibodies to voltage-gated calcium channels are observed in at least some patients with sporadic ALS and such antibodies may affect intracellular Ca^{2+} homeostasis in motor neurons *(26,27)*.

Mutant Cu/Zn Sodium Dismutase

In the 1–2% of ALS cases with a mutation of Cu/Zn-SOD a "gain of adverse function," such as the overproduction of hydroxyl radicals, peroxidase activity or an increased ability to react with peroxynitrite ($ONOO^-$) to form nitrated tyrosine residues on specific proteins have been proposed *(7,28–35)*. There is considerable controversy regarding the role of hydroxyl radicals *(36,37)*, and it is suggested that the gain of adverse function is the reduced affinity for zinc in the mutant enzyme that will convert peroxynitrite more readily into nitronium ions, increasing nitration of tyrosine residues

(16). Regardless of the origin, indisputable signs of oxidative damage or sensitivity to oxidizing agents have been demonstrated in several studies of mutant SOD1 cells in animals and in patients *(38–41).* Further supporting a role for oxidative damage in the pathogenesis of ALS is the demonstration of protective effects of antioxidative treatment in the experimental setting. In SOD1 mutants, various antioxidant compounds including vitamin E, selenium, carboxyfullerenes, D-penicillamine and *N*-acetyl-L-cysteine have been tested with varied effectiveness *(42–46).*

Some of these special features of motor neurons are likely related to physiological compensatory mechanisms connected with the special metabolic demands on the motor neuron but may at the same time render them vulnerable in situations of inherited or acquired dysfunction.

The Mitochondrial Hypothesis

Much evidence supports a central and crucial role for mitochondrial dysfunction in the chain of events leading to selective motor neuron death in experimental and human ALS. The current view favors a large heterogeneous group of primary disturbances (which includes mitochondrial defects) of cellular function leading to an increase in free-radical activity, mitochondrial dysfunction (and permeability transition), and subsequent execution of apoptotic cell death.

Experimental Evidence of Mitochondrial Involvement in the Pathogenesis of ALS

FALS mouse mitochondria have prominent pathological features of microvacuolarization, swelling, and distortion *(47)* and the demonstration of a marked increase in this vacuolization coincident with rapid motor decline suggests that mitochondrial function is directly linked to neuronal death *(48).* In G93A FALS mice there is a significant loss of mitochondrial membrane potential, an increased sensitivity toward the potassium ionophore valinomycin and a parallel increase in cytosolic Ca^{2+} concentration *(49).*

Bcl-2 is a mitochondrial outer membrane protein. It inhibits both apoptosis and necrosis, through prevention of the stress-triggered mitochondrial permeability transition (see below) and release of apoptogenic factors *(50–53).* Overexpressing Bcl-2 prolonged survival in FALS mutant mice by 12.5% *(54).* Supporting a notion of apoptotic cell death with mitochondrial origin in ALS is the finding that the proapoptotic proteins Bax and Bak are elevated and the protective Bcl-2 is decreased in the mitochondrial-enriched membrane compartment of vulnerable regions in ALS *(55).*

Further supporting an important role for the mitochondrial permeability transition in ALS is the demonstration by Klivenyi and colleagues *(43)* that oral administration of creatine (which stabilizes the mitochondrial creatine kinase and inhibits opening of the mitochondrial transition pore) produced a dose-dependent improvement in motor performance and extended survival in FALS mice.

Human Data Supporting Mitochondrial Involvement in the Pathogenesis of ALS

Reports of alterations in the function of the mitochondrial electron-transport chain include an increase in complex I and II–III activities in FALS *(56)*. In skeletal muscle homogenates derived from patients with sporadic ALS, an approximately twofold lower specific activity of complex I was found. The finding was confirmed by detailed analysis of mitochondrial oxidative phosphorylation using permeabilized muscle fibers and functional imaging of mitochondria which demonstrated partially respiratory chain inhibited mitochondria *(57)*. Furthermore, in sporadic ALS a selective decrease in the activity of the mitochondrial DNA-encoded complex IV in human spinal cord motor neurons has been demonstrated *(58–60)*.

Motor nerve terminals from human ALS specimens display increased calcium and increased mitochondrial volume compared to disease control groups *(61)*. In addition, increased basal oxygen consumption rate, induced by an uncoupler of oxidative phosphorylation, was depressed and the resting level of free cytosolic calcium was higher in lymphocytes from patients with the sporadic form of ALS *(62)*.

In a study designed to address whether aberration of mitochondrial DNA could play a role in the pathogenesis of ALS, mitochondrial DNA from ALS subjects was transferred to human neuroblastoma cells depleted of mitochondrial DNA. The resulting ALS cytoplasmic hybrids (cybrids) exhibited abnormal electron-transport chain functioning, increases in free radical scavenging enzyme activities, perturbed calcium homeostasis, and altered mitochondrial ultrastructure *(63)*.

In an early study, ultrastructural changes of hepatocytes were studied in liver biopsy specimens from ALS patients. Some of the pathological findings were bizarre giant mitochondria and intramitochondrial paracrystalline inclusions. The mitochondrial inclusions appeared to be a highly specific finding in ALS *(64)*.

CYCLOSPORIN A

A Powerful Neuroprotective Agent

Cyclosporin A (CsA) is a cyclic polyamino acid molecule, consisting of 11 amino acids. The molecule is highly lipophilic, and virtually insoluble in water. CsA is a well-known immunosuppressive agent and has been used for over two decades for organ transplantation and exerts this effect by binding to intracellular cyclophilins, and inhibiting the calcium-dependent serine–threonine protein phosphatase calcineurin within immune cells leading to suppression of cytokine gene expression and inhibition of T-lymphocyte action. However, it has been demonstrated that cyclophilins are highly enriched in neuronal cells, especially the motor nuclei of the brainstem and the spinal anterior horn *(65)*, and furthermore, CsA has recently been found to be a potent neuroprotective agent in animal models of global ischemia *(66–68)*, focal ischemia *(69–71)*, and traumatic brain injury *(72–76)* in situations where it can penetrate the blood–brain barrier. In addition cyclosporin has been shown to be protective in models of neurodegeneration: Parkinson's disease *(77–84)* and Huntington's disease *(85)*. The powerful neuroprotective effect of CsA is clearly separated from its actions on white blood cells and is attributed to its effect of stabilizing mitochondrial membranes (*see* below) and inhibiting neuronal calcineurin. This is demonstrated in experiments performed with nonimmunosuppressive analogs of CsA and FK506 (an immunosuppressive calcineurin inhibitor) in focal ischemia, hypoglycemic coma, and cortical impact models *(69,73,86)*.

Mitochondrial Permeability Transition

It is well established that CsA prevents the assembly of the mitochondrial permeability transition (mPT) pore. The assembly mechanisms as well as the constituents of the mPT pore remain unclear but it has been suggested that the pore forms at contact sites between the two mitochondrial membranes and proposed primary components include the adenine nucleotide transporter (ANT) in the inner mitochondrial membrane, matrix cyclophilin D and the voltage-dependent anion channel (VDAC) in the outer membrane *(87,88)*. The likelihood of pore formation is enhanced by mitochondrial depolarization, increased mitochondrial Ca^{2+} concentration, and oxidizing agents *(89–91)*. When formed, it allows rapid egress of solutes with a molecular mass of up to 1.5 kDa. The mPT disrupts oxidative phosphorylation and initiates release of mitochondrial calcium. In addition, the extrusion of apoptogenic factors such as cytochrome *c*, procaspase 9, and apoptosis-inducing factor (AIF) from the mitochondrial intermembrane space is facilitated. Cyclosporin A prevents the interaction of cyclophilin D with the ANT, powerfully blocks the formation of the mPT pore and thereby stabilizes neuronal mitochondrial membranes and function (oxidative phosphorylation) allowing for cell survival.

Blood–Brain Barrier Penetration

Under normal conditions CsA does not cross the blood-brain barrier despite its highly lipophilic nature. It is actively blocked from entering the brain by the P-glycoprotein (P-gp), an ATP-dependent multidrug efflux pump expressed in the luminal surface of brain capillary endothelial cells *(92,93)*. High intravenous doses are needed to completely overcome the P-glycoprotein transport *(94)*. There are several ways to deliver CsA across the blood–brain barrier and in the study described below we chose the most direct route, of direct intracerebroventricular (intrathecal) injection.

CYCLOSPORIN A AND ALS: WORK IN PROGRESS

Since mitochondrial dysfunction has been convincingly implicated in nerve cell degeneration in ALS, the hypothesis that CsA as a potent blocker of mitochondrial permeability transition might slow progression of motor neuron death and paralysis and prolong survival was created. Many people that are diagnosed with ALS are already in relatively advanced stages. The objective of this initial study was therefore to evaluate the effect of CsA on progression to limb paralysis and survival in late stage ALS mice.

Materials and Methods

SOD1 transgenic mice were purchased from Jackson Laboratory (Bar Harbor, ME). The strain designated B6SJL-TgN(SOD1-G93A)2Gur was maintained by breeding homozygous carriers to B6SJLF1 hybrids. A standard PCR protocol using two sets of primers was used as confirmatory genotyping *(95)*. All procedures complied with federal guidelines and the experimental protocol was approved by the University of Hawaii Institutional Animal Care and Use Committee. Transgenic mice at 3 mo of age were anesthetized with ketamine (60 mg/kg, ip) and placed in a Kopf stereotacic frame. A 24-gauge guide cannula (Plastics One, Roanoke, VA) was implanted into the right lateral ventricle (coordinates from bregma: AP = 0.0 mm, ML = +1.0 mm, DV = – 2.5 mm; toothbar = 0.0 mm) in all animals and was secured to the skull with a jeweler's screw and dental cement. Following surgery the mice were placed in individual cages with free access to water and food on a 12-h light/dark cycle. Mice were examined every 2 d for irregularity of gait, limping, or dragging of hindlimbs and were weighed. Spasticity was sought in the form of crossed hindlimbs on suspending the mouse by the tail, and by observing tonic elevation of the tail either spontaneously or on stroking. Strength and agility of the hindlimbs were tested by the ability to grasp the cage top bars and walk upside down. Loss of the ability to use hindlimbs to grasp the cage bars while upside-down was the criterion for late-stage disease. Diagnosis was confirmed by a second examiner. Following diagnosis, mice were examined daily and randomized to CsA ($n = 7$) and vehicle ($n = 5$) infusions every other day: 5 µL (25 µg CsA, 0.5% CsA in 20% soybean oil and lecithin oil-in-water emulsion) (CicloMulsion AG, Germany) was injected intrathecally using a Hamilton syringe and a 30-gauge inner cannula. Three mice were inadvertently given CsA on two consecutive d (instead of every 2 d), of which one died 2 d later (d 3 following diagnosis) and was excluded. Paralysis of both hindlimbs or inability to eat with resultant pronounced weight loss was defined as the end point (time of death) and the animals were euthanized with an overdose of ketamine and transcardially perfused in buffered 4% PFA. Brains were removed and postfixed in 4% PFA. The implanted cannula was found to extend to the lateral ventricle in all operated animals. Unpaired Student's *t*-test was used to compare time to endpoint between the groups. Data are presented as mean ±SEM.

Results

Mice receiving intrathecal vehicle infusions reached end point 11.8 ± 1.7 d after diagnosis with a range of 8–18 d (Fig. 1) and behaved and progressed neurologically in a manner identical to nontreated ALS mice (data not shown). Hindlimbs slowly became paralyzed and demonstrated markedly increased tone. Forepaws became weak, but not paralyzed. The spine developed kyphotic arch and tail tone dramatically increased causing a 90° elevation. Stroking the tail induced reflex elevation of the tail. Mice were completely alert with heads moving normally and would eat from a pellet placed in the forepaws up until the time of euthanasia. Stool would collect in a pile because of immobility on the last day prior to euthanasia.

Mice receiving CsA infusions behaved and progressed in a markedly different way. Two mice displayed asymmetry of motion. The left side became more robust and active. The mouse leaned with the right side against the cage wall and moved robustly in a counterclockwise direction. When placed with the left side against the wall, the mouse would fall onto the right and turn in circles propelled with the left legs until able to again orient with the weaker side against the cage wall and would resume propulsion in a counterclockwise fashion. The mice became gradually weaker with a pattern different from the vehicle-treated mice. The hindlimbs weakened and finally paralyzed, but did not increase in tone or spasticity. The spinal column did not become arched. Ambulation was closer to the ground, with the back straight, more like a lizard slither. The tail became less active, but remained supple without increased tone and would not become erect, even with stroking. Mice receiving CsA infusions lived 24.2 ± 4.1 d after diagnosis with a range of 16 through 37 d (Fig. 1). Two mice that reached end point at 17 and 19 d did so without paralysis. They seemed lethargic, but arousable. The lethargy led to decreased feeding and drinking causing weight loss and triggering euthanasia. This lethargy is not seen in nontreated or vehicle mice, suggesting an overdose or toxic

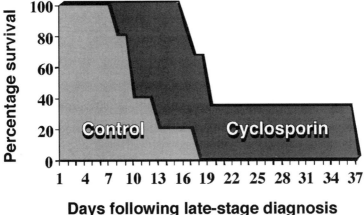

Fig. 1. Survival times following diagnosis of late-stage amyotrophic lateral sclerosis (ALS) in G93A mice carrying the mutant Cu/Zn superoxide dismutase (SOD1) gene. Mice were diagnosed as late-stage when they were no longer able to use their hindlimbs to climb upside down. At diagnosis intracerebroventricular injections of cyclosporin A ($n = 6$) or its vehicle ($n = 5$) were started. The end point was paralysis of both hindlimbs. Values are presented as mean ±SEM. $*p < .05$; Student's unpaired t-test.

effect of CsA at this dose. One mouse (CsA-treated) was euthanized at 37 d when its skull cannula dislodged, even though still active and had not yet reached the criteria for euthanasia.

CONCLUDING REMARKS

About 90% of ALS patients have the sporadic form of the disease and have no early warning as potentially do those with FALS. Thus it is not an option for them to be "pretreated" with a medication before they develop weakness. Drugs that slow mouse disease when given a month before weakness develops, and increase total life span by 27 d for caspase inhibitors *(96)*, 26 d for 2% creatin *(43)*, 9 d for carboxyfullerenes *(44)*, 10 d for penicillamine *(42)* are of uncertain utility for humans but may shed important light on the pathogenesis. For a drug to be useful in treating humans with ALS, it must halt disease when given after first symptoms are diagnosed.

The intrathecal dose of CsA given here (25 µg every other day) seems to be tolerated by most ALS transgenic mice but is likely at the upper threshold. This represents approximately a 18 mg/kg/d CsA dose seen by the craniospinal neuroaxis. One mouse in three that inadvertently received 25 µg doses on two consecutive d died shortly thereafter. The two mice that survived went on to live the longest of the mice, both 37 d. Two CsA mice succumbed at d 17 and d 19, not from paralysis but loss of interest in eating or drinking. The doses given seemed to have a paradoxical energizing and also mild "taming" effect, the later not unlike major tranquilizers. Pilot high-dose intrathecal CsA made animals initially hyperactive, then dazed, docile and uninterested in eating (data not shown).

The disease was chosen at a late stage, when the mice could no longer grasp the cage roofbars with hindpaws while hanging upside down. From this point, the normal course is rapid progression to hindlimb paralysis in 11 ± 1 d *(97)* or 12 ± 2 d *(98)*. Our vehicle mice lived 11.8 ± 2 d, demonstrating that the surgery and intrathecal lipid emulsion injections did not influence survival.

Mice receiving CsA lived 24.2 ± 4 d, 12 d longer than vehicle controls. This survival at even late-stage administration is comparable to extensions in survival seen with long-term riluzole pre-treatment *(45)*. One study of cell cultures transfected with mutant SOD demonstrated increased cell death when CsA was added to the culture medium *(99)*. However, the transfected cells were hippocampal pyramidal neurons and therefore the results are difficult to extrapolate to in vivo administration of CsA and degenerating motor neurons in FALS mice.

In 1988 a human double-blind CsA study attempted treating ALS on the hypothesis that ALS was an autoimmune disease. Patients received 10 mg/kg systemic CsA for up to 40 wk. The same motor decline was seen for both placebo and CsA-treated patients *(100,101)*. The conclusion was that ALS is not affected by immunosuppressive treatment. Possible direct neuroprotective effects could not be evaluated because CsA does not cross the intact blood–brain barrier and was not able to reach the CNS of the patients *(see* ref. *102)*.

More work is currently underway to define the therapeutic and toxic windows for intrathecal CsA administration as well as to carefully evaluate possible CsA effects on spinal motor neuron loss at defined stages of the disease. In addition, to determine the importance of calcineurin inhibition in the beneficial effect, a study with FK506 and nonimmunosuppressive analogues of CsA is underway. In conclusion, CsA treatment positively influences the survival of late stage ALS transgenic mice and further implicates mitochondrial function in the pathogenesis of amyotrophic lateral sclerosis.

ACKNOWLEDGMENTS

This study was supported by the Victoria S. and Bradley L. Geist Foundation, the Restorative Neurosurgery Foundation and Maas BiolAB, LLC.

Maas BiolAB, LLC intellectual property includes the use of cyclosporin for neurological indications. Cyclosporin-A in lipid emulsion was kindly provided by CicloMulsion AG, Germany.

REFERENCES

1. Oppenheimer DR, Esiri MM. (1992) In: Adams JH, Duchen LW, eds. Greenfield's Neuropathology. Arnold, New York, 1992, pp. 988–1045.
2. Charcot JM. Prog Med 1874;2:325–327.
3. Williams DB, Windebank AJ. Motor neuron disease (amyotrophic lateral sclerosis). Mayo Clin Proc 1991;66:54–82.
4. Hirano A, Kurland LT, Sayre GP. Familial amyotrophic lateral sclerosis. A subgroup characterized by posterior and spinocerebellar tract involvement and hyaline inclusions in the anterior horn cells. Arch Neurol 1967;16:232–243.
5. Cudkowicz ME, McKenna-Yasek D, Sapp PE, et al. Epidemiology of mutations in superoxide dismutase in amyotrophic lateral sclerosis. Ann Neurol 1997;41:210–221.
6. Crapo JD, Oury T, Rabouille C, et al, Copper,zinc superoxide dismutase is primarily a cytosolic protein in human cells. Proc Natl Acad Sci USA 1992;89:10,405–10,409.
7. Liu R, Althaus JS, Ellerbrock BR, et al. Enhanced oxygen radical production in a transgenic mouse model of familial amyotrophic lateral sclerosis. Ann Neurol 1998;44:763–770.
8. Pardo CA, Xu Z, Borchelt DR, et al. Superoxide dismutase is an abundant component in cell bodies, dendrites, and axons of motor neurons and in a subset of other neurons. Proc. Natl. Acad. Sci. USA 1995;92:954–958.
9. Gurney ME, Pu H, Chiu AY, et al. Motor neuron degeneration in mice that express a human Cu,Zn superoxide dismutase mutation. Science 1994;264:1772–1775.
10. Dal Canto MC. Comparison of pathological alterations in ALS and a murine transgenic model: pathogenetic implications. Clin Neurosci 1995;3:332–337.
11. Dal Canto MC, Gurney ME. Development of central nervous system pathology in a murine transgenic model of human amyotrophic lateral sclerosis. Am J Pathol 1994;145:1271–1279.
12. Chiu AY, Zhai P, Dal Canto MC, et al. Age-dependent penetrance of disease in a transgenic mouse model of familial amyotrophic lateral sclerosis. Mol Cell Neurosci 1995;6:349–362.
13. Dal Canto MC, Gurney ME. Neuropathological changes in two lines of mice carrying a transgene for mutant human Cu,Zn SOD, and in mice overexpressing wild type human SOD: a model of familial amyotrophic lateral sclerosis (FALS). Brain Res 1995;676:25–40.
14. Kaal EC, Vlug AS, Versleijen MW, et al. Chronic mitochondrial inhibition induces selective motoneuron death in vitro: a new model for amyotrophic lateral sclerosis. J Neurochem 2000;74:1158–1165.
15. al-Chalabi A, Powell JF, Leigh PN. Neurofilaments, free radicals, excitotoxins, and amyotrophic lateral sclerosis. Muscle Nerve 1995;18:540–545.

16. Crow JP, Ye YZ, Strong M, et al. Superoxide dismutase catalyzes nitration of tyrosines by peroxynitrite in the rod and head domains of neurofilament-L. J Neurochem 1997;69:1945–1953.
17. Collard JF, Cote F, Julien JP. Defective axonal transport in a transgenic mouse model of amyotrophic lateral sclerosis (see comments). Nature 1995;375:61–64.
18. Julien JP. A role for neurofilaments in the pathogenesis of amyotrophic lateral sclerosis. Biochem Cell Biol 1995;73:593–597.
19. Straube-West K, Loomis PA, Opal P, Goldman RD. Alterations in neural intermediate filament organization: functional implications and the induction of pathological changes related to motor neuron disease. J Cell Sci 1996;109, 2319–2329.
20. Tu PH, Gurney ME, Julien JP, et al. Oxidative stress, mutant SOD1, and neurofilament pathology in transgenic mouse models of human motor neuron disease. Lab Invest 1997;76, 441–456.
21. Williams TL, Day NC, Ince PG, et al. Calcium-permeable alpha-amino-3-hydroxy-5-methyl-4-isoxazole propionic acid receptors: a molecular determinant of selective vulnerability in amyotrophic lateral sclerosis. Ann Neurol 1997;42, 200–207.
22. Rothstein JD. Excitotoxicity hypothesis. Neurology 1996;47, S19–S25; discussion S26.
23. Shaw PJ, Ince PG. Glutamate, excitotoxicity and amyotrophic lateral sclerosis. J Neurol 1996;244:S3–S14.
24. Pellegrini-Giampietro DE, Gorter JA, Bennett MV, Zukin RS. The GluR2 (GluR-B) hypothesis: Ca(2+)-permeable AMPA receptors in neurological disorders. Trends Neurosci 1997;20:464–470.
25. Alexianu ME, Ho BK, Mohamed AH, et al. The role of calcium-binding proteins in selective motoneuron vulnerability in amyotrophic lateral sclerosis. Ann Neurol 1994;36:846–858.
26. Smith RG, Siklos L, Alexianu ME, et al. Autoimmunity and ALS. Neurology 1996;47:S40–S45; discussion S45–S46.
27. Engelhardt JI, Siklos L, Komuves L, et al. Antibodies to calcium channels from ALS patients passively transferred to mice selectively increase intracellular calcium and induce ultrastructural changes in motoneurons. Synapse 1995;20:185–199.
28. Beckman JS, Carson M, Smith CD, Koppenol WH. ALS, SOD and peroxynitrite. Nature 1993;364:584.
29. Parge HE, Hallewell RA, Tainer JA. Atomic structures of wild-type and thermostable mutant recombinant human Cu,Zn superoxide dismutase. Proc Natl Acad Sci USA 1992;89:6109–6113.
30. Wiedau-Pazos M, Goto JJ, Rabizadeh S, et al. Altered reactivity of superoxide dismutase in familial amyotrophic lateral sclerosis. Science 1996; 271:515–518.
31. Bredesen DE, Wiedau-Pazos M, Goto JJ, et al. Cell death mechanisms in ALS. Neurology 1996;47:S36–S38; discussion S38–S39.
32. Yim MB, Kang JH, Yim HS, et al. A gain-of-function of an amyotrophic lateral sclerosis-associated Cu,Zn- superoxide dismutase mutant: An enhance-

ment of free radical formation due to a decrease in Km for hydrogen peroxide. Proc Natl Acad Sci USA 1996;93:5709–5714.

33. Yim MB, Chock PB, Stadtman ER. Enzyme function of copper, zinc superoxide dismutase as a free radical generator. J Biol Chem 1993;268:4099–4105.

34. Yim HS, Kang JH, Chock PB, et al. A familial amyotrophic lateral sclerosis-associated A4V Cu, Zn-superoxide dismutase mutant has a lower Km for hydrogen peroxide. Correlation between clinical severity and the Km value. J Biol Chem 1997;272:8861–8863.

35. Bogdanov MB, Ramos LE, Xu Z, Beal MF. Elevated "hydroxyl radical" generation in vivo in an animal model of amyotrophic lateral sclerosis. J Neurochem 1998;71:1321–1324.

36. Singh RJ, Karoui H, Gunther MR, et al. Reexamination of the mechanism of hydroxyl radical adducts formed from the reaction between familial amyotrophic lateral sclerosis-associated Cu,Zn superoxide dismutase mutants and H2O2. Proc Natl Acad Sci USA 1998;95:6675–6680.

37. Bruijn LI, Beal MF, Becher MW, et al. Elevated free nitrotyrosine levels, but not protein-bound nitrotyrosine or hydroxyl radicals, throughout amyotrophic lateral sclerosis (ALS)- like disease implicate tyrosine nitration as an aberrant in vivo property of one familial ALS-linked superoxide dismutase 1 mutant. Proc Natl Acad Sci USA 1997;94:7606–7611.

38. Ferrante RJ, Browne SE, Shinobu LA, et al. Evidence of increased oxidative damage in both sporadic and familial amyotrophic lateral sclerosis. J Neurochem 1997;69:2064–2074.

39. Hall ED, Andrus PK, Oostveen JA, et al. Relationship of oxygen radical-induced lipid peroxidative damage to disease onset and progression in a transgenic model of familial ALS. J Neurosci Res 1998;53:66–77.

40. Andrus PK, Fleck TJ, Gurney ME, Hall ED. Protein oxidative damage in a transgenic mouse model of familial amyotrophic lateral sclerosis. J Neurochem 1998;71:2041–2048.

41. Mena MA, Khan U, Togasaki DM, et al. Effects of wild-type and mutated copper/zinc superoxide dismutase on neuronal survival and L-DOPA-induced toxicity in postnatal midbrain culture. J. Neurochem. 1997;69:21–33.

42. Hottinger AF, Fine EG, Gurney ME, et al. The copper chelator d-penicillamine delays onset of disease and extends survival in a transgenic mouse model of familial amyotrophic lateral sclerosis. Eur J Neurosci 1997;9:1548–1551.

43. Klivenyi P, Ferrante RJ, Matthews RT, et al. Neuroprotective effects of creatine in a transgenic animal model of amyotrophic lateral sclerosis. Nat Med 1999;5:347–350.

44. Dugan LL, Turetsky DM, Du C, et al. Carboxyfullerenes as neuroprotective agents. Proc Natl Acad Sci USA 1997;94:9434–9439.

45. Gurney ME, Cutting FB, Zhai P, et al. Benefit of vitamin E, riluzole, and gabapentin in a transgenic model of familial amyotrophic lateral sclerosis. Ann Neurol 1996;39:147–157.

46. Andreassen OA, Dedeoglu A, Klivenyi P, et al. *N*-Acetyl-L-cysteine improves survival and preserves motor performance in an animal model of familial amyotrophic lateral sclerosis. Neuroreport 2000;11:2491–2493.

47. Gurney ME. Transgenic-mouse model of amyotrophic lateral sclerosis. N Engl J Med 1994;331:1721–1722.

48. Kong J, Xu Z. Massive mitochondrial degeneration in motor neurons triggers the onset of amyotrophic lateral sclerosis in mice expressing a mutant SOD1. J Neurosci 1998;18:3241–3250.

49. Carri MT, Ferri A, Battistoni A, et al. Expression of a Cu,Zn superoxide dismutase typical of familial amyotrophic lateral sclerosis induces mitochondrial alteration and increase of cytosolic Ca^{2+} concentration in transfected neuroblastoma SH-SY5Y cells. FEBS Lett 1997;414:365–368.

50. Reed JC. Cytochrome *c*: can't live with it—can't live without it. Cell 1997; 91:559–562.

51. Kharbanda S, Pandey P, Schofield L, et al. Role for Bcl-xL as an inhibitor of cytosolic cytochrome *C* accumulation in DNA damage-induced apoptosis. Proc Natl Acad Sci USA 1997;94:6939–6942.

52. Prehn JH, Bindokas VP, Marcuccilli CJ, et al. Regulation of neuronal Bcl2 protein expression and calcium homeostasis by transforming growth factor type beta confers wide-ranging protection on rat hippocampal neurons. Proc Natl Acad Sci USA 1994;91:12,599–12,603.

53. Miller RG. New approaches to therapy of amyotrophic lateral sclerosis. West J Med 1998;168:262–263.

54. Kostic V, Jackson-Lewis V, de Bilbao F et al. Bcl-2: prolonging life in a transgenic mouse model of familial amyotrophic lateral sclerosis. Science 1997;277:559–562.

55. Martin LJ. Neuronal death in amyotrophic lateral sclerosis is apoptosis: possible contribution of a programmed cell death mechanism. J. Neuropathol. Exp Neurol 1999;58:459–471.

56. Browne SE, Bowling AC, Baik MJ, et al. Metabolic dysfunction in familial, but not sporadic, amyotrophic lateral sclerosis. J Neurochem 1998;71: 281–287.

57. Wiedemann FR, Winkler K, Kuznetsov AV, et al. Impairment of mitochondrial function in skeletal muscle of patients with amyotrophic lateral sclerosis. J Neurol Sci 156:65–72.

58. Fujita K, Yamauchi M, Shibayama K, et al. Decreased cytochrome *c* oxidase activity but unchanged superoxide dismutase and glutathione peroxidase activities in the spinal cords of patients with amyotrophic lateral sclerosis. J Neurosci Res 1996;45:276–281.

59. Borthwick GM, Johnson MA, Ince PG, et al. Mitochondrial enzyme activity in amyotrophic lateral sclerosis: implications for the role of mitochondria in neuronal cell death. Ann Neurol 1999;46:787–790.

60. Vielhaber S, Kunz D, Winkler K, et al. Mitochondrial DNA abnormalities in skeletal muscle of patients with sporadic amyotrophic lateral sclerosis. Brain 2000;123:1339–1348.

61. Siklos L, Engelhardt J, Harati Y, Smith RG, Joo F, Appel SH. Ultrastructural evidence for altered calcium in motor nerve terminals in amyotrophic lateral sclerosis. Ann. Neurol. 1996;39:203–216.

62. Curti D, Malaspina A, Facchetti G, et al. Amyotrophic lateral sclerosis: oxidative energy metabolism and calcium homeostasis in peripheral blood lymphocytes. Neurology 1996;47:1060–1064.

63. Swerdlow RH, Parks JK, Cassarino DS, et al. Mitochondria in sporadic amyotrophic lateral sclerosis. Exp Neurol 1998;153:135–142.

64. Nakano Y, Hirayama K, Terao K. Hepatic ultrastructural changes and liver dysfunction in amyotrophic lateral sclerosis. Arch Neurol 44:103–106.

65. Lad RP, Smith MA, Hilt DC. Molecular cloning and regional distribution of rat brain cyclophilin. Mol Brain Res 9:239–244.

66. Li PA, Uchino H, Elmér E, Siesjö BK. Amelioration by cyclosporin A of brain damage following 5 or 10 min of ischemia in rats subjected to preischemic hyperglycemia. Brain Res 1997;753:133–140.

67. Uchino H, Elmér E, Uchino K et al. Cyclosporin A dramatically ameliorates CA1 hippocampal damage following transient forebrain ischaemia in the rat. Acta Physiol Scand 1995;155:469–471.

68. Uchino H, Elmér E, Uchino K, et al. Amelioration by cyclosporin A of brain damage in transient forebrain ischemia in the rat. Brain Res 1998;812: 216–226.

69. Matsumoto S, Friberg H, Ferrand-Drake M, Wieloch T. Blockade of the mitochondrial permeability transition pore diminishes infarct size in the rat after transient middle cerebral artery occlusion. J Cereb Blood Flow Metab 1999;19:736–741.

70. Yoshimoto T, Siesjö BK. Posttreatment with the immunosuppressant cyclosporin A in transient focal ischemia. Brain Res 1999;839:283–291.

71. Kuroda S, Janelidze S, Siesjö BK. The immunosuppressants cyclosporin A and FK506 equally ameliorate brain damage due to 30-min middle cerebral artery occlusion in hyperglycemic rats. Brain Res 1999;835:148–153.

72. Sullivan PG, Thompson M, Scheff SW. Continuous infusion of cyclosporin A postinjury significantly ameliorates cortical damage following traumatic brain injury. Exp Neurol 2000;161:631–637.

73. Scheff SW, Sullivan PG. Cyclosporin A significantly ameliorates cortical damage following experimental traumatic brain injury in rodents. J Neurotrauma 1999;16:783–792.

74. Okonkwo DO, Povlishock JT. An intrathecal bolus of cyclosporin A before injury preserves mitochondrial integrity and attenuates axonal disruption in traumatic brain injury. J Cereb Blood Flow Metab 1999;19:443–451.

75. Okonkwo DO, Buki A, Siman R, Povlishock JT. Cyclosporin A limits calcium-induced axonal damage following traumatic brain injury. NeuroReport 1999;10:353–358.

76. Buki A, Okonkwo DO, Povlishock JT. Postinjury cyclosporin A administration limits axonal damage and disconnection in traumatic brain injury. J Neurotrauma 1999;16:511–521.

77. Borlongan CV, Freeman TB, Hauser RA, et al. Cyclosporine-A increases locomotor activity in rats with 6-hydroxydopamine-induced hemiparkinsonism: relevance to neural transplantation. Surg Neurol 1996;46:384–388.

78. Matsuura K, Kabuto H, Makino H, Ogawa N. Cyclosporin A attenuates degeneration of dopaminergic neurons induced by 6-hydroxydopamine in the mouse brain. Brain Res 1996;733:101–104.

79. Matsuura K, Makino H, Ogawa N. Cyclosporin A attenuates the decrease in tyrosine hydroxylase immunoreactivity in nigrostriatal dopaminergic neurons and in striatal dopamine content in rats with intrastriatal injection of 6-hydroxydopamine. Exp Neurol 1997;146:526–535.

80. Seaton TA, Cooper JM, Schapira AH. Cyclosporin inhibition of apoptosis induced by mitochondrial complex I toxins. Brain Res 1998;809:12–17.

81. Tatton WG, Chalmers-Redman RM. Mitochondria in neurodegenerative apoptosis: an opportunity for therapy? Ann Neurol 1998;44:S134–S141.

82. Cassarino DS, Parks JK, Parker D Jr, Bennett JP Jr. The parkinsonian neurotoxin MPP+ opens the mitochondrial permeability transition pore and releases cytochrome c in isolated mitochondria via an oxidative mechanism. Biochim. Biophys. Acta 1999;1453:49–62.

83. Borlongan CV, Stahl CE, Fujisaki T, et al. Cyclosporine A-induced hyperactivity in rats: is it mediated by immunosuppression, neurotrophism, or both? Cell Transplant 1999;8:153–159.

84. Berman SB, Hastings TG. Dopamine oxidation alters mitochondrial respiration and induces permeability transition in brain mitochondria: implications for Parkinson's disease. J Neurochem 1999;73:1127–1137.

85. Petersen A, Castilho RF, Hansson O, et al. Oxidative stress, mitochondrial permeability transition and activation of caspases in calcium ionophore A23187-induced death of cultured striatal neurons. Brain Res 2000;857:20–29.

86. Friberg H, Ferrand-Drake M, Bengtsson F, et al. Cyclosporin A, but not FK 506, protects mitochondria and neurons against hypoglycemic damage and implicates the mitochondrial permeability transition in cell death. J Neurosci 1998;18:5151–5159.

87. Crompton M, Virji S, Ward JM. Cyclophilin-D binds strongly to complexes of the voltage-dependent anion channel and the adenine nucleotide translocase to form the permeability transition pore. Eur J Biochem 1998;258:729–735.

88. Crompton M. The mitochondrial permeability transition pore and its role in cell death. Biochem J 1999;341:233–249.

89. Chen QX, Perkins KL, Choi DW, Wong RKS. Secondary activation of a cation conductance is responsible for NMDA toxicity in acutely isolated hippocampal neurons. J Neurosci 1997;17:4032–4036.

90. Lemasters JJ. V. Necrapoptosis and the mitochondrial permeability transition: shared pathways to necrosis and apoptosis. Am J Physiol 1999;276:G1–G6.

91. Kristal BS, Dubinsky JM. Mitochondrial permeability transition in the central nervous system: induction by calcium cycling-dependent and -independent pathways. J Neurochem 1997;69:524–538.

92. Begley DJ, Squires LK, Zlokovic BV, et al. Permeability of the blood brain barrier to the immunosuppressive cyclic peptide cyclosporin A. J Neurochem 1990;55:1222–1230.

93. Tsuji A. P-glycoprotein-mediated efflux transport of anticancer drugs at the blood-brain barrier. Ther Drug Monit 1998;20:588–590.

94. Lemaire M, Bruelisauer A, Guntz P, Sato H. Dose-dependent brain penetration of SDZ PSC 833, a novel multidrug resistance-reversing cyclosporin, in rats. Cancer Chemother Pharmacol 1996;38:481–486.

95. Gurney ME. Transgenic animal models of familial amyotrophic lateral sclerosis. J Neurol 1997;244:S15–S20.

96. Li M, Ona VO, Guegan C, et al. Functional role of caspase-1 and caspase-3 in an ALS transgenic mouse model. Science 2000;288:335–339.

97. Pedersen WA, Mattson MP. No benefit of dietary restriction on disease onset or progression in amyotrophic lateral sclerosis Cu/Zn-superoxide dismutase mutant mice. Brain Res 1999;833:117–120.

98. Friedlander RM, Brown RH, Gagliardini V, et al. Inhibition of ICE slows ALS in mice. Nature 1997;388:31.

99. Lee JP, Palfrey HC, Bindokas VP, et al. The role of immunophilins in mutant superoxide dismutase-1linked familial amyotrophic lateral sclerosis. Proc Natl. Acad Sci USA 1999;96:3251–3256.

100. Appel SH, Stewart SS, Appel V, et al. A double-blind study of the effectiveness of cyclosporine in amyotrophic lateral sclerosis. Arch Neurol 1988; 45:381–386.

101. Tindall RS. Immunointervention with cyclosporin A in autoimmune neurological disorders. J Autoimmun 1992;5:301–313.

102. Lensmeyer GL, Wiebe DA, Carlson IH, Subramanian R. Concentrations of cyclosporin A and its metabolites in human tissues postmortem. J Anal Toxicol 1991;15:110–115.

19

Psychological Effects of Cyclosporin A

Shigeru Watanabe

INTRODUCTION

One of the most widely used immunosuppressive drugs is cyclosporin A. This fungal metabolite extracted from Tolypocladium inflatum Gams was introduced in early 1970s and has been used in organ transplantation. Recently, neural transplantation became a potential treatment for neurodegenerative disorders such as Parkinson's disease, Alzheimer's disease and Huntington's disease. Because these diseases are associated with cognitive disorder, examination of possible effects of cyclosporin A upon cognitive ability is an important topic. There is no direct evidence demonstrating that cyclosporin A passes the blood–brain barrier, but several experimental data suggest CNS effects after systemic injection of cyclosporin A (e.g., *1,2*). Even though psychological effects of cyclosporin A may be principally mediated by peripheral mechanisms, it is also essential to identify the brain processes accompanying such effects. Elucidation of neural mechanisms underlying cyclosporin A will allow not only a better understanding of central action of the drug in producing psychological effects, but also draw attention to the potential use of cyclosporin A as a therapeutic agent for brain dysfunctions.

COGNITIVE FUNCTION

One of the most basic functions of cognitive ability is memory. In the laboratory, cognitive ability has been analyzed using retention, a rather simple memory that can be formed using a passive avoidance paradigm. Our group and several others have demonstrated that rats acquire and retain memory of a passive avoidance task *(3)*. Many investigators have used a test chamber that consists of a dark and a white compartment. We have used this passive avoidance paradigm in investigating the effects of cyclosporin A on retention in adult Wistar rats. Animals were first placed in the white compartment and received an electric shock from the floor when they entered the dark com-

From: *Immunosuppressant Analogs in Neuroprotection*
Edited by: C. V. Borlongan, O. Isacson, and P. R. Sanberg © Humana Press Inc., Totowa, NJ

partment. This training continued until the animals stayed in the white compartment for 3 min. Then, the experimental group received daily injections of cyclosporin A (10 mg/kg) for 26 d and retention was tested on every fourth day. No electric shock was given in the retention tests. The control group received the same tests except that they were injected the vehicle (peanut oil) instead of cyclosporin A. Figure 1 shows latencies to enter the dark compartment during the seven tests. Both control and experimental groups stayed at the white compartment for more than 2 min until the third test. That is, they maintained their memory for around 10 d and no difference between the cyclosporin A-treated and vehicle-treated animals.

No deficits in retention of memory in this experiment might be caused by systemic injection of cyclosporin A. Because abundant cyclosporin A binding sites exist in the whole blood, only very limited cyclosporin A was available to the brain, therefore the drug did not produce detectable changes in brain functions. Moreover, these results might simply reflect the absence of cyclosporin A in the brain because of the blood–brain barrier. However, several studies, such as enhancement of neurotoxicity of N-methyl-4-phenyl-1,2,3,4-tetrahydropyridine (MPTP) by cyclosporin A *(1)*, suggest that systemic injection of cyclosporin A affects the central nervous system. Chronic treatment with cyclosporin A also caused side effects on the brain functions in human patients *(2)*. These results suggest that cyclosporin A can affect the brain only when the drug is able to pass the blood–brain barrier, that is, when the barrier is compromised (as in MPTP intoxication) or when the drug is given chronically and at high dose.

In order to clarify the central effects of cyclosporin A, we examined the effects of the drug in rats with a compromised blood–brain barrier to *(4)*. To break the blood–brain barrier, we employed intraparenchymal microinjection of saline into the brain. Disruption of the blood–brain barrier after the micro-injection of the saline into the brain starts as early as 3 d after the surgery and continued up to 7–8 d *(5)*. The rats were initially trained on the passive avoidance described above, then received stereotaxic injection of the saline into the brains. After that, the experimental groups were injected intraperitoneally with 5, 10, or 20 mg/kg cyclosporin A daily for 9 d and received the retention test on every other day. The control group was injected intraperitoneally with the vehicle. The results support our previous finding; that is, cyclosporin A injection did not impair retention of the memory.

Previous reports using animals with intact blood–brain barrier suggested impairment of memory *(6,7)*, but higher than 20 mg/kg dose of cyclosporin A was injected in these experiments. Of note, the toxicity of high-dose cyclosporin A (e.g., 20 mg/kg and higher) has been well documented *(8,9)*. In fact, five of eight rats injected with 20 mg/kg cyclosporin A died in our

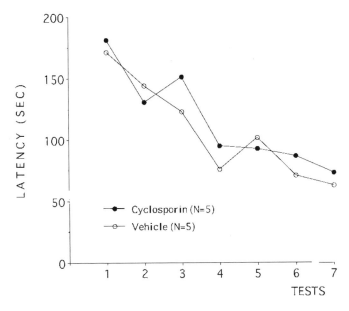

Fig. 1. Retention curves of passive avoidance in rats. Chronic treatment with cyclosporin does not impair the retention. (Modified from ref. *3*).

experiment and the performance of the survivors was worst among the cyclosporin A-injected groups, although not significantly different from the control groups. Thus, apparent impairment in the previous studies might reflect unhealthy condition of the subjects. Another set of data showing memory deficits by cyclosporin A was obtained from chicks. Intracranial injection of cyclosporin A did, however, produce memory deficits of one-trial passive avoidance in day-old chicks *(10)*. The deficits could not be observed until 85-min after the training, thus the effects were time-dependent. Cyclosporin A inhibits peptidylprolyl-*cis-trans*-isomerase (PPIlase) activity of cyclophilin and intracranial injection of nonimmunosuppressive cyclosporin A analogs that have the PPIlase-inhibiting effects also cause retention deficits in retention of the passive avoidance *(11)*. The authors claimed that cyclophilin had a crucial role in memory formation. In addition to the species difference and procedural difference, the chick experiments demonstrated deficits in memory formation, whereas ours demonstrated no impairment in retention of already consolidated memory.

REINFORCING PROPERTIES

From the preceding section, it is clear that cyclosporin A affects retention of a passive avoidance task in rats. The next problem is whether cyclosporin

A produces reinforcing or aversive effects. It is also of clinical importance to clarify these psychological properties of cyclosporin A. Thorndike *(12)* provided the first behavioral definition of "satisfaction" a long time ago (1913). According to him, "by a satisfying state of affairs is meant one which the animal does nothing to avoid, often doing things which maintain or renew it." He postulated the well-known law of effect, that is, "of several responses made to the same situation those which are accompanied or closely followed by satisfaction to the animal will be more firmly connected with the situation." Since then, psychologists have defined satisfaction, pleasure, reward, and reinforcement in several different ways. However, the definition by Thorndike is still useful to measure what the animal likes.

Measurement of Reinforcing Property

Reinforcing properties of an event can be demonstrated in many animals, including birds, by measuring the staying time of the animals in an environment associated with the event. For example, reinforcing property of music for Java sparrows was examined by measuring the staying time of the bird in a chamber *(13)*. The experimental chamber was a modified cage for small birds. There were three perches in the cage and perching at each perch was detected by a photosensor. Perching on one of the end perches connected a line from a CD player that continuously played French suite by J. S. Bach to a speaker. Perching on the other end perch connected a line from another CD-player playing suite for piano by A. Schoenberg to a speaker. So, if a bird prefers a specific music, it should stay on the perch connected with that music. Each music was presented continuously as long as the subject stayed at each perch and loudness of the music was adjusted at approximately the same.

The birds significantly stayed longer on the perch associated with Bach music and remained their preference of Bach to Schoenberg when other kind of music by Bach and Schoenberg were used. These birds also preferred Vivaldi to Carter, suggesting preference for classic music over modern music. These results suggest that Java sparrows have musical preference and the preference can be measured by staying time.

Conditioned Place Preference with Methamphetamine

The experiments described above are direct measurement of rewarding effect in which staying at one place directly rewarded by events such as play of music or visual stimulation. The procedure can be expanded to conditioning experiment, in which one particular space and rewarding events are paired. This method, called conditioned place preference, has been widely used in pharmacological research. The standard method consisted of three phases; habituation or baseline phase in which animals can stay at either of two environments and their initial preference is measured. Then, in conditioning phase animals are injected with a drug and confined in one environment on one day and are injected with vehicle and confined in another environment on the next day. Usually, the conditioning is repeated three times each. After the conditioning, preference is measured again as the first phase. If the drug has reinforcing properties, the animals should stay longer at the environment associated with the drug.

The strongest way to demonstrate reinforcing properties of a drug is, however, self-administration experiment in which animals received intravenous injections of drug through a flexible tube just after operant response. This method is identical to usual operant conditioning in which occurrence of operant response followed presentation of food reinforcement and directly measures the reinforcing effect of drugs. On the other hand, conditioned place preference measures conditioned reinforcing properties of the drug. Staying at particular environment can be considered as an operant, but the reinforcer contingent upon that operant is a conditioned reinforcer (environment) formed through respondent conditioning. In general, results of conditioned place preference agree well to those of self-administration.

One advantage of conditioned place preference is its applicability to species that cannot perform self-administration, for example, fish and invertebrates. One interesting phenomenon in investigations of reinforcing properties of drugs is their cross-species universality. Drugs that are abused in humans have reinforcing properties in animals, although some drugs, such as hallucinogens, do not show clear reinforcing properties in animals (14). These observations suggest common phylogenetic origin of the reinforcing properties or "pleasure." Comparative study of reinforcing properties of drugs makes it possible to trace evolutionary history of drug-seeking behavior. One of the most powerful drugs that causes addiction is the dopaminergic agonist, such as amphetamine and cocaine. Figure 2 presents dose-response curves of reinforcing properties of methamphetamine obtained from mice, quails, goldfish, and planarians (15,16). For vertebrates, conventional conditioned place preference procedure was employed. Intramuscular injection of methamphetamine HCl was paired with one side of the two compartments conditioned place preference box. The methamphetamine increased staying time at the drug-associated compartment dose-dependently. The maximum effect of the methamphetamine is approximately the same among the species. The gold fish shows the curve with the highest potency among the vertebrates. These results clearly demonstrate that these animals share reinforcing property of the methamphetamine.

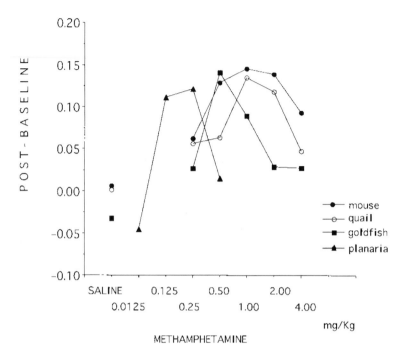

Fig. 2. Cross-species comparison of reinforcing properties of methamphetamine. The vertical axis indicates relative change before and after the conditioning. Data of mice, quails and fish from ref. *15* and planarians from ref. *16*.

The planarians appeared on the earth a billion years ago and are considered to be the ancestor of all *Bilateria (17,18)*. They have well-developed brains *(19)*. In addition to dopaminergic receptors, the planarian possesses opiate *(20)*, serotonin *(21)*, and acetylcholine receptors *(22)*. For conditioned place preference in planarians, we used a Petri dish in which quadrants a plain paper and a filter paper were alternately floored. Planarians were first measured for their initial preference between a plain paper and a filter paper in a Petri dish. In drug-treatment sessions, a drop of methamphetamine solution was dropped on the center of the dorsal surface of the planarian. In vehicle treatment sessions, a drop of distilled water was similarly dropped on the body surface of the planarian. After this conditioning, the preferential behavior was measured again. As shown in Fig. 2, the conditioning with 0.125 and 0.5 mg/kg methamphetamine increased the staying time on the nonpreferred paper, but 0.0125 or 1.0 mg/kg did not produce any observable effects on preference. These results indicate that methamphetamine has reinforcing effects dose-dependently in simple invertebrates such as planarians.

The haloperidol antagonized the reinforcing effect of the methamphetamine in planarians. Also both the D_1-selective antagonist, SCH23390, and the D_2-selective antagonist, sulpiride antagonized the reinforcing effects of the methamphetamine. Therefore both D_1 and D_2 receptors are involved in the dopaminergic reinforcing system of the planarians. These results suggest that our drug-seeking behavior probably originated one billion years ago. In other words, we share some aspects of "pleasure" with planarians.

A previous study in planarians demonstrated that D_1 agonists produced a screwlike hyperkinetic response, while D_2 agonists induced a C-like tonic curling postures, and these behaviors are selectively inhibited by pretreatment with D_1 and D_2 antagonists, respectively *(2,3)*. Thus, D_1 and D_2 receptors may have different functions in the planarian motor system, but the present results showed that both D_1 and D_2 receptors share a similar function in reinforcing mechanism of methamphetamine.

Conditioned Place Preference/Aversion with Cyclosporin A

Cyclosporin A protects against dopaminergic depletion in parkinsonian animal models *(24,25)*. It increased locomotor activity in rats *(26,27)*. Cyclosporin A alters the plasma and platelet catecholamine levels in cyclosporin A-induced hyperactive rats *(28)*. These results suggest that cyclosporin A affects preferential behavior in animals through modulation of the dopaminergic system because dopamine is strongly involved in the preferential behavior.

One method to measure reinforcing or aversive effect is a taste aversion procedure. If animals become unpleasantly conditioned after consumption of novel flavored water, they avoid the flavored water. This conditioning has peculiar features, that is, the taste is selectively associated with the aversive state, especially illness. Visual or auditory stimulus cannot associate with the illness and electric shock cannot be associated with taste. Usually, this procedure is employed to detect aversive properties of drugs not reinforcing effect. Klosterhalfen and Klosterhalfen *(29)* did not find conditioned taste aversion to cyclamate or vinegar after association with cyclosporin A injection in rats. On the other hand, they observed conditioned inhibition of experimentally induced arthritis. Thus, this experiment suggests dissociation between psychological and immune functions in conditioning. However, taste aversion experiments in which drinking saccharin associated with cyclosporin A injection demonstrated that cyclosporin A caused conditioned taste aversion *(30)*. Although there are procedural differences, such as strains of rats and kinds of conditioned stimuli, in these two experiments, cyclosporin A causes aversive effects at least under some conditions.

We tried to examine possible aversive effects of cyclosporin A in a conditioned place preference experiment. We used male Wistar rats and measured their preference in a two-compartment (black and white) test chamber *(31)*. Then, the animals were alternately injected with cyclosporin A (5, 10, 20, and 30 mg/kg) and vehicle (peanut oil) for 6 d. After the injection of cyclosporin A, the animals were placed in their preferred compartment, whereas they were placed in their nonpreferred compartment after the vehicle injection. As shown in Fig. 3, the conditioning with cyclosporin A resulted in decreased staying time in a previously preferred compartment. The strongest inhibiting effect was obtained from the 10 mg/kg injection group. Thus, cyclosporin A antagonized the spontaneous preferential behavior. One interesting point in this experiment is the correlation between preconditioning preference and postconditioning preference. The postconditioning preference was inversely correlated with the preconditioning preference ($r = -0.62$) indicating that the higher the preference at the preconditioning, the more effective the inhibiting action of cyclosporin A conditioning. The results agree with those by Exton and colleagues *(30)*.

Modulation of Conditioned Place Preference by Cyclosporin A

Cyclosporin A attenuated formation of physical dependence on morphine and withdrawal syndrome in morphine-dependent rats *(32,33)*. However, using suppression of lever pressing for food by naloxone as an index of withdrawal in morphine-dependent rats, Dantzer and colleagues *(34)* did not find behavioral effects of cyclosporin A injection. On the other hand, they observed enhancing effects on reducing body temperature induced by naloxone. Thus, effects of cyclosporin A on behavior mediated by morphine have not been well clarified.

Using the conditioned place preference paradigm, Suzuki and colleagues *(35)* injected cyclosporin A (10, 30, 50 mg/kg) into mice 2 h before injection of morphine (5 mg/kg). The mice were confined to one compartment after the morphine injection and to the other compartment after saline injection. In the control animals without pretreatment with cyclosporin A, the morphine injection produced preference for the drug-associated compartment, while the animals pretreated with cyclosporin A did not show the conditioned place preference in a dose-dependent manner. But as demonstrated by the taste aversion experiments and conditioned place preference with cyclosporin A, injection of cyclosporin A itself may have aversive effects. Because injection of cyclosporin A was paired with injection of morphine in this experiment, apparent suppression of the preferential behavior might simply reflect the aversive effect of the cyclosporin A. Interestingly, μ receptor-deficient CXBK

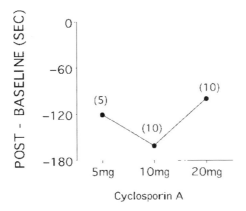

Fig. 3. Conditioned aversion by cyclosporin A. Numbers in the graph indicate the number of rats in each condition. Modified from ref. *31*.

mice did not show suppression of morphine-induced place preference by cyclosporin A treatment. These results suggest that the suppression of conditioned place preference by cyclosporin A may be mediated by μ receptor.

We chronically injected cyclosporin A into rats with damaged blood–brain barrier and carried out single-trial conditioned place preference with methamphetamine *(36)*. In single trial conditioned place preference, animals receive one injection with a drug and confined in a white compartment, then their preference between the white and black compartments was examined on the next day *(37)*. Because rats have some preference for the dark area, preference for the white compartment should, if observed, show conditioned reinforcing effects of the drug. The single-trial conditioned place preference training is suitable for examination of drugs that cause tolerance or sensitization by repeated injection. Because cyclosporin A was not associated with a specific compartment in the conditioned place-preference apparatus, the results were not contaminated with possible aversive effects of cyclosporin A. Although individual differences were observed, single injection of methamphetamine produced the conditioned place preference in control rats to which vehicle (peanut oil) was chronically injected. This conditioned preference was severely suppressed by injection of dopamine antagonist haloperidol. Cyclosporin A also suppressed the conditioning in the experimental group. The results suggest that cyclosporin A modified reinforcing properties of methamphetamine, not through its possible direct aversive effects, but through modulation of dopaminergic system.

MOOD MODIFICATION

The results of conditioned place preference suggest a mood-modifying factor of cyclosporin A. The main immunosuppressive effects of cyclosporin A are reduction of IL-2 production and there are several studies suggesting that IL-2 modify "mood." For examples, intraventricular injection of IL-2 increase 5-HT and noraderenaline and reduced behavioral changes induced by olfactbulblectomy in rats *(38)*, and treatment with IL-2 injection induced depressive state in human patients dose-dependently *(39)*. These observations indicate that cyclosporin A changes depressive state by modulating production of 5-HT mediated through its effects on IL-2 production.

There are several procedures to measure "depressive" state of animals. One most common procedure is a forced swimming test in which animals are placed in a jar with water and the depressive animals show longer immobilized time in the water. Another common procedure is an emergence box test where the depressive animals take longer time to enter a bright area from a dim box. In our laboratory, effects of cyclosporin A on stress-induced depressive state was examined by the forced swimming and the emergence box tests *(40)*. Male Fisher rats were exposed to "unpredictable long-term" stress consisted of rotation, water deprivation, hypotemperature, physical restriction, hypertemperature, food deprivation, and tail pinch for 3 wk. As shown in Fig. 4, this treatment induced stress and resulted in longer latency in the emergence box and longer immobilized time in the forced swimming test. Imipramine (10 mg/kg), a typical tricyclic antidepressant clearly reduced such stress induced depressive state. Chronic injection of cyclosporin A also reduced the immobilized time in the forced swimming task and latency in the emergence box (Fig. 5). In other words, cyclosporin A can mimic antidepressive effects of imipramine. However, the mechanisms by which cyclosporin A and imipramine produced antidepressive effects may be different. Imipramine reversed the stress-induced shrinkage of thymus, but cyclosporin A injection did not. In fact, cyclosporin A injection caused a reduction in thymus weight *(30)*. Cyclosporin A injection itself did not cause increment of adrenal organ weights, but cyclosporin A injection during exposure to the stressful experience resulted in increment. These results suggest that cyclosporin A modified depressive state induced by a stressful experience via a mechanism different from imipramine.

CONCLUSION

There have been many studies demonstrating interaction between nervous and immune systems (for example, *see* ref. *41*). Although there are some controversial data, the effects of immunosuppressants, that is,

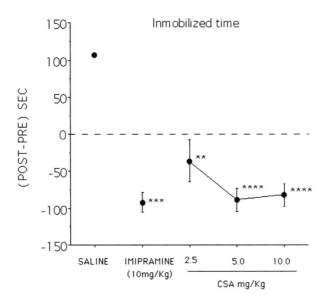

Fig. 4. Immobilized time in the forced swimming test. The vertical axis indicates change between before and after the chronic stress exposure. The number of rats in each group is 9 except for the cyclosporin 2.5 mg/kg group ($n = 8$). Both imipramine and cyclosporin A reduce the stress-induced depressive state. $**p < 0.05$, $***p < 0.001$, $****p < 0.0001$ (two-tailed t-test) Modified from ref. *40*.

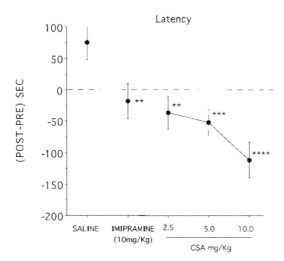

Fig. 5. Latency in the emergence box test. The vertical axis indicates change between before and after the chronic stress exposure The number of rats in each group is 9 except for the cyclosporin 2.5 mg/kg group ($n = 8$). Both imipramine and cyclosporin A reduce the stress-induced depressive state. $**p < 0.05$, $***p < 0.001$, $****p < 0.0001$ (two-tailed t-test) Modified from ref. *40*.

cyclosporin A, on memory function are slight, if any. On the other hand, recent results suggest that cyclosporin A induces change of psychological states. The direct CNS mechanism underlying such psychological effects is not well clarified at present; several views have been proposed, including the interaction of cyclosporin A and calcineurin, as well as the trophic factor effects of cyclosporin A on specific neurotransmitter systems (e.g., dopaminergic and cholinergic; *see* refs. *42* and *43*). While additional studies are needed to relate these brain alterations with psychological and/or memory effects of cyclosporin A, accumulating evidence strongly indicates that cyclosporin A can produce psychological effects.

REFERENCES

1. Hagihara M, Fujishiro K, Takahashi A, et al. Cyclosporin A, an immune suppressor, enhanced neurotoxicity of *N*-methyl-4-phenyl-1,2,3,4-tetra hydropyridine (MPTP) in mice. Neurochem Int 1989;15:249–254.
2. Berden JHM, Hottsuma AJ, Merx JL, Keyser A. Severe central nervous system toxicity associated with cyclosporin. Lancet 1985;219–220.
3. Borlongan CV, Fujisaki T, Watanabe S. Chronic administration of cyclosporin-A does not impair memory retention in rats. NeuroReport 19978:673–676.
4. Borlongan CV, Fujisaki T, Watanabe S. Chronic cyclosporin-A injection in rats with damaged blood–brain-barrier does not impair retention of passive avoidance. Neurosci Res 1998;32:195–200.
5. Brundin P, Widner H, Nilsson OG, et al. Experimental intracerebral xenografts of dopamine neurons: the role of immunosuppression and the blood brain barrier. Brain Res 1989;75:195–207.
6. Famiglio L, Racusen L, Fivush B, et al. Central nervous system toxicity of cyclosporin in a rat model. Transplantation 1989;48:316–321.
7. Racusen LC, Famiglio LM, Fivush BA, et al. Neurologic abnormalities and mortality in rats treated with cyclosporin A. Transplant Proc 1988;20: 934–936.
8. Racusen LC, Solez K. Cyclosporin nephrotoxicity. Int Rev Exp Pathol 1988;30:107–157.
9. de Mattos AM, Olyaei AJ, Bennett WM. Nephrotoxicity of immunosuppressive drugs: long-term consequences and challenges for the future. Am J Kidney Dis 2000;35:333–346.
10. Bennett PC, Zhao W, Lawen A, Ng KT. Cyclosporin A, a inhibitor of calcineurin, impairs memory formation in day-old chicks. Brain Res 1996; 730:107–117.
11. Bennett PC, Singaretnam LG, Zhao W, Lawen A, Ng KT. Peptidyl-prolyl-cis/trans-isomerase activity may be necessary for memory formation. FEBS Lett 1998;431:386–390.
12. Thorndike EL. The law of effect. Amer J Psychol 1927;39:212–222.
13. Watanabe S, Nemoto M. Reinforcing property of music in Java sparrows (*Padda oryzivora*). Behav Proc 1998;43:211–218.

14. Hoffmeister F. Negative reinforcing properties of some psychotropic drugs in drug-naive rhesus monkeys. J Pharmacol Exp Ther 1976;192:468–477.
15. Tuazon DB. The neuropsychopharmacological bases of reward: A view from the conditioned place preference paradigm. Ph.D. thesis, Keio University, 1993.
16. Kusayama T, Watanabe S. Reinforcing effects of methamphetamine in planarians. NeuroReport 2000;11:2511–2513.
17. Johnston RN, Shaw C, Halton DW, et al. GYIRFamide: a novel FMRFamide-related peptide FaRP) from the triclad turbellarian, Dugesia tigrina.1995 Biochem Biophys Res Commun 1995;209:689–697.
18. Sarnat HB, Netsky MG. The brain of the planarian as the ancestor of the human brain. Can J Neurol Sci 1985;12:296–302.
19. Schaeffer DJ. Planarians as a model system for in vivo tumorigenesis studies. Ecotoxicol Environ Safety 1993;25:1–18.
20. Venturini G, Carolei A, Palladini G, et al. Radioimmunological and immuno-cyochemical demonstration of Met-enkephalin in planaria. Comp Biochem Physiol 1983;74:23–25.
21. Franquinet R. The role of serotonin and catecholamines in the regeneration of the Planaria polycelis tenvis. J Embryol Exp Morphol 1979;51:85–95.
22. Tiras KP. Acetylcholinesterase activity in the nervous system of normal planaria and during regeneration. Ontogenez 1978;9:262–268.
23. Venturini G, Stocchi F, Margotta M, et al. A pharmacological study of dopaminergic receptors in planaria. Neuropharmacology 1989;28:1377–1382.
24. Matsuura K, Kakubo H, Makino H, Ogawa N. Cyclosporin A attenuates degeneration of dopaminergic neurons induced by 6-hydroxydopamine in the mouse brain. Brain Res 1996;733:101–104.
25. Matsuura K, Makino H, Ogawa N. Cyclosporin A attenuates the decrease in tyrosine hydroxylase immunoreactivity in nigrostraital dopaminergic neurons and in striatal dopamine contents in rats with intrastriatal injection of 6-hydroxydopamine. Exp Neurol 1997;146:526–535.
26. Borlongan CV, Freeman TB, Hauser RA, et al. Cyclosporin-A increases locomotor activity in rats with 6-hydroxydopamine-induced hemiparkinsonism: relevance to neural transplantation. Surg Neurol 1996;46:384–388.
27. Borlongan CV, Freeman TB, Scorcia TA, et al. Cyclosporin-A increases spontaneous and dopamine agonist-induced locomotor behavior in normal rats. Cell Transplant 1995;4:65–73.
28. Reis F, Tavares P, Teixeira F. The distribution of catecholamines between plasm and platelets in cyclosporin A-induced hyperactive rats. Pharmacol Res 2000;41:129–135.
29. Klosterhalfen S, Klosterhalfen W. Conditioned cyclosporin effects but not conditioned taste aversion in immunized rats. Behav Neurosci 1990;104:716–724.
30. Exton MS, Von Horsten S, Voge J, et al. Conditioned taste aversion produced by cyclosporin A: concomitant reduction in lymphoid organ weight and splenocyte proliferation. Physiol Behav 1998;63:241–247.
31. Borlongan CV, Kwanbara Y, Fujisaki T, Watanabe S. Cyclosporin-A reduces spontaneous place preference in adult rats. Neurosci Lett 1999;267:169–172.

32. Dafny N. Modification of morphine withdrawal by interferon. Life Sci 1983;32:303–305.
33. Dafny N, Wagle VG, Drath DB. Cyclosporin A alters opiate withdrawal in rodents. Life Sci 1985;36:1721–1726.
34. Dantzer R, Satinoff E, Kelley KW. Cyclosporin A and alpha-interferon do not attenuate morphine withdrawal in rats but do impair thermoregulation. Physiol Behav 1987;39:593–598.
35. Suzuki T, Yoshiike M, Funada M, et al. Effect of cyclosporin A on the morphine-induced place preference. Neurosci Lett 1993;160:159–162.
36. Watanabe S, Ikeda M, Ezawa K, Kosaki Y. Suppression of reinforcing properties of methamphetamine by chronic administration of cyclosporin-A in rats. Paper read at the 30th Annual Congress of Japanese Neuropsychopharmacology, 2000.
37. Bardo MT, Valone JM, Bevins RA. Locomotion and conditioned place preference produced by acute intravenous amphetamine: role of dopamine receptors and individual differences in amphetamine self-administration. Psychopharmacology 1999;143:39–46.
38. Song C, Leonard BE. Interleukin-2-induced changes in behavioural, neurotransmitter, and immunological parameters in the olfactory bulbectomized rat. Neuroimmunomodulation 1995;2:263–273.
39. Krigel RL, Padavic-Shaller KA, Rudolph AR, et al. A phase I study of recombinant interleukin 2 plus recombinant beta-interferon. Cancer Res 1988;48: 3875–3881.
40. Fujisaki T. Anti-depressive effects of cyclosporin-A in rats (in Japanese). Master's thesis, Keio University, 1997.
41. Schedlowski M, Tewes U. Psychoneuroimmunology. Kluwer Academic/Plenum, New York, 1999.
42. Borlongan CV, Stahl CE, Fujisaki T, et al. Cyclosporin A induced hyperactivity in rats: is it mediated by immunosuppression, neurotrophism, or both? Cell Transplant 1999;8:153–159.
43. Borlongan CV, Stahl CE, Keep MF, Elmer E, Watanabe S. Cyclosporine-A enhances choline acetyltransferase immunoreactivity in the septal region of adult rats. Neurosci Lett 2000;279:73–76.

Index